ANESTHETIC MANAGEMENT OF ACUTE HEAD INJURY

ANESTHETIC MANAGEMENT OF ACUTE HEAD INJURY

Editor

Arthur M. Lam, M.D.

Professor of Anesthesiology and Neurological Surgery
Department of Anesthesiology
University of Washington School of Medicine
Harborview Medical Center
Seattle, Washington

**RETURN
TO
DEPARTMENT OF ANAESTHETICS
ROYAL UNITED HOSPITAL
BATH**

McGraw-Hill, Inc.
Health Professions Division

New York   St. Louis   San Francisco   Auckland
Bogotá   Caracas   Lisbon   London   Madrid
Mexico City   Milan   Montreal   New Delhi
San Juan   Singapore   Sydney   Tokyo   Toronto

Anesthetic Management of Acute Head Injury

1234567890 KGPKGP 987654

ISBN 0-07-036127-4

This book was set in ITC Galliard by TCSystems, Inc. The editors were Michael J. Houston and Steven Melvin; the production supervisor was Richard Ruzycka; the cover designer was Marsha Cohen/Parallelogram; the index was prepared by Lillian Rodberg.

Quebecor Printing/Kingsport was printer and binder.

This book is printed on acid-free paper

Library of Congress Cataloging-in-Publication Data

Anesthetic management of acute head injury / editor, Arthur M. Lam.
    p. cm.
    Includes bibliographical references and index.
    ISBN 0-07-036127-4
    1. Brain damage—Surgery. 2. Head—Wounds and injuries.
3. Anesthesia I. Lam, Arthur M.
    [DNLM: 1. Brain Injuries—surgery. 2. Brain Injuries—
physiopathology. 3. Anesthesia—methods. 4. Anesthetics—
pharmacology. WL 354 A579 1994]
RD594.A54 1994
617.9'67481—dc20
DNLM/DLC
for Library of Congress   93-49496

*To my wife Annie and my children Derek,
Jessica, and Michelle*

C O N T E N T S

CONTRIBUTORS

Alan A. Artru, M.D.
Professor of Anesthesiology
University of Washington Medical
  Center
University of Washington
Seattle, Washington [7]

Wendy A. Cohen, M.D.
Associate Professor of Radiology
Harborview Medical Center
University of Washington
Seattle, Washington [4]

Karen B. Domino, M.D.
Associate Professor of Anesthesiology
  and Neurological Surgery
Harborview Medical Center
University of Washington
Seattle, Washington [3]

M. Sean Grady, M.D.
Associate Professor of Neurological
  Surgery
Harborview Medical Center
University of Washington
Seattle, Washington [1,2,5]

Mark M. Harris, M.D.
Associate Clinical Professor of
  Anesthesiology
University of Virginia
Charlottesville, Virginia [9]

Arthur M. Lam, M.D.
Professor of Anesthesiology and
  Neurological Surgery
Harborview Medical Center
University of Washington
Seattle, Washington [5,8,10,12]

Peter D. LeRoux, M.D.
Instructor of Neurological Surgery
Harborview Medical Center
University of Washington
Seattle, Washington [1,6]

Teresa S. Mayberg, M.D.
Assistant Professor of Anesthesiology and
  Neurological Surgery
Harborview Medical Center
University of Washington
Seattle, Washington [8]

David W. Newell, M.D.
Associate Professor of Neurological
  Surgery
Harborview Medical Center
University of Washington
Seattle, Washington [10,11]

Yoram Shapira, M.D.
Associate Professor of Anesthesiology
Ben Gurion University of the Negev
Medical School
Soroka Medical Center
Beer Sheva, Israel [2,12]

H. Richard Winn, M.D.
Professor and Chairman of Neurological
  Surgery
Harborview Medical Center
University of Washington
Seattle, Washington [6]

Numbers in brackets refer to chapters written or cowritten by the contributors.

F O R E W O R D

Of all the injuries sustained in a traumatic event, head injury is frequently associated with the most devastating outcome. Although the patient may survive the accident, he or she may do so with a major loss of neurologic function or, worse yet, remain in a vegetative state. However, the outcome of patients who have sustained a head injury need not necessarily be so grim.

There have been several major advances in the care of the head-injured patient. These include the regionalization of trauma care and the institution of trauma centers with ready availability of imaging equipment, neuroradiologists, neurosurgeons, and neuroanesthesiologists. Perhaps one of the most effective measures for early treatment of the head-injured patient has been the improvement of prehospital care with tracheal intubation, oxygenation, and hyperventilation taking place at the scene of the accident.

Improvements have also been achieved for the in-hospital care of the trauma patient. These include routine use of sophisticated new imaging techniques, ready availability and routine use of sophisticated devices for monitoring the status of the brain, the availability of new pharmacologic agents for treatment of the injured brain, plus development of intensive care units intended only for patients with neurologic problems. Lastly, improved outcome from head injury can be attributed to active research programs, better training of physicians in the care of head-injured patients, and to improved collaboration between the various specialists involved in the care of the head-injured patient.

The Trauma Center at Harborview Medical Center in Seattle is respected locally, nationally, and internationally. Dr. Lam is to be congratulated for gathering a number of experts from this institution to serve as his panel of authors for this authoritative and unique treatise on the *Anesthetic Management of Acute Head Injury*. Although there are sections in anesthesiology textbooks that consider the subject, including textbooks devoted to neurosurgical anesthesia, there are no books devoted exclusively to anesthetic management of acute head injury. Dr. Lam and his colleagues have composed an important book that can serve as a reference for other physicians who participate in the care of the head-injured patient. It is hoped that, by reading the book and utilizing the information contained within it, readers will improve their expertise and, ultimately, the outcome of their patients.

BRUCE F. CULLEN, M.D.
Professor, Department of Anesthesiology
University of Washington
Anesthesiologist-in-Chief
Harborview Medical Center
Seattle, Washington

P R E F A C E

Head injury remains an epidemic in North America and represents an enormous drain on health care resources. The economic cost to society is staggering, because a large proportion of the patients affected are young people in their most productive years. Although the most severe injuries are often fatal, and the only treatment for these is preventative, the importance of secondary injury as a determinant of outcome has only recently been recognized.

Although much of the information in this book can be garnered from different sources, there is currently no other textbook that encompasses the variety of materials covered in this text. This book is intended to provide a concise review of the pathophysiology of head injury and a practical approach to the anesthetic management of the head-injured patient. While this book is intended primarily for the trainee and practicing anesthesiologist, it is my hope it will be useful to anyone participating in the acute care of the head-injured patient.

This book clearly would not have been possible without the many laboring hours put in by the contributing authors, nor without the patience and assistance from the Medical Editor, Mr. Michael Houston of McGraw-Hill. Last, but definitely not least, I would like to express my sincere gratitude to my secretary, Karen Rutherford, who carefully read through every manuscript and kept track of the progress of the project.

ANESTHETIC MANAGEMENT OF ACUTE HEAD INJURY

Epidemiology of Head Injury

Peter D. LeRoux and M. Sean Grady

Head injury in the United States is a poorly recognized epidemic. Over 500,000 U.S. citizens are evaluated in emergency rooms each year for a traumatic loss of consciousness. Furthermore, 50,000 individuals die annually from traumatic brain injury. This chapter will review the populations at risk, and the causes, incidence, severity and outcome of head injury. In the past two decades, a number of thorough national and international epidemiologic studies of head injury have been performed; however, these reports have methodological biases that should be recognized before an adequate perspective on the epidemiology of head injury can be achieved.

> "When I use a word," Humpty Dumpty said in rather a scornful tone, "it means just what I choose it to mean—nothing more nor less."
> *Alice's Adventures in Wonderland,* Lewis Carroll

CASE DEFINITION

Definitions are the starting point for any epidemiologic study. An investigator poses certain questions, and the readers must understand what the investigator means. When readers review epidemiologic studies of head injury, they should ask, "What condition constitutes a head injury in this study? Does the study include only those individuals with injury to the brain, or are individuals with skull fracture, but with no evidence of neurologic involvement by history or examination, also included?" For example, Annegers and coworkers include patients suffering a skull fracture, but with no evidence of neurologic injury.[1] In contrast, other investigators define "head injury" as being synonymous with "traumatic brain injury" (TBI).[2-4] The latter is manifested, at least, by a transient alteration in consciousness or posttraumatic amnesia. TBI is a more specific characterization than head injury and will be used preferentially in this chapter.

CASE COLLECTION

Once the injury to be studied is specifically defined, the scope of the data base requires clarification. For example, will the data on all patients suffering TBI, including those who die at the scene, be collected, or will data be included on only those patients admitted to or evaluated at a hospital? Some studies are comprehensive and collect data from both the medical examiner's office to identify those patients who die before reaching a hospital, and hospital records to identify all patients evaluated in the hospital.[1,4-6] These studies permit determination of the incidence of moderate or severe TBI; however, they may underestimate the number of minor traumatic brain injuries because many of the second group of patients may not seek medical evaluation at a hospital. Nonhospitalized individuals with head injury are more common than hospitalized patients; therefore, a more accurate assessment of the incidence of minor head injury may be provided by studies such as the Health Interview Survey of the National Center for Health Statistics, which relies on a telephone or mail survey of the general population and includes hospitalized and nonhospitalized patients with TBI.[7] To generalize study findings to the population as a whole, it is important to define the population base from which the data base is drawn. As will be discussed in a later section, the population group studied can significantly skew results.

CASE IDENTIFICATION

Hospital statistics on TBI can be obtained from many sources. Therefore, it is important to recognize the criteria used to identify the cases included in a study. For example, some studies rely on hospital-derived data bases, using International Classification of Disease codes.[8] The investigator, therefore, depends on accurate recognition of the exact extent of the injury by hospital personnel. This method has some limitations, and clinical correlation using hospital records may be necessary to confirm that coding was accurately performed. In the National Head and Spinal Cord Injury study, hospital records were not cross-checked; therefore, patients could have been included who may not have suffered a TBI but instead suffered an injury to the skull only.[8]

Other parameters, such as the clinicopathologic type of TBI, may be included in the study. By design, some studies exclude penetrating injury or are limited to patients suffering either mild or severe TBI. Furthermore, some investigations are confined to a particular cause of TBI; for example, those injuries resulting only from motor vehicle accidents. Other studies have focused on a specific pathologic feature of TBI, such as subdural hematomas or diffuse axonal injury. In general, the methodology is well described so readers can understand each study's parameters.

Despite these study limitations, there is more similarity than difference among epidemiologic studies evaluating TBI. To provide an overview of this public health problem, the remainder of this chapter will concentrate on a number of recently published studies that describe the epidemiology of head injury in the United States.

Incidence

The approximate incidence of TBI in the United States is 200 cases per 100,000 people. The highest incidence of TBI, 367 cases per 100,000 people, was identified by Whitman, and coworkers in their study of Chicago's inner city; however, the determined incidence was not adjusted for age or race of the U.S. population and therefore may not accurately reflect the general population.[9] In contrast with the Whitman study, Fife and coworkers and MacKenzie and coworkers determined incidences of TBI of 136 and 132 cases per 100,000 people, respectively.[4,7] Fife and coworkers' study population is derived from the National Health Interview Survey. In this data base, 40,000 U.S. households were surveyed through a questionnaire about health events in the 2 weeks prior to the survey. The data base was accumulated over 5 years, thereby providing information from 200,000 U.S. households. A positive response was counted if there was a skull or intracranial injury that required a minimum of one physician visit or resulted in 1 day of disability. In contrast, the study population used by MacKenzie and coworkers was derived from data in the hospital discharge summary of all nonfederal hospitals in Maryland, but the data is not adjusted for age and does not include patients who died at the scene of the accident or during transport to the hospital.

In general, the incidence of TBI reported in other studies resembles that quoted in a retrospective review of Mayo Clinic records.[1] In this report, Annegers and coworkers reported a head injury incidence of 193 cases per 100,000 residents of Olmstead County, Minnesota. This figure was derived from inpatient records, emergency department and outpatient visits, and medical examiner records. However, patients with skull fractures but with no evidence of concussion or posttraumatic amnesia were also included in this report. In two reports from San Diego County in 1978 and 1981, only patients with a traumatic loss of consciousness were included.[5,6] In these reports, incidences of 294 and 180 cases per 100,000 patients, respectively, were estimated. The discrepancies in incidence of TBI among these studies can be accounted for by variability in operational definitions, failure to adjust for age, or fluctuations in population base. Nevertheless, if an approximate incidence of TBI is 200 cases per 100,000 patients, then, based on U.S. population of approximately 250 million in 1990, an estimated 500,000 patients suffer TBI each year.

Age/Gender/Socioeconomic Status

In the majority of studies, the peak age for TBI is 15 to 25 years. Secondary peaks are recognized in infants and in the elderly (>65 years). Discrepancies between studies examining peak ages can be ascribed to differences in the study populations. For example, TBI in an inner city population is more likely to result from interpersonal violence and as a result tends to occur in an older age group than TBI resulting from motor vehicle accidents, which tends to occur more in younger age groups.[9] This point reemphasizes the importance of understanding the population base from which a study is drawn. All studies report a higher number of head injuries in males, the incidence being twice that in females. Socioeconomic status, determined on the basis of median family income, though examined to a limited extent, appears to play a role in TBI.[9] People in lower socioeconomic groups apparently are at higher risk. It is unclear how an individual's family is a risk factor, but this effect may be due partly to the increased rates of interpersonal violence in lower income, inner city populations.

Mechanism of Injury

The majority of brain injuries result from motor vehicle accidents; however, the mechanism of injury is often reported in a nonuniform manner. For example, an injury may be classified as a motor vehicle accident when the victim was either (1) a motorcycle rider (2) a motor vehicle occupant or (3) a pedestrian struck by a vehicle. Fortunately, overall trends can be discerned. The majority of individuals are injured in automobile accidents.[1,3,6,10] Motorcycle or bicycle riders form a smaller but significant group. Falls, particularly in the elderly, constitute the second leading cause of TBI. In the urban population, TBI resulting from assault or firearms are more common than motor vehicle accidents.[2] Participation in certain sports may also result in TBI, although such injury is uncommon. Boxing, in particular, is associated with TBI, but other contact sports are well recognized as rare causes of TBI.

Severity and Outcome

Accurate determination of the outcome following TBI, particularly the effects of treatment, requires an objective classification of the severity of head injury. This classification is achieved most frequently using the Glasgow Coma Scale (GCS).[11] This simple system is widely recognized and grades TBI based on neurologic tests involving motor, verbal, and eye responses to verbal command or painful stimulus. The score ranges from 3, a very severe brain injury, to 15, which is normal. Operational definitions of the severity of TBI have been developed using the GCS, and are widely accepted.[11] A severe TBI is defined as a GCS of 3 through 8; a moderate TBI, a GCS of 9 through 12; and mild TBI, a GCS of 13 through 15. By using this guide, most of the studies have found approximately 60 to 80 percent of head injuries in the United States can be considered mild; 10 to 20 percent, moderate; and the remainder, about 10 percent, severe (Fig. 1-1). However, in a study from north central Virginia evaluating TBI at a neurosurgery center, 25 percent of patients suffered severe injuries.[10] This data likely reflects the experience at a tertiary care referral center where the incidence of severe TBI may be higher because patients with less severe TBI are often treated at local hospitals. Using the numbers determined in most of the studies, 10 percent of all patients suffering brain injury sustain a severe TBI. This percentage means that 50,000 patients with severe brain injury will be seen annually in the United States.

The incidence of death resulting from TBI ranges from 22 to 30 cases

Incidence of TBI by Severity

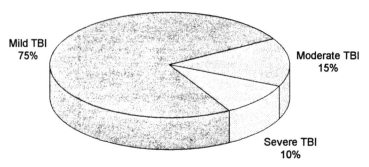

Figure 1-1 Average incidence of severity of TBI.

per 100,000 population, or between 50,000 to 75,000 deaths annually. In-hospital deaths account for a small part of this—about 8 cases per 100,000 population or 20,000 deaths annually. Most deaths from TBI occur at the scene of the accident or during transport. Therefore, to accurately calculate fatality rates of TBI, these deaths must be included.

Whereas the severity of the initial TBI is relatively simple to determine, defining the outcome after TBI has been difficult for any result other than a persistent vegetative state or death. To overcome these difficulties, researchers have frequently used the Glasgow Outcome Scale.[12] This scale consists of five categories: (1) dead, (2) persistent vegetative, (3) severe disability, (4) moderate disability and (5) good recovery. As might be anticipated, inter-observer variability is a significant factor, particularly when categorizing patients as "good recovery" or "moderate disability." This variability is true also of other functional outcome measurements. Any classification of outcome should not be decided for at least 6 months after injury to permit recovery to occur.[13,14] Finally, the extent of disability after head injury can be difficult to define, as it may include physical, neurologic or neurobehavioral deficits. Because of these limitations, no study to date has followed up a sufficiently broad group of brain-injured patients from injury through recovery to provide detailed information relating outcome to severity of head injury. Nevertheless, if certain reasonable assumptions are allowed, then an estimate of the extent of disability after TBI can be made.

The Traumatic Coma Data Bank reported a survival rate of 67 percent, excluding gunshot wounds (GSW), in all patients admitted to a hospital with a diagnosis of severe TBI.[15] Only 7 percent of these patients could subsequently be classified as a "good recovery" at the time of hospital discharge. Therefore, nearly all survivors of severe TBI are left with some degree of neurologic disability. About 50,000 individuals are admitted to a hospital each year with a diagnosis of severe TBI. Of these patients 15,000 die, therefore more than 30,000 individuals annually leave the hospital with a neurologic deficit, ranging from vegetative to moderate disability. This number does not include those individuals with moderate or mild TBI, many of whom suffer disabling neurobehavioral problems for weeks or months after their injury.

Cost and Prevention

The cost of TBI, in both economic and social terms, is immense. In 1985, the cost of a motor vehicle-caused TBI fatality averaged $110,000.[16] This figure represents only medical costs and does not take into account the lifetime loss of earnings or goods and services that are not produced. Because TBI is most common in young people, the loss of these lifetime factors represents a significant loss to society. Direct and indirect costs for survivors of severe TBI, including the expense of extended acute care, rehabilitation care, and wages lost by the inability to return to a prior job can easily exceed the medical cost of a fatal TBI. When critically examined, the cost of preventing TBI pales when compared to the cost of treating patients with TBI. Prevention requires a concerted effort from a broad spectrum of groups.

Alcohol remains a significant factor in motor vehicle accidents.[17] Public education combined with enforcement of drunk driving laws has reduced alcohol-related motor vehicle accidents, from 60 to 40 percent of all accidents. The use of three-point belt restraints and air bags have clearly demonstrated

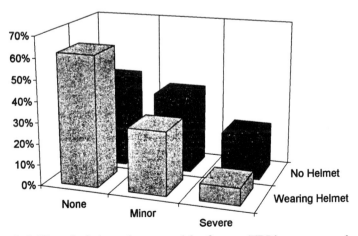

Influence of Helmet Use on Head Injury in MCAs

Figure 1-2 Use of a helmet decreases risk of severe TBI in a motorcycle accident. [*From Harborview Medical Center Trauma Data Base, 1988–1992*]

Effect of Motorcycle Helmet Law on Head Injuries

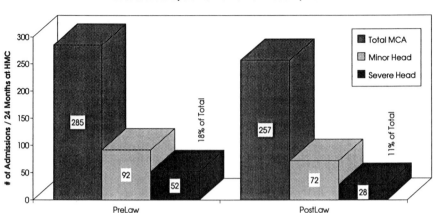

Figure 1-3 Helmet legislation and reduction in severity of TBI in motorcycle accidents is directly correlated. A significant reduction in severe TBI was seen in accidents involving motorcycle riders admitted to Harborview Medical Center after mandatory helmet legislation was enacted. [*From Harborview Medical Center Trauma Data Base, 1990–1992*]

efficacy in decreasing the mortality and morbidity of TBI in motor vehicle accidents.[18] The use of helmets by motorcycle and bicycle riders has also been shown to significantly reduce the risk of TBI in accidents (Figs. 1-2, 1-3). Simple measures such as these, in addition to firearm legislation and public education programs such as *Think First,* can produce significant cost savings for a low investment.

REFERENCES

1. Annegers JF, Grabow HD, Kurland LT, et al: The incidence, causes, and secular trends in head injury in Olmsted County, Minnesota, 1935–1974. *Neurology* 30:912, 1980.

2. Cooper JD, Tabaddor K, Hauser WA: The epidemiology of head injury in the Bronx. *Neuroepidemiol* 2:70, 1983.

3. Kraus JF, Black MA, Hessol N, et al: The incidence of acute brain injury and serious impairment in a defined population. *Am J Epidemiol* 119:196, 1984.

4. Mackenzie EJ, Edelstein SL, Flynn JP: Hospitalized head-injured patients in Maryland: Incidence and severity of injuries. *Maryland Med J* 38:725, 1989.

5. Klauber MR, Barrett-Connor E, Marshall LF, et al: The epidemiology of head injury. A prospective study of an entire community: San Diego County, California, 1978. *Am J Epidemiol* 113:500, 1981.

6. Klauber MR, Marshall LF, Barrett-Connor E: Prospective study of patients hospitalized with head injury in San Diego County, 1978. *Neurosurgery* 9:235, 1981.

7. Fife D: Head injury with and without hospital admission: Comparisons of incidence and short-term disability. *Am J Public Health* 77:810, 1987.

8. Anderson DW, Kalsbeck WD, Hartwell TD: The national head and spinal cord injury survey: Design and methodology. *J Neurosurg* 53:11, 1980.

9. Whitman S, Coonley-Hoganson R, Desai BT: Comparative head trauma experiences in two socioeconomically different Chicago-area communities: A population study. *Am J Epidemiol* 119:570, 1984.

10. Jagger J, Levine J, Jane J, et al: Epidemiologic features of head injury in a predominantly rural population. *J Trauma* 24:40, 1984.

11. Jennett B, Teasdale G: *Management of Head Injuries.* Philadelphia, FA Davis, 1981:77.

12. Jennett B, Bond MR: Assessment of outcome after severe brain damage: A practical scale. *Lancet* i:480, 1975.

13. Bowers S, Marshall L: Outcome in 200 consecutive cases of severe brain injury treated in San Diego County: A prospective analysis. *Neurosurgery* 6:237, 1980.

14. Eisenberg H: Outcome after head injury: General considerations. *Central Nervous System Status Report,* 1985. National Institutes of Health, National Institute of Neurological Disorders and Stroke. Washington, DC, US Government Printing Office, 1988.

15. Foulkes MA, Eisenberg HM, Jane JA, et al: The Traumatic Coma Data Bank: Design, methods, and baseline characteristics. *J Neurosurg* 75(S):8, 1991.

16. Rice DP, MacKenzie EJ, Jones AJ: *Cost of Injury in the United States: A Report to Congress,* San Francisco, CA. Institute for Health and Aging, University of California and Injury Prevention Center, the Johns Hopkins University, 1989, p. 37.

17. Honkanen R, Smith G: Impact of acute alcohol intoxication on the severity of injury: A cause-specific analysis of non-fatal trauma. *Injury* 21:353, 1990.

18. Kraus JF, Black MA, Hessol N, et al: The incidence of acute brain injury and serious impairment in a defined population. *Am J Epidemiol* 119:186, 1984.

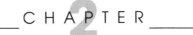

Pathophysiology of Head Injury

Primary Central Nervous System Effects

M. Sean Grady and Yoram Shapira

MECHANISMS OF INJURY
PATHOLOGIC AND BIOCHEMICAL CHANGES
CEREBRAL BLOOD FLOW AND METABOLISM

Traumatic brain injury (TBI) causes a broad spectrum of effects that may be divided into direct and indirect consequences on the central nervous system. Direct consequences of TBI are those attributable to brain trauma, i.e., cerebral contusions, intracerebral hemorrhages, and axonal injury. These pathologic findings cause immediate tissue death or may result in progressive neuronal cell loss due to axonal disruption. Alternatively, indirect consequences of TBI may cause cell death through biochemical processes initiated by trauma or resultant ischemia. Trauma alone may precipitate this molecular cascade of events leading to cell death, but ischemia usually plays the major role in initiation. These biochemical processes involve metabolic pathways that either regulate intracellular Ca^{2+} concentration or are important for membrane stabilization. The pathways are linked to excitatory amino acids, such as glutamate and highly reactive free radical molecules. Trauma-induced causes of ischemia may be multiple: increased intracranial pressure, cardiovascular collapse, hypoxia, or other events that result in inadequate cerebral perfusion. These secondary biochemical events are amenable to intervention and have provided most of the basis for the improved outcome in TBI, from early "in-field" resuscitation efforts to pharmacologic manipulation.[1,2] This chapter will focus on three aspects of the pathophysiology of TBI: (1) mechanisms of injury, (2) pathologic and biochemical changes, and (3) changes in cerebral blood flow and metabolism.

MECHANISMS OF INJURY

The mechanisms of injury can be major determinants in the resultant pathologic findings of TBI. The majority of cases of severe TBI in the United States are vehicular related, with automobile accidents as the primary cause.[3,4] Falls are the leading minority cause of TBI. The biomechanical effects on the brain after these two different injuries result in different pathologic findings. High-speed motor vehicle accidents result more frequently in diffuse axonal injury without major intracerebral hemorrhage. In contrast, falls result more frequently in subdural and intracerebral hematomas. Several reasons may explain these findings.[5-10]

First, the elderly are more prone to falls and generally have more cerebral atrophy than the young, who are more likely to be in a motor vehicle accident. Second, in the older individual, atrophy permits a greater shift of the brain within the cranial vault, thereby increasing the possibility of a vascular injury. Third, subdural veins are more liable to rupture in a rapid deceleration injury such as a fall or assault, compared with the longer period of deceleration in a motor vehicle accident. Finally falls or assaults were the mechanisms of injury in 72 percent of patients with acute subdural hematoma.[3,5] Comparatively, 89 percent of patients in prolonged coma who did not exhibit a mass lesion as seen by CT scan were involved in a motor vehicle accident.

Aside from the direct mechanisms of brain injury, other factors, such as hypoxia and hypertension, can be considered as indirect mechanisms of cerebral injury. As will be discussed later, TBI is frequently associated with global or regional ischemia due to changes in cerebral blood flow. Global cerebral ischemia can be initiated by high intracranial pressure, or cardiovascular and/ or respiratory compromise. Increased pressure in brain tissue adjacent to a mass lesion can cause hypoperfusion to that particular area; therefore, ischemia in TBI can be as important a mechanism of the outcome as the injury itself. A significant body of work has described the gross and microscopic pathologic findings in TBI. Recently, the biochemical basis of cell death after ischemia has shed new light on the ischemic processes that follow TBI.

PATHOLOGIC AND BIOCHEMICAL CHANGES

Gross and microscopic pathologic changes following TBI in humans have been well described.[5,6,11,12] These changes include intracranial hematomas, contusions, and diffuse axonal injury. Other pathologic findings may also be dependent on an indirect consequence of TBI, i.e., ischemia.[13–16] These findings include selective neuronal loss in brain regions particularly susceptible to ischemia (hippocampus, cerebellum), focal neural tissue loss in regions adjacent to hematomas or contusions, and diffuse neural loss due to poor cerebral perfusion. Neural tissue loss may occur in specific vascular patterns, such as the result of an infarct in the posterior cerebral artery (PCA) distribution from occlusion of the PCA by uncal herniation, or tissue loss may also occur in vascular watershed regions. Discerning the direct pathologic effects of TBI from those due to ischemia may be a difficult task.

Intracranial hematomas are defined by their anatomic distribution: extradural, subdural and intracerebral. Extradural hematomas (EDH) originate from the rupture of a meningeal artery and constitute about 15 percent of intracranial hemorrhages. They are frequently associated with skull fracture and tend to be associated with little direct neural injury. Much of the morbidity and mortality of EDH is derived from the consequences of an expanding mass lesion in the confinement of the cranial cavity.[17] The mass lesion may cause a displacement of brain structures (uncal herniation) or an increase in intracranial pressure, which may cause poor cerebral perfusion. In contrast, subdural hematomas (SDH) originate from venous or arterial hemorrhage in the cerebral cortex and are frequently associated with direct brain injury in addition to the consequences of acting as a mass lesion. The incidence of SDH in brain injury varies, depending on the study, from 30 percent of patients with a severe brain injury to 63 percent of patients with a fatal TBI.[6,10] Finally, intracerebral hematomas (ICH) occur in about 15 percent of fatal TBI. Such hematomas vary significantly in size, from small petechial hemorrhages to large clots that can act as mass lesions.

Although cerebral contusions may be found throughout the brain, they are most frequently found along the basal surfaces adjacent to areas of brain herniation through the tentorium and falx, and over the cortical surface. Generally, contusions are related to points of direct impact. For example, contusions are frequently found on the basal surface of the frontal lobe, resulting from impact of these brain surfaces against the rough anterior skull base as the brain shifts during deceleration. These points of impact will cause a contusion that can be grossly differentiated from ischemic hemorrhages. Generally, traumatic contusions spare the portion of the gyrus that is hidden deep in the sulcus, whereas ischemic hemorrhages involve superficial and deep parts of the gyrus.

Finally, diffuse axonal injury (DAI) is a microscopic diagnosis made by identifying the pathologic consequences of axonal disruption (Figs. 2-1, 2-2). Typically, axon retraction balls form at sites of axonal injury. Although

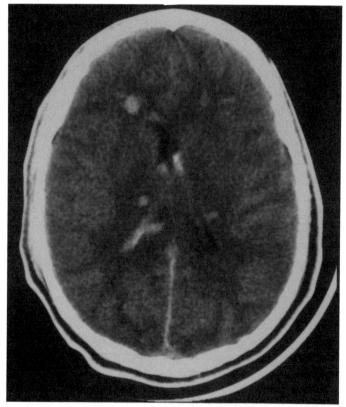

Figure 2-1 CT scan of patient with severe TBI, demonstrating multiple punctate hemorrhages in deep white matter and corpus callosum. This patient died 5 days after injury.

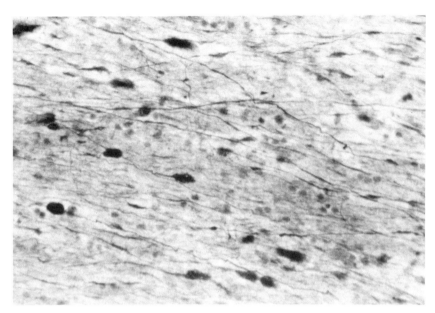

Figure 2-2 Photomicrograph of section taken from corpus callosum of patient illustrated in Fig. 2-1, demonstrating axon retraction balls. Palmgren, 69 ×.

these balls can be identified throughout the brain, they may be concentrated within long, white-matter tracts that curve abruptly, such as in the corpus callosum or brainstem.[11] DAI may be diagnosed with certainty only by pathologic examination but may be inferred in either (1) those patients with both a prolonged coma and no identifiable abnormality in CT or (2) patients whose CT scans show cerebral edema or punctate hemorrhages in subcortical white matter, corpus callosum or brainstem.[18] DAI can be a particularly morbid consequence of brain injury, resulting in prolonged coma and a poor clinical outcome. A spectrum of DAI appears to exist and is likely to occur in all degrees of severity of brain injury.

The pathologic effects of ischemia on neural tissue are not particularly characterized to one brain region, although certain regions may be more susceptible than others. Pathologic changes of ischemia on the neuron are best described on the molecular and biochemical level.[19]

Biochemical changes usually develop within minutes to hours following initial TBI and represent a cascade of pathophysiologic changes prompted by the initial injury.[16,20] There are many factors contributing to cerebral ischemia. Any cause of increased intracranial pressure, such as hemorrhage or edema, may affect cerebral perfusion resulting in ischemia. Noncerebral contributing factors include hypoxia, hypotension, or both due to many reasons, including chest, abdominal, or pelvic trauma. Severe TBI is associated with hypoxia and hypotension caused by extracranial events in almost half of all cases.[21,22] Postmortem studies show that diffuse or regional areas of cerebral ischemia and even infarctions occur in as many as 91 percent of patients with TBI.[13] The ischemic process is accompanied by increased cerebral synthesis of injury mediators or markers, such as catecholamines, excitatory amino acids, arachidonic acid and its metabolites, in addition to other less-defined mediators.[23,24] The end result of the ischemia and the consequent release of these compounds is a cellular damage cascade.

The ischemic damage cascade results in a significant influx of calcium ions into intracellular spaces.[25,26] This increase is due to three factors:

1. The decrease in the transmembrane potential during ischemia opens voltage-dependent calcium gates and the decrease in the transmembrane sodium gradient slows the outward transport of Ca^{2+}.
2. Ca^{2+} is released from the endoplasmic reticulum due to a decrease in adenosinetriphosphate (ATP) levels as a result of ischemia.
3. Excitatory amino acid levels increase during ischemia, causing an overstimulation of the glutamate receptors and the consequent opening of N-methyl-D-aspartate (NMDA), kainate-and quisqualate-gated sodium and calcium channels.

The increase in intracellular Ca^{2+} impacts the cell in several ways.[27–30] High intracellular Ca^{2+} concentration arrests the phosphorylation processes in the mitochondria and thus prevents production of ATP. Ca^{2+} forms a complex with inorganic phosphates, which not only decreases intracellular Ca^{2+} but also inhibits ATP renewal. The loss of ATP through the activation of cell processes, overactivation of various ionic pumps, and the reduction in ATP production causes a drastic decrease in ATP to a level at which the cell can no longer function. The mechanism by which these effects occur may be described as a positive feedback loop in which an initial rise in intracellular Ca^{2+} due to ischemia causes an additional increase in intracellular Ca^{2+} levels, which leads to a constantly increasing cascade of Ca^{2+} influx, ultimately resulting in metabolic failure and cell death (Fig. 2-3).

The increase in intracellular Ca^{2+} also affects cell membranes by activating phospholipase A_2 (PLA_2) and phospholipase C (PLC), resulting in the hydrolysis of membrane phospholipids and the release of free fatty acids, including arachidonic acid.[23,24,31–33] Reesterification of the fatty acids does not occur in ischemia because these processes are energy dependent.[34] The decrease in membrane phospholipid content and the increase in the free fatty-acid content lead to irreversible cell membrane damage. Furthermore, the loss of membrane phospholipids disturbs the balance between membrane proteins and lipids causing a considerable increase in calcium penetration into the cell.

The release of free fatty acids (arachidonic acid and others) damages a cell in other ways. Arachidonic acid acts as a substrate in two major distinct metabolic pathways: (1) oxidation by cyclooxygenase results in the production of prostaglandins, and (2) oxidation by lipoxygenase yields leukotrienes. Both of these classes of compounds play an important role in the severity of edema

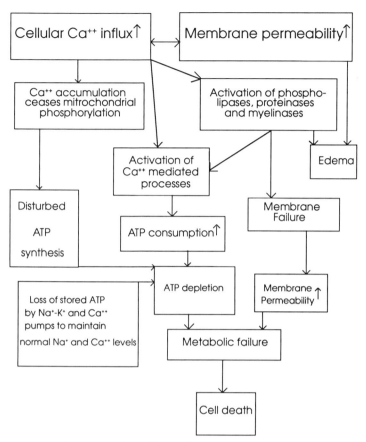

Figure 2-3 Scheme showing effects of membrane permeability changes and increased intracellular Ca^{2+}.

formation.[35-37] The thromboxanes, also formed by the cyclooxygenase pathway, cause vasoconstriction and platelet aggregation. The combination of cerebral edema, vasoconstriction, and platelet aggregation exacerbate any problems with cerebral perfusion, thus increasing ischemic damage.

Recently, the role that excitatory amino acids play in ischemia has been examined. High levels of extracellular glutamate and aspartate have been identified in animal models of ischemia. Beneviste and coworkers has suggested that the high-affinity uptake system of these neurotransmitters fails during ischemia, resulting in the elevated concentrations of these excitatory amino acids.[38] Glutamate produces a toxic Ca^{2+} influx into the neurons through channels opened by the NMDA receptor, which is also highly permeable to Na^+. These channels have a greater Ca^{2+} conductance than the voltage-dependent Ca^{2+} channels, which can be blocked by the dihydropyridine family of Ca^{2+} channel blockers. Choi suggests that NMDA receptor-mediated neuronal injury can be separated into two components: an acute Na^+-dependent component marked by immediate cell swelling, and a delayed Ca^{2+}-dependent component marked by delayed cell degeneration.[25] Both components, at least in vitro where cell swelling is unlimited, are alone capable of producing irreversible neuronal injury. However, with lower toxic influxes, the Ca^{2+}-dependent component probably predominates. The nature of this component reflects the outcome of ischemic neuronal injury, which demonstrates substantial delayed cell degeneration.[39]

Globus and coworkers recently introduced the concept of the *excitotoxic index*.[40] Ischemia-induced glutamate release alone does not explain the pattern of selective neuronal vulnerability. One possible mechanism underlying the selective vulnerability of neurons to transient ischemia is an imbalance between excitation and inhibition during the recirculation period, such as is seen in the rat hippocampus. Other neurotransmitters such as glycine (excitatory) and gamma-aminobutyric acid (inhibitory) may be involved in the mediation of ischemic neuronal damage. The excitotoxic index reflects the composite magnitude of changes in extracellular levels of excitatory and inhibitory neurotransmitters.

Recent pharmacologic treatment strategies are based on the recognition of calcium's role in neuronal injury.[2,16,29,41–43] As a result, drug development and testing has been targeted at several cellular sites. A class of drugs that selectively blocks the NMDA channel is in development and has been considered for treatment in disorders characterized by a release of excitatory neurotransmitters, such as epilepsy, stroke, and trauma. In addition, methylprednisolone and derivative compounds such as the 21-aminosteroids prevent cell membrane decomposition by free radicals formed under conditions of ischemia. Free radical formation is promoted by the shutdown of the normal cell metabolism by calcium influx. To reduce the formation of these free radicals, naturally occurring cellular antioxidants such as superoxide dismutase (SOD) can be supplemented parenterally. In the next section, the role of cerebral blood flow and metabolism as a cause of ischemia during TBI will be examined.

CEREBRAL BLOOD FLOW AND METABOLISM

Cerebral blood flow (CBF) is tightly regulated in the brain. The brain is a stable consumer of oxygen under normal conditions, increasing its global demands only during pain and anxiety.[44] There may be regional variations that are dependent on function. For example, there is an increase in CBF to the Rolando's cortex when the opposite side of the body is voluntarily moved, but global measurements of CBF do not fluctuate because of a decrease in CBF to other brain regions.[45–47] CBF is kept constant over a wide range of arterial pressures by autoregulation, a mechanism by which the tone of the cerebral microvasculature changes to accomodate systemic arterial pressure flux. Autoregulation of CBF can be disturbed under a variety of abnormal conditions including trauma. Normal levels of CBF are 50 ml/100g per min, clinical evidence of cerebral ischemia occurs at 20 ml/100g per min, and neuronal death is imminent at 10–15 ml/100g per min. These figures assume normal brain metabolism, a condition that may not be present after trauma.

There is a substantial body of indirect evidence that indicates a major role for ischemia in the pathophysiologic mechanisms of TBI. Direct clinical documentation of cerebral ischemia after cerebral injury is less extensive, for technical and logistic reasons.[48,49] Neuronal ischemia is initiated when CBF fails to meet metabolic demands. In order to diagnose ischemia, therefore, CBF and cerebral metabolism must be measured. Techniques and timing become critical rate-limiting steps in these measurements.

The most common technique for CBF measurement relies on either radioactive xenon 133 or "cold" (nonradioactive) xenon.[50–52] Xenon is a small, lipophilic molecule that readily crosses the blood-brain barrier, acting as a contrast agent in a manner similar to the more frequently used iodinated or gadolinium-tagged agents. Xenon can be injected or inhaled, and it has an advantage over the conventional agents in that it rapidly and directly passes into the brain parenchyma independent of the state of the blood-brain barrier. Therefore, measurement of xenon in the brain parenchyma provides an estimate of the amount of perfusion (CBF) to that tissue. Detection and measurement of xenon can be accomplished in several ways. Xenon 133 can be measured by collimators placed around the skull to detect photons of released radioactivity. This technique is precise but has poor spatial resolution. Alternatively, cold xenon can be detected by CT, a method that provides better spatial resolution but is time consuming, is less quantitative and is unable to be performed at the bedside.

Newer techniques of CBF measurement include single photon emission computed tomography (SPECT) and magnetic resonance imaging (MRI).[41,53] SPECT relies on iodoamphetamine I^{123} as a tracer, and in the early minutes after intravenous injection can be detected as a marker of CBF.[54] Iodoamphetamine I^{123} binds to parenchymal receptors and can be used as a marker of metabolism when imaged several hours after injection. Spatial resolution is not equal to that of CT and presently is less quantitative. MRI has great potential for imaging both CBF and metabolism but is not clinically available at the present time. Use of this tool is limited by its lack of bedside availability. Bedside measurement is particularly important because ischemic conditions may fluctuate significantly, dependent on arterial blood pressure, ventilation parameters, and brain metabolism.

The other half of the equation that determines the occurrence of ischemia is the metabolic state of the brain. Oxygen demands of the brain may decrease under certain conditions. Drowning in warm versus cold water provides an excellent illustration. Good clinical outcome is well known after prolonged cold-water immersion, unlike that reported in warm-water drowning. Lowering brain temperature reduces cellular metabolic demands, enabling longer neuronal survival even after extremely low levels of CBF. Therefore, before conditions of ischemia can be diagnosed, brain metabolism must be determined.

Cellular metabolism is indirectly measured by subtracting the jugular venous oxygen content from the arterial content. The result is known as the arteriovenous oxygen content difference (AVD_{O_2}). This calculation indicates the amount of oxygen extracted by the brain. Arteriovenous oxygen differences above normal values imply that the brain is operating under conditions of ischemia because more oxygen than the normal amount is being extracted. Levels of AVD_{O_2} below normal imply that the brain is receiving sufficient oxygenation. As with CBF measurment, this technique measures global metabolism and is not reflective of regional variations. Coma occurs when the cerebral metabolic rate falls below 2.0 ml/100g per min. The calculation of cerebral metabolic rate (CMR_{O_2}) is found in the following equation:

$$CMR_{O_2} = CBF \times AVD_{O_2}/100$$

It is readily apparent that CBF and oxygen extraction are directly linked, and determination of cerebral metabolism is dependent on knowing both figures. It is also clear that normal cerebral metabolism may occur under conditions of low CBF if the brain can extract sufficient oxygen from the blood and, conversely, if the blood has sufficient oxygen to supply the brain. Another way of looking at this equation is from a therapeutic standpoint. When the AVD_{O_2} is high and the brain is ischemic because of inadequate CBF, normal metabolism can be restored by increasing CBF.

Measurement of arterial and venous oxygenation is straightforward; however, venous oxygenation must be measured at the jugular bulb, requiring placement of a retrograde jugular catheter. Present methods rely on intermittent measurement of oxygenation concentration, an unsatisfactory limitation under rapidly changing conditions. Continuous monitoring of venous oxygenation may be possible with recent technical advances in fiberoptic catheters.

The actual occurrence of ischemia after TBI has been very difficult to document, for all of the previous reasons.[49,55–58] However, the weight of evidence continues to indicate that ischemia does occur at very early time points, usually within the first 6 h after TBI. This conclusion is consistent with results from drug trials in the treatment of brain trauma-induced central nervous system (CNS) injury; i.e., drug intervention is only useful early in the course of the injury. Most of the past clinical reports were unable to determine CBF or AVD_{O_2} until 24 h after injury. However, investigators at the Medical College of Virginia have scrupulously documented the occurrence of an ischemic state within 6 h of admission in 30 percent of their patients with severe TBI.[48] In contrast, CBF values obtained after 24 h uniformly failed to support the presence of ischemia, as has also been demonstrated in numerous other studies.[57,58] Furthermore, condition of early ischemia portended a poor clinical outcome.

In summary, ischemia appears to be a common entity after TBI. The outcome after TBI is clearly affected by the perfusion state of the brain, because systemic hypotension is adversely linked with good recovery. Meticulous attention should be paid to optimizing cerebral perfusion as soon as possible after injury and to continuing that level of care throughout the operative and postoperative periods. Cerebral perfusion pressure is easily calculated by subtracting intracranial pressure from mean arterial pressure. Fiberoptic intracranial pressure monitors are rapidly and easily inserted in most environments (emergency dept, ICU or OR). The more complicated CBF measurement techniques are likely to be supplanted by use of thermal diffusion flow probes or transcranial Doppler methods, thereby making CBF determination broadly available and part of the routine management of TBI.

REFERENCES

1. Cottrell JE: Brain protection. *ASA Annual Refresher Course Lectures* 1990:252.

2. Latchaw RE, Eelkema EA, Hecht ST: Imaging methods: CT, MR, xenon enhanced CT and SPECT. In Weinstein PR, Faden AI (eds): *Protection of the Brain from Ischemia*. Baltimore, Williams & Wilkins, 1990:81.

3. Baker CC, Oppenheimer L, Stephens B, et al: Epidemiology of trauma deaths. *Am J Surg* 140:144, 1980.

4. Goris RJ, Draaisma J: Causes of death after blunt trauma. *J Trauma* 22:141, 1982.

5. Adams JH, Graham DI, Gennarelli TA: Head injury in man and experimental animals—neuropathology. *Acta Neurochir* 32(suppl):15, 1983.

6. Freytag E: Autopsy findings in head injuries from blunt forces. *Arch Pathol* 75:402, 1963.

7. Gennarelli TA: Head injury in man and experimental animals—clinical aspects. *Acta Neurochir* 32(suppl):1, 1983.

8. Gennarelli TA, Thibault LE: Biomechanics of acute subdural hematoma. *J Trauma* 22:680, 1982.

9. Gennarelli TA, Thibault LE, Adams JH, et al: Diffuse axonal injury and traumatic coma in the primate. *Ann Neurol* 12:564, 1982.

10. Maloney AJF, Whatmore WJ: Clinical and pathological observations in fatal head injuries—a 5 year study of 172 cases. *Br J Surg* 56:23, 1969.

11. Adams JH, Doyle D, Ford I, et al: Diffuse axonal injury in head injury: definition, diagnosis and grading. *Histopathology* 15:49, 1989.

12. Strich SJ: The pathology of brain damage due to blunt head injuries. In Walker AE, Caveness WF, Critchley M (eds): *The Late Effects of Head Injury.* Springfield, IL, Charles C. Thomas, 1969:501.

13. Graham DI, Adams JH, Doyle D: Ischemic brain damage in fatal non-missile head injuries. *J Neurol Sci* 39:213, 1978.

14. Graham DI, Ford I, Adams JH, et al: Ischemic brain damage is still common in fatal non-missile head injury. *J Neurol Neurosurg Psychiatry* 52:346, 1989.

15. Jennett B, Graham DI, Adams H, et al: Ischemic brain damage after fatal blunt head injury. In McDowall FH, Brennan RW (eds): *Cerebrovascular Diseases, Eighth Princeton Conference.* New York, Grune & Stratton, 1973:163.

16. Miller JD: Head injury and brain ischemia—implications for therapy. *Br J Anaesth* 57:120, 1985.

17. Bricolo AP, Pasut LM: Extradural hematoma: Toward zero mortality. A prospective study. *Neurosurgery* 14:8, 1984.

18. Zimmerman RA, Bilaniuk LT, Gennarelli TA: Computed tomography of shearing injuries of the cerebral white matter. *Radiology* 127:393, 1978.

19. Farber JL, Chien KR, Mittnacht SJR: The pathogenesis of irreversible cell injury in ischemia. *Am J Pathol* 102:271, 1981.

20. Raichle ME: The pathophysiology of brain ischemia. *Ann Neurol* 13:2, 1983.

21. Foukles MA, Eisenberg HM, Jane JA, et al: The Traumatic Coma Data Bank: Design, methods, and baseline characteristics. *J Neurosurg* 75:508, 1991.

22. Rose J, Valtones S, Jennett B: Avoidable factors contributing to death after head injury. *Br Med J* 2:615, 1977.

23. Abe K, Kogure K, Yamamoto H, et al: Mechanism of arachidonic acid liberation during ischemia in gerbil cerebral cortex. *J Neurochem* 48:503, 1987.

24. Edgar AD, Strosznjder J, Horrocks LA: Activation of ethanolamine phospholipase A_2 in brain during ischemia. *J Neurochem* 39:1111, 1982.

25. Choi WD: Calcium mediated neurotoxicity: Relationship to specific channel types and role in ischemic damage. *Trends Neurosci* 11:465, 1988.

26. Nowycky MC, Fox AP: Three types of neuronal calcium channel with different calcium agonist sensitivity. *Nature* 316:440, 1985.

27. Bygrave FL: Calcium transport in mitochondria isolated from normal and injured tissue. In Anghileri LJ, Tuffet-Anghileri AM (eds): *The Role of Calcium in Biological Tissues,* Vol 1. Boca Raton, CRC Press, 1982:122.

28. Meech RW: Intracellular calcium and the control of membrane permeability. *Symp Soc Exp Biol* 30:161, 1976.

29. Rasmussen H. The calcium massenger system. *N Engl J Med* 314:1094, 1986.

30. Shapira Y, Yadid G, Cotev S, et al: Accumulation of calcium in the brain following head trauma. *Neurol Res* 11:169, 1989.

31. Shohami E, Shapira Y, Yadid G, et al: Brain phospholipase A$_2$ is activated after experimental closed head injury in the rat. *J Neurochem* 53:1541, 1989.

32. Unterberg A, Wahl M, Hammersen F, et al: Permeability and vasomotor response of cerebral vessels during exposure to arachidonic acid. *Acta Neuropathol* 73:209, 1987.

33. Van den Bosch H: Phospholipase. In Hawthorne JN, Ansell GB (eds): *Phospholipids*. Amsterdam: Elsevier, 1982:313.

34. Wei EP, Lamb RG, Kontos HA: Increased phospholipase C activity after experimental brain injury. *J Neurosurg* 56:695, 1982.

35. Klatzo I: Brain edema following brain ischemia and the influence of therapy. *Br J Anaesth* 57:18, 1985.

36. Klatzo I: Pathophysiological aspects of brain edema. *Acta Neuropathol* 72:236, 1987.

37. Wahl M, Unterberg A, Beathmann A, et al: Mediators of blood brain barrier dysfunction and formation of vasogenic brain edema. *J Cereb Blood Flow Metab* 8:621, 1988.

38. Beneviste H, Drejer J, Schousboe A, et al: Elevation of extracellular concentration of glutamate and aspartate in rat hippocampus during transient ischemia monitored by intracerebral microdialysis. *J Neurochem* 43:1369, 1984.

39. Kirino T: Delayed neuronal death in the gerbil hippocampus following ischemia. *Brain Res* 239:57, 1982.

40. Globus MY-T, Ginsberg MD, Busto R: Excitotoxic index—A biochemical marker of selective vulnerability. *Neurosci Lett* 127:39, 1991.

41. Brant-Zawadzki M, Norman D (eds.): *Magnetic Resonance Imaging of the Central Nervous System*. New York, Raven Press, 1987:221.

42. Miller RJ. Calcium signalling in neurons. *Trend Neurosci* 11:415, 1988.

43. Zivin JA, Choi DW: Stroke therapy. *Sci Am* 265:56, 1991.

44. Kety SS: Round table discussion: psychoactive drugs and anxiety, their influence on cerebral circulation and metabolism. In Ingvar DH, Lassen NA (eds): *Brain Work*. Copenhagen, Munksgaard, 1975:472.

45. Olesen J: Contralateral focal increase of cerebral blood flow in man during arm work. *Brain* 94:635, 1971.

46. Raichle ME, Grubb RL, Mohktar HT, et al: Correlation between regional cerebral blood flow and oxidative metabolism. *Acta Neurol* 33:523, 1976.

47. Siesjo BK: Ischemia. In Siesjo BK (ed): *Brain Energy Metabolism*. New York, John Wiley, 1978:453.

48. Bouma GJ, Muizelaar JP, Choi SC, et al: Cerebral circulation and metabolism after severe traumatic brain injury: The elusive role of ischemia. *J Neurosurg* 75:685, 1991.

49. Dickman CA, Carter LP, Bladwin HZ, et al: Continuous regional cerebral blood flow monitoring and intracranial pressure monitoring in acute craniocerebral trauma. *Neurosurgery* 28:467, 1991.

50. Obrist WD, Thompson H-K Jr, Wang HS, et al: Regional cerebral blood flow estimated by 133-Xenon inhalation. *Stroke* 6:245, 1975.

51. Yonas H, Good WF, Gur D, et al: Mapping cerebral flow by xenon-enhanced computed tomography: Clinical experience. *Radiology* 152:435, 1984.

52. Yonas H, Gur D, Latchaw RE, et al: Xenon computed tomographic blood flow mapping. In Wood JH (ed): *Cerebral Blood Flow*. New York, McGraw-Hill, 1987:220.

53. Hilal SK, Maudsley AA, Simon HE, et al: In vivo NMR imaging of tissue sodium in the intact cat before and after acute cerebral stroke. AJNR *Am J Neuroradiol* 4:245, 1983.

54. Holman BL, Hill TC: Perfusion imaging with single photon emission computed tomography. In Wood JH (ed): *Cerebral Blood Flow*. New York, McGraw-Hill, 1987:243.

55. Jaggi JL, Obrist WD, Gennarelli TA, et al: Relationship of early cerebral blood flow and metabolism to outcome in acute head injury. *J Neurosurg* 72:176, 1990.

56. Muizelaar JP, Marmarou A, DeSalles AAF, et al: Cerebral blood flow and metabolism in severely head-injured children: I. Relation with GCS, outcome, ICP and PVI. *J Neurosurg* 71:63, 1989.

57. Obrist WD, Gennarelli TA, Segawa H, et al: Relation of cerebral blood flow to neurological status and outcome in head-injured patients. *J Neurosurg* 51:292, 1979.

58. Obrist WD, Langfitt TW, Jaggi JL, et al: Cerebral blood flow and metabolism in comatose patients with acute head injury: Relationship to intracranial hypertension. *J Neurosurg* 61:241, 1984.

CHAPTER 3

Pathophysiology of Head Injury: Secondary Systemic Effects

Karen B. Domino

There are numerous systemic sequelae of head trauma, including pulmonary abnormalities, cardiovascular changes, fluid and electrolyte derangements, and alterations of coagulation and gastrointestinal function. This chapter will review the secondary multisystem effects of head injury, as these additional disorders may exacerbate neurologic injury and contribute to the morbidity and mortality from head trauma.

PULMONARY EFFECTS

Arterial hypoxemia occurs commonly in patients with head injuries.[1–5] Up to 65 percent of spontaneously breathing head trauma patients may be hypoxemic, even though they do not appear to be in respiratory distress.[1,4,6] The cause of the decrease in arterial blood oxygenation is multifactorial and may reflect direct lung trauma; pulmonary causes, such as aspiration or fat embolism; or processes that are secondary effects of the brain injury (Table 3-1). Hypoxemia following head trauma is associated with a poorer neurologic outcome[5,6]; therefore, prompt recognition of hypoxemia, determination of its cause, and prompt treatment are important.

Table 3-1 Pulmonary Effects of Head Trauma

Pulmonary Etiologies
Flail chest
Pneumothorax
Hemothorax
Pulmonary contusion
Aspiration
Atelectasis
Cardiogenic pulmonary edema
Fat embolism syndrome
Adult respiratory distress syndrome (ARDS)
Pneumonia

Neurogenic Etiologies
Abnormal respiratory patterns
Reduced functional residual capacity
Neurogenic alterations in ventilation/perfusion
  matching
Neurogenic pulmonary edema

Pulmonary Causes

Because head trauma victims may have other injuries, pulmonary damage may result from either direct trauma to the chest wall and lung or from secondary lung injuries, such as gastric aspiration and pulmonary edema. Acute traumatic injuries of the chest that may contribute to impaired pulmonary function include chest wall injuries (flail chest), pneumothorax, hemothorax, pulmonary contusion, tracheobronchial disruptions, and diaphragmatic disruption. Secondary pulmonary injuries include aspiration of gastric contents, atelectasis, fat embolism syndrome associated with long-bone fractures, cardiogenic pulmonary edema, and the adult respiratory distress syndrome (ARDS). Fat embolism commonly accompanies long-bone fractures, but only 2 to 10 percent of patients with long-bone fractures develop fat embolism syndrome.[7] The diagnosis is made by the development of respiratory insufficiency, neurological defects, and a petechial rash that occurs in 50 to 60 percent of patients. In the initial 24 h after injury, a decrease in arterial blood oxygenation may occur, as fat globules become lodged in the pulmonary microvasculature. However, severe pulmonary failure and subsequent development of ARDS do not result until 24 to 72 h later. An inflammatory response occurs after lipase breaks down the fat globules into free fatty acids, an effect which may damage the pulmonary capillary membrane.

Many head trauma patients with multiple injuries are at high risk for the development of ARDS. Risk factors include aspiration of gastric contents, pulmonary contusion, multiple emergency transfusions, and sepsis syndrome.[8] An increase in fibrin degradation products may also identify patients with head injury who are at high risk for ARDS.[9] Sixty to 70 percent of patients develop ARDS within the first 24 h after trauma, although few patients become manifest within 6 h of injury.

The most common pulmonary complication in the head-injured patient is pneumonia.[10, 11] Pneumonia develops in 20 to 70 percent of patients with severe head injury.[10–12] The major cause is believed to be aspiration of oral pharyngeal secretions that are colonized by pathogenic bacteria. Profound coma depresses the gag reflex and impairs the cough reflex. Impairment in mucociliary clearance; abnormalities in surfactant metabolism; impairment in alveolar macrophage function; and iatrogenic insults, such as endotracheal intubation, mechanical ventilation, and suctioning in an intensive care unit contribute to the development of pneumonia.[13, 14] Neutrophil function and cell-mediated immunity are also impaired after head trauma, especially in patients treated with corticosteriods.[15] Fifty percent of head-injured patients who were intubated for longer than 5 days developed bacterial pneumonia.[14] Use of cimetidine[13, 16] and antacids[16] has been shown to increase the likelihood of a bacterial pneumonia. Elevation of gastric pH may enhance the risk of nosocomial pneumonia by causing gastric bacterial colonization.[16] Steroid and prophylactic antibiotics may also increase the risk of pneumonia, whereas aggressive pulmonary toilet and postural drainage may reduce the risk.[10]

Fatal pulmonary embolism may occur in 2 to 3 percent of head-injured patients.[17] Thirty to 40 percent of such patients are at high risk for development of deep vein thrombosis because of prolonged bed rest, hemiparesis, long operations, and disseminated intravascular coagulation.[18]

Neurogenic Causes of Pulmonary Dysfunction

Abnormal Respiratory Patterns

Impaired ventilation is common after head injury. Variations in the depth and the rate of spontaneous respirations occur in 60 percent of patients with brain injury.[6, 19, 20] Cheyne-Stokes respiration, irregular breathing, and tachypnea are among the patterns commonly observed.[20] Cheyne-Stokes respiration is periodic breathing in which tidal volume waxes and wanes separated by periods of apnea. It is associated with bilateral destructive lesions in the cerebral hemispheres or basal ganglia, and the prognosis is poor (mortality >50 percent).[6] Spontaneous tachypnea with hyperventilation to a Pa_{CO_2} less than 30 mmHg is also associated with a reduced survival rate.[19] Irregular respiration, such as ataxic and apneustic breathing is seen with medullary and pontine lesions.[19] Hypoventilation with hypercarbia is usually seen only as a terminal event.

Reduced Functional Residual Capacity

The functional residual capacity (FRC), or the amount of gas present in the lungs at the end of a normal expiration, is reduced after isolated head injury. Cooper and Boswell[21] found a 32 percent reduction in FRC, increased pulmonary shunt (19.6 ± 9.9 percent), and decreased lung and chest wall compliance in 24 comatose mechanically ventilated head-injured patients. Seven patients with the largest shunts had severe reductions in FRC to less than 55 percent of predicted values. The pulmonary shunting and decreases in FRC were not correlated with the level of intracranial pressure (ICP) nor the presence of pulmonary disease as seen on chest x-ray. The reduction in FRC was large enough to expect closure of small airways and significant ventilation/perfusion (V_A/Q) mismatch. The cause of the reduction in FRC in severe head injury is unclear. It may be related to chest wall changes due to neuromuscular blockade or a comatose state or both, as the reduction in FRC is similar in magnitude to that observed under general anesthesia.

Neurogenic Alterations in Ventilation/Perfusion Matching

Hypoxemia and increased pulmonary shunting have been observed in animals and patients with increased ICP in the absence of pulmonary edema or any pulmonary disease. Marked reversible increases in pulmonary shunt occur with very high ICPs (>100 mmHg) in animals with normal lungs.[22,23] Unexplained increases in pulmonary shunt have been reported in patients in the absence of intracranial hypertension after head trauma[24] and intraoperatively during biopsy of hypothalamic lesions.[25] Increased perfusion of shunt and low $\dot{V}A/\dot{Q}$ areas have been observed in patients with isolated head trauma and normal lungs, especially in those with high cardiac output and low pulmonary vascular resistance.[26,27]

The cause of the above changes in $\dot{V}A/\dot{Q}$ matching is not known. It may be related to CNS modulation of $\dot{V}A/\dot{Q}$ regulatory mechanisms. Hypoxic pulmonary vasoconstriction (HPV) is an important regulatory mechanism that preserves oxygenation by maintaining matching of perfusion to ventilation in the lung. The pulmonary vasculature constricts in areas that are hypoxic or atelectactic, resulting in diversion of blood flow to well-ventilated, normoxic lung regions. Hypoxic pulmonary vasoconstriction was attenuated by marked increases in ICP in dogs, predominately due to the effect of accompanying hemodynamic changes on HPV.[28] It has been speculated that intravascular release of brain thromboplastin may contribute to abnormal $\dot{V}A/\dot{Q}$ matching in head trauma.[27] Thromboplastin initiates the coagulation cascade and causes deposition of fibrin microemboli and platelet aggregates in the pulmonary capillaries. Neutrophil accumulation and release of vasoactive substances may subsequently cause abnormalities of local ventilation and perfusion. In fact, patients with increased fibrin-split products are more likely to develop respiratory failure after head trauma.[9]

Neurogenic Pulmonary Edema

On rare occasions, acute pulmonary edema may develop after severe head trauma.[29] Neurogenic pulmonary edema (NPE) also occurs in patients after a variety of other CNS disorders, including subarachnoid hemorrhage,[30] intracranial hemorrhage,[31] spinal cord trauma,[32] acute hydrocephalus,[33] colloid cyst of the third ventricle,[34] seizures,[35] and hypothalamic lesions.[36] An acute rise in ICP often, but not always, accompanies the development of pulmonary edema. Increases in ICP may elicit only the sympathetic activation and cardiopulmonary responses that are essential for the development of NPE.

Classic NPE has an immediate onset and becomes clinically recognizable 2 to 12 h after injury; however, in some patients, the onset is delayed from 12 h to several days. Neurogenic pulmonary edema is generally of short duration. If the patient survives, it resolves within hours to days. Longer episodes of edema may represent ARDS, fat embolism, or some other cause. The usual clinical findings are dyspnea, tachypnea, hypoxemia, reduced pulmonary compliance, and bilateral "fluffy" alveolar infiltrates on the chest x-ray (Fig. 3-1).

Little is known about the CNS structures that mediate NPE.[37,38] Stimulation, distortion, and destruction of anatomically discrete centers in the medulla (Areas A1 and A5, nuclei of the solitary tract, and area postrema) can cause

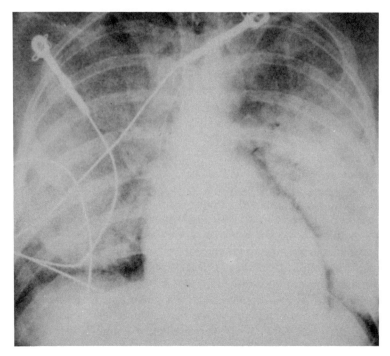

Figure 3-1 Chest x-ray of a patient with neurogenic pulmonary edema. Characteristic bilateral fluffy alveolar infiltrates are evident.

pulmonary edema. These areas activate preganglionic sympathetic and parasympathetic outflow tracts in the cervical spine. Hypothalamic centers may contribute but are not essential to the development of edema. Experimentally induced NPE can be blocked either by section of the cervical spinal cord or by beta-adrenergic blockade.

The study of NPE has been hindered by the lack of good animal models. NPE is only variably induced in animals by acute elevation of ICP.[14,39] Intracisternal injection of various substances, such as veratrine alkaloids in dogs[40,41] and fibrinogen in rabbits[42] has been more successfully used to induce NPE. Intracisternal injection transiently and markedly increases systemic mean arterial pressure (MAP), pulmonary arterial pressure (PAP), and left ventricular end-diastolic pressure (LVEDP).[40] The animals that developed gross alveolar flooding had higher PAP and LVEDP than those that developed only interstitial edema. The ratio of airway fluid-to-plasma protein concentrations (0.48–0.84) ranged between the ratio observed in hydrostatic edema (0.54) and that observed in alloxan-induced permeability edema (0.98).[41] Variable amounts of airway fluid protein have also been observed in patients with NPE.

The pathogenesis of NPE is complex and is not completely understood. Both hydrostatic and increased permeability mechanisms may play a role in the cause of NPE. Sympathetic activation, especially beta-adrenergic discharge, is believed to be essential for the development of NPE (Fig. 3-2). The CNS insult activates the central sympathetic nervous system causing release of catecholamines from the adrenal medulla.[43] This effect results in an increase of systemic vascular resistance, MAP, and LVEDP. Blood, shunted from the systemic to the pulmonary circulation, increases venous return and left atrial pressure and reduces pulmonary vascular and lung compliance. Pulmonary artery pressure is increased, and pulmonary venous vasoconstriction[44] may increase the pulmonary venous to arterial resistance ratio, the pulmonary microvascular pressure, and the pulmonary fluid filtration.[45,46] Pulmonary capillary permeability also may be increased as a result of pulmonary endothelial injury (e.g., stretched pores) and direct increases in pulmonary capillary permeability. McClelland and coworkers[47] found that raising ICP in dogs

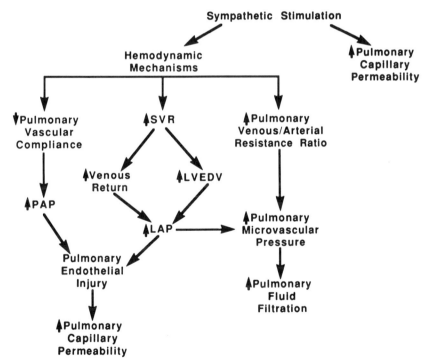

Figure 3-2 Hypothesized mechanism in the pathogenesis of neurogenic pulmonary edema. SVR = systemic vascular resistance; PAP = pulmonary artery pressure; LVEDV = left ventricular end-diastolic volume; LAP = left atrial pressure.

increased their pulmonary vascular permeability to protein, an effect which could not be reproduced with similar increases in PAP or cardiac output by either infiltration of a left atrial balloon or infusion of isoproterenol. The hemodynamic changes resolve quickly, so normal pressures are observed when measurements are made in patients. However, the increases in pulmonary capillary permeability may persist, and edema can develop later. Sympathetic-induced constriction of pulmonary lymphatics may reduce the ability of the lung to compensate for increased edema formation.[38,42]

Treatment of Hypoxemia in Head-Injured Patients

Prompt and aggressive treatment of hypoxemia is imperative in head-injured patients because hypoxemia is associated with a worse neurologic outcome.[4,5] Hypoxemia results in a vicious cycle of increases in cerebral blood flow including arterial oxygen tensions less than 50 mmHg; increases in ICP, neuronal swelling and dysfunction; and greater systemic hypoxemia, ultimately resulting in death.

Positive end-expiratory pressure (PEEP) may be required for head-injured patients with lung disease to improve oxygenation and reduce the inspired oxygen tension. The concern is that PEEP may increase ICP in patients with head injuries. PEEP increases the superior vena cava pressure by increasing intrapleural pressure. Cerebral venous outflow is decreased, which may result in increases in ICP, especially in patients with a brain mass. The most recent studies suggest that 10 cmH_2O of PEEP improves oxygenation and usually causes clinically inconsequential increases in ICP in patients with severe head trauma.[21,48,49] For instance, Cooper and coworkers[49] found that application of 10 cmH_2O of PEEP only increased ICP from 13 ± 8 mmHg (SD) to 14 ± 8 mmHg in 33 patients with severe head trauma. Furthermore, eight patients with elevated baseline ICP did not experience a significant increase in ICP. Up to 20 cmH_2O of PEEP has been used to treat hypoxemia with minimal adverse effect on ICP.[48] However, because larger, potentially serious increases in ICP in addition to clinical deterioration have been observed in some head-injured patients with PEEP,[50,51] ICP should be monitored when possible.

The variable clinical responses to PEEP in head-injured patients may be secondary to PEEP's effect on other hemodynamic and respiratory variables (Table 3-2). Factors that modify the effect of PEEP on ICP include (1) the amount of PEEP, (2) the patient's preexisting ICP and brain elastance, (3) the degree of respiratory disease indicated by lung compliance and intrapulmonary shunt, (4) the intravascular volume loading, (5) the patient position, (6) the effect of PEEP on Pa_{CO_2}, and (7) the adequacy of sedation. PEEP therapy may cause a more serious increase in ICP in patients with reduced

Table 3-2 Factors Affecting the Change in ICP
with PEEP

Amount of PEEP
Pre-existing ICP and brain elastance
Lung compliance
Patient position
Intravascular volume loading
Mannitol
Increase in dead space and Pa_{CO_2}
Coughing and struggling by the patient

intracranial compliance.[50,52] The magnitude of the increase in ICP is greater when higher amounts of PEEP[53] are applied and when the intravascular volume is expanded with saline, than when blood pressure is allowed to fall.[54,55] PEEP occasionally increases Pa_{CO_2} because it increases physiologic dead space.[49,56] Increases in ICP due to PEEP can be reduced by elevating the head 30° and by concurrent mannitol administration.[49] Abrupt removal of PEEP may result in increases in ICP.[57]

PEEP may affect ICP less in patients with the stiffest lungs, who usually are the ones most in need of PEEP. Both animal[53,57] and human[49,52] studies found that the increase in ICP with PEEP was attenuated as pulmonary compliance was reduced. Burchiel and coworkers[52] evaluated the effects of PEEP on ICP in 18 brain-injured patients who required PEEP therapy to treat hypoxemia. PEEP increased ICP in five patients who had reduced intracranial compliance and normal lung compliance, but did not increase it in patients with reduced lung compliance (≤ 30 ml/cmH$_2$O). In the presence of stiff lungs, changes in airway pressure have less effect on intrapleural pressure and jugular venous return. However, reduced pulmonary compliance does not always prevent PEEP-induced increases in ICP. Cooper and coworkers[49] found that PEEP resulted in ICP increases greater than 5 mmHg in two patients with reduced pulmonary compliance. They found that PEEP tended to elevate ICP in respiratory disorders characterized by an increased pulmonary shunt but with normal lung compliance, suggested clinically by the presence of low peak airway pressures.

Therefore, PEEP should be administered as required to treat hypoxemia in the head trauma patient; 10 cmH$_2$O is generally well tolerated. ICP should be monitored if higher amounts of PEEP are required to preserve oxygenation with a safe inspired oxygen tension.

CARDIOVASCULAR EFFECTS

Hyperdynamic Cardiovascular Response

A hyperdynamic cardiovascular state is the most common hemodynamic response to severe head trauma (Table 3-3).[58] The score on the Glasgow Coma Scale (GCS) and the level of serum catecholamines are inversely related; i.e., serum catecholamine levels are higher in more severely injured patients.[59,60] The hyperdynamic cardiovascular state is responsible for producing hypertension, cardiac arrhythmias, and electrocardiogram (ECG) changes that are commonly observed in patients with severe head injuries and are indicative of myocardial ischemia.

Table 3-3 Cardiovascular Effects of Head Trauma

Hyperdynamic Cardiovascular State
  Hypertension
    Increased cardiac output
    Increased intracranial pressure (Cushing response)
  Cardiac arrhythmias
    Bradycardia
    Nodal rhythms
    Sinus tachycardia
    Sinus arrhythmia
    Atrial fibrillation
    Premature ventricular contraction
    Heart block
    Ventricular tachycardia (*torsade de pointes* arrhythmia)
  Electrocardiogram changes of myocardial ischemia
    Peaked P waves
    Prolonged QT intervals, corrected for heart rate
    Depressed ST segments
    Inverted/flattened T waves
    Prominent U waves
  Focal areas of myocardial necrosis

Hypotension
  Uncommon, must rule out other causes
  May occur with brain decompression

Hypertension

Hypertension is common following head trauma. Systolic blood pressures greater than 160 mmHg have been reported on admission in 25 percent of head-injured patients.[61] Most of the increase in systemic blood pressure is due to increased cardiac output rather than increased systemic vascular resistance[58,60,62]; however, cardiac output is not invariably elevated in severe head trauma. It may be decreased in some head-injured patients because of hypovolemia, due to diuretics and blood loss, and because of decreased venous return, due to mechanical hyperventilation used to reduce Pa_{CO_2}.[61,63]

Severe elevation of systemic blood pressure may also result from increased ICP, brain stem compression, or medullary ischemia. These conditions decrease cerebral perfusion pressure and distort the brain stem which activates medullary sympathetic and vagal centers.[64,65] Cushing[64,66,67] in his classic papers described an increase in systemic blood pressure in response to increases in ICP. However, the presence of severe hypertension does not invariably signify the presence of increased ICP because the stress response to any severe injury may elicit release of catecholamines and may cause hypertension.[68] In fact, the magnitude of the hypertension does not correlate well with either ICP, GCS score, or computerized tomography findings.[58] Hypertension is associated with poor neurological outcome in animals[69] and humans after acute brain injury[68,70]; therefore, severe hypertension should be treated in the head-injured patient.

Cardiac Arrhythmias

Cardiac arrhythmias are common after severe head injury. Bradycardia,[64] tachycardia,[61] nodal rhythms,[71] sinus arrhythmia,[72] atrial fibrillation,[73] premature ventricular contractions,[74] heart block,[71] and ventricular tachycardia[75-77] may occur. The arrhythmias are mediated by changes in sympathetic and vagal tone. Bradycardia has been classically described as part of the Cushing response to increases in ICP.[64,66,67] Bradycardia results from direct and indirect (via the baroreceptors) stimulation of brain stem parasympathetic neurons in the cardioinhibitory center of the medulla. Although the bradycardic response is a part of the classic Cushing triad, it is a more variable accompaniment of increased ICP than hypertension.[66] In fact, there is a poor correlation between elevated ICP and decreases in heart rate in head trauma patients.[78] Heart rate may be influenced by many factors, including the type of drugs administered (e.g., pancuronium), the presence of hypovolemia, or the degree of pain experienced. The most common heart rate response in severely head-injured patients is tachycardia.[61,71] Heart rates over 120 beats per minute have been reported at time of hospital admission in over 30 percent of brain-injured patients.[61] Although ventricular arrhythmias are rare, they are serious for they are life-threatening. One such reported arrhythmia is the *torsade de pointes* arrhythmia, a form of ventricular tachycardia (Fig. 3-3).[77]

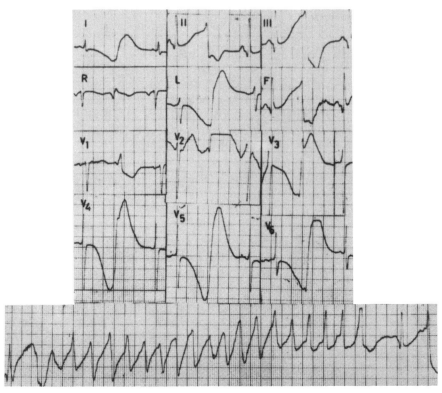

Figure 3-3 *Torsade de pointes* arrhythmia after head trauma. In the 12-lead ECG (*top*), interpolated nodal escape beats are superimposed at the end of the previous T waves. The QT interval is prolonged. The *bottom* rhythm strip (lead II) shows that the *torsade de pointes* ventricular arrhythmia reverts spontaneously to sinus rhythm at the end of the strip. The arrhythmia is precipitated when the second sinus beat is superimposed on the previous T wave. (*Reprinted from Rotem M et al.,[77] with permission of publisher*).

Electrocardiogram (ECG) Changes

Electrocardiogram changes are common in head-injured patients. When compared to normal subjects or other patients with limb trauma, patients with severe head injuries had a greater prevalence of ECG abnormalities, especially peaked P waves and prolonged QT invervals.[71,72,76,79] All severely injured patients had an increased prevalence of depressed ST segments, inverted T waves, and large U waves.[72] The T wave flattening or inversion and ST-segment abnormalities resemble those seen in myocardial ischemia (Fig. 3-4). These ECG changes have been observed in other patients with acute cerebral lesions, such as subarachnoid hemorrhage,[74,80–86] meningitis,[80] and stroke.[87] Prolonged QT intervals, T wave inversions, and ST-segment abnor-

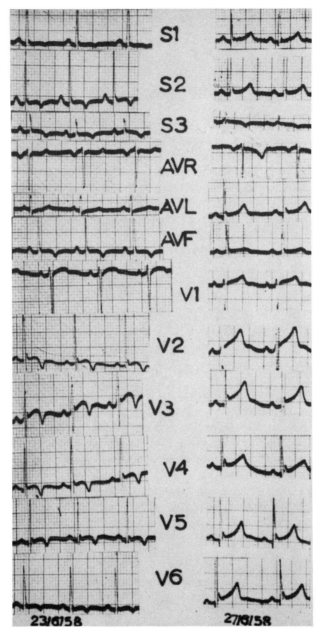

Figure 3-4 ECG changes in head trauma. *Left* shows inverted T waves. *Right,* performed 4 days later, shows that the T waves became upright except in lead III and the ST segments were elevated. (*Reprinted from Hersch C,*[72] *with permission of publisher*).

malities have been induced in experimental models of head trauma and subarachnoid hemorrhage.[88,89] The ECG changes have also been induced experimentally in animals by the exogenous administration of high doses of catecholamines.[90,91]

Increases in the myocardial isoenzyme of creatine kinase (CK-MB) have also been frequently observed in patients with severe head trauma,[92] subarachnoid hemorrhage,[93,94] and stroke.[87] The elevation of CK-MB is highly correlated with abnormal ECGs in these patients. Hackenberry and coworkers[92] found elevations of CK-MB in 28 of 30 comatose head-injured patients with a mean age of 27 years. Ninety percent of these patients had a prolonged QT interval, while 53 percent had nonspecific ST and T wave changes, especially T wave inversions and ST depression. No patient had ECG evidence of a massive myocardial infarction. The CK-MB remained elevated for 3 days after injury, in contrast to the time observed after an acute myocardial infarction, when CK-MB usually returns to normal after 24 to 36 h.

The abnormal ECGs and release of CK-MB may be attributable to the development of focal areas of myocardial necrosis in patients with severe head trauma. Myocardial lesions have been found in patients with lethal head injuries (Fig. 3-5).[75,95,96] Kolin and coworkers[96] found that foci of damaged myocardial fibers were more prevalent at autopsy in patients who died of intracranial mass lesions (62 percent) than control patients who died of other causes (26 percent). The myocardial damage that was present in the control subjects occurred in patients who died of either shock, acute circulatory failure, or metabolic failure. No victims of sudden violent death exhibited these lesions. Similar areas of focal myocardial damage have been described in association with the administration of catecholamines[97] and the induction of experimental intracerebral hemorrhage in animals.[98] The cardiac damage in experimental intracerebral hemorrhage was prevented by prior adrenalectomy or beta-adrenergic blockade.[88,98] Similar lesions in humans may also be prevented by sympathetic blockade.[99]

Causes of Hyperdynamic Cardiovascular Response

Although the sympathetic nervous system is implicated in the causes of the ECG changes and myocardial damage, the exact neuronal pathways mechanism of the damage is not known. The hyperdynamic cardiovascular response to head trauma is mediated by the central stimulation of the sympathetic nervous system, which is mediated by structures in the hypothalamus, nuclei of the solitary tract, area postrema, and areas A1 and A5 of the medulla.[83] These areas stimulate preganglionic sympathetic outflow tracts that activate the sympathetic nervous system and cause the release of catecholamines.[59,60] Ischemic stimulation of the posterior hypothalamus or insula cortex may be responsible for an abrupt increase in sympathetic tone.[83,100] Stimulation of the posterior hypothalamus resulted in marked hypertension, T wave changes, QT prolongation, and arrhythmias.[83] Neil-Dwyer and coworkers[99] found a

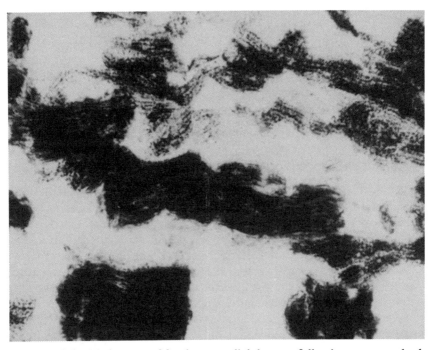

Figure 3-5 Example areas of focal myocardial damage following acute cerebral lesion. Focal damage characterized by granular staining pattern in upper third of picture. A band of normal myocardium characterized by myofibrillar staining is shown in the center. A histochemical method for succinic dehydrogenase activity using nitroblue tetrazolium was used. (*Reprinted from Kolin A, Norris JW,*[96] *with permission of publisher*).

high correlation between the presence of ischemic lesions in the hypothalamus and the presence of necrotic lesions in the myocardium in 54 patients who died following a subarachnoid hemorrhage.

Much of the evidence in support of the role of abnormal sympathetic nervous system activity and the release of catecholamines is derived from the similarity of the ECG changes and myocardial lesions to those induced by excessive amounts of catecholamines.[83,100] In contrast, administration of beta-adrenergic blockers reduced the myocardial damage in experimental models of intracerebral hemorrhage[88,98] and in head-injured patients.[86] The prevalence of T wave inversions and CK-MB levels was reduced in head-injured patients who were beta-blocked with atenolol compared with those who received a placebo.[86,99] Sympathetic blockade with stellate ganglion block reduced cardiac arrhythmias in patients with acute brain injuries.[101] Abnormal activation of the central sympathetic pathways may alter regional myocardial perfusion[76,83,100] and coronary vasospasm.[84] Sympathetic nervous system modulation is probably of more importance in causing the cardiovascular changes than the release of high levels of catecholamines.[102]

Electrolyte disturbances may also contribute to the ECG abnormalities and arrhythmias observed in head-injured patients. Hypokalemia may cause inverted T waves, ST depression, and prominent U waves. Hypocalcemia may increase the duration of the QT interval. Although these electrolyte disorders are common in the head-injured patient, the ECG changes usually correlate poorly with reduced electrolyte levels.[81]

Prognosis of Hyperdynamic Cardiovascular Changes

The significance of ECG changes and how such changes as well as the presence of myocardial lesions influence the outcome following head trauma is unclear. Although there are areas of focal myocardial necrosis, cardiac function assessed by an echocardiogram is generally normal. A poor correlation was found between the presence of ECG changes and wall motion abnormalities in patients following subarachnoid hemorrhage.[85] Wall motion abnormalities were observed in only a few patients and this occurrence correlated highly with the presence of severe neurological dysfunction. The incidence of potentially life-threatening arrhythmias may be increased in the presence of the ECG abnormalities. Prolongation of QT intervals, T wave flattening or inversion, and ST segment alterations represent repolarization abnormalities. In patients, following subarachnoid hemorrhage, serious ventricular arrhythmias, such as bigeminy or multifocal premature ventricular contractions, were accompanied by an increase in the QT interval.[74] Prolonged QT intervals have been associated with the *torsade de pointes* arrhythmia, a form of ventricular tachycardia.[77] This abnormality has been detected in 4 percent of patients with subarachnoid hemorrhage[103] and also occurs in patients with severe head trauma. It is initiated as a reentry mechanism when there is prolonged ventricular repolarization.

Treatment of Hyperdynamic Cardiovascular State

Because excessive sympathetic nervous system activity is implicated in both the cause of the ECG changes and the hyperdynamic cardiovascular state in head trauma patients, consideration should be given to the administration of beta-adrenergic blockers in the treatment of hypertension. If other causes of hypertension such as increased ICP and light anesthesia are first ruled out, beta-adrenergic blockers should be used to treat hypertension. Preliminary evidence also suggests that prophylactic beta-blockade may be helpful in reducing ECG changes indicative of myocardial ischemia and focal areas of myocardial necrosis and in preventing arrhythmias secondary to impaired ventricular repolarization.[99] In a randomized, double-blind study of 114 hemodynamically stable head trauma patients, Cruickshank and coworkers[86] found that the beta-blocker, atenolol, reduced the likelihood of supraventricular tachycardia, ST segment and T wave changes, and also prevented cardiac necrosis, as determined in the postmortem examination of six patients. Thirty percent of the placebo group, in contrast to 7.4 percent of the atenolol group had pathologically elevated CK-MB levels. Their findings are suggestive that beta 1-selective blockade might reduce catecholamine-induced myocardial necrosis. However, whether prophylactic beta-blockade actually improves outcome has not been studied; therefore, definite recommendations regarding the efficacy of beta-blockade of all patients cannot be made at this time.

Hypotension

In most situations, hypotension in the patient with an acute brain injury is due to a cause other than the head injury. In young children, blood loss from the scalp lacerations and within the expansible skull may lead to hypotension; however, in adults, isolated head injury is usually not associated with hypotension, as the blood loss from the head wound is usually insufficient to cause hypotension. If the patient is hypotensive, other sources of blood loss (e.g., pelvic, thoracic, abdominal, long bone) or causes of impaired cardiac output (e.g., tension pneumothorax) should be ruled out. A brain injury that would be severe enough to cause hypotension by itself would involve destruction of the vasomotor center in the medulla and is universally fatal.[95] Hypotension should be promptly treated as it may exacerbate neurologic damage.[104]

When an acute intracranial mass is decompressed and ICP is suddenly reduced to normal, hypotension may occur. Cushing[66] observed a marked (150–200 mmHg) decrease in systemic blood pressure following the removal of an intracranial blood clot in humans and reported the same observation in animals following the prompt reduction of ICP after artificial elevation. In most patients, the blood pressure falls from high to normal levels. However, a head-injured patient may have normal blood pressure if the increase in ICP is accompanied with hypovolemia resulting from blood loss or administration of mannitol. Such a patient may exhibit a severe hypotension with surgical compression of the brain, whereby the sympathetic tone is suddenly reduced, systemic vascular resistance decreases, and hypovolemia becomes manifest. Large amounts of intravenous fluids and vasopressors may be required to support the blood pressure in such patients.

FLUID AND ELECTROLYTE EFFECTS

Hypokalemia

The head-injured patient may develop hypokalemia in response to stress and trauma.[105] Beta-adrenergic stimulation from epinephrine causes a decrease in serum potassium by driving potassium into the cells.[106] Similarly when pH is elevated, as is common in the head-injured patient where hyperventilation is used to reduce ICP, potassium is driven intracellularly as hydrogen ions are released. Aldosterone secretion from the stress of trauma may also cause hypokalemia. Decreases in serum potassium associated with acute hyperventilation and stress do not need to be treated because total body potassium is unchanged. However, diuretic-induced renal losses of potassium require replacement in order to avoid complications of acute intracellular potassium depletion, including the potentiation of neuromuscular blockade and cardiac arrhythmias. Often in the patient with an acute brain injury, the cause of hypokalemia is multifactorial (Table 3-4). Initiation of treatment depends upon the prevailing clinical circumstances.

Hyponatremia

Hyponatremia may also occur in the patient with an acute brain-injury. Antidiuretic hormone (ADH) and aldosterone are released in response to the stress of the head trauma. Hyponatremia may be associated with three categories of extracellular fluid volumes (Table 3-4): (1) diminished (e.g., diuretic usage, adrenal insufficiency, natriuresis), (2) expanded (e.g., congestive heart failure, renal failure), and (3) normal [e.g., hypothyroidism, syndrome of inappropriate antidiuretic hormone (SIADH)]. Rapid reduction of serum sodium to less than 125 to 130 meq/liter may cause changes in mental status and seizures. The first step in diagnosis and treatment of hyponatremia is to establish the category to which the patient belongs.

Table 3-4 Fluid and Electrolyte Effects

Hypokalemia
    Stress and trauma (beta-adrenergic stimulation)
    Stress-induced aldosterone secretion
    Hyperventilation to lower Pa_{CO_2} and raise pH
    Renal losses due to diuretics or steroids

Hyponatremia
    Diminished volume
        (e.g., diuretics, adrenal insufficiency,
        CNS natriuresis)
    Normal volume
        (e.g., hypothyroidism, SIADH)
    Expanded volume
        (e.g., congestive heart failure, renal failure)

Hyperglycemia

Hypernatremia: Diabetes insipidus

Hyponatremia due to SIADH is fairly common in head-injured patients.[107] The diagnosis of SIADH should be made only after excluding other causes. Modest cases of SIADH are treated with fluid restriction. Demeclocycline, which impairs the effect of ADH on the kidney, is used to treat chronic SIADH.[108] Hypertonic saline is used only to correct particularly severe and symptomatic hyponatremia (serum sodium concentration <120 meq/liter). Judiciously rapid correction of such low concentrations by hypertonic saline until levels are mildly hyponatremic (serum sodium concentration, 121–134 meq/liter) is generally not harmful.[109] However, overzealous correction with rapid conversion of hyponatremia to normal levels of serum sodium concentration or hypernatremia may produce cerebral demyelinating lesions and death.[109]

In neurosurgical patients, hyponatremia may also be associated with intravascular volume depletion due to diuretic administration or a loss of sodium by the kidney. Following subarachnoid hemorrhage, patients may have a primary natriuresis ("cerebral salt wasting"), which unlike SIADH, is associated with a decreased intravascular volume.[110] Elevation of plasma and cerebrospinal atrial natriuretic factor, which regulates intravascular volume and sodium balance, have been observed in subarachnoid hemorrage[111,112]; however, the relationship between atrial natriuretic factor and hyponatremia remains unclear.[111] Cerebral salt wasting may also occur with head injury. In contrast to SIADH, aggressive fluid therapy, rather than fluid restriction, may be indicated to maintain a normal intravascular volume.

Hyperglycemia

Hyperglycemia often accompanies significant head trauma.[113–115] Increases in blood glucose levels may occur in response to increases in circulating catecholamines[60] and cortisol levels[116] that occur after head trauma. Insulin release is diminished by high catecholamine levels, and steroids promote gluconeogenesis. Hyperglycemia may reflect the extent and severity of the initial neurologic injury. The more severe the injury, the greater the increase in serum catecholamines, as an inverse relationship exists between the GCS score and the level of serum catecholamines.[60] The presence of hyperglycemia also correlates highly with the ultimate neurologic outcome following head injury.[114,115] In severely injured patients with a GCS score ≤8, an elevated blood glucose level greater than 200 mg/dl was associated with a significantly worse neurologic outcome. The increase in blood glucose may be both the cause and the effect of a worse neurologic outcome. Administration of glucose-containing solutions exacerbated the severity of ischemic brain injury in animals,[117] although hyperglycemia did not affect neurologic outcome in rats subjected to head trauma.[118] However, patients with persistent hyperglycemia had poorer outcome than patients with temporary hyperglycemia, and patients who had normal blood glucose levels on admission to hospital but who subsequently developed hyperglycemia, had a worse outcome than patients who remained normoglycemic.[115] These results suggest that a causal relationship may exist between hyperglycemia and poor outcome.

Hypernatremia: Diabetes Insipidus

Diabetes insipidus may occur in approximately 1 percent of head trauma patients. Patients with basilar skull fractures or severe head injuries involving the hypothalamus, pituitary stalk, or neurohypophysis, are at higher risk of incurring this disease.[119] Antidiuretic hormone (ADH) is synthesized in the hypothalamus and secreted by the posterior pituitary gland.[120] ADH enhances the permeability of free H_2O in the distal convoluted tubule and collecting duct of the kidney. Patients with diabetes insipidus can lose large volumes (25 liters/day) of dilute urine, resulting in marked increases in serum sodium and osmolality.

Diabetes insipidus should be considered in the differential diagnosis of polyuria in any patient with head trauma. The differential diagnosis of intraoperative polyuria includes (1) excessive fluid administration, (2) osmotic agents (e.g., hyperglycemia with glucose >180 mg/dl, mannitol), (3) use of diuretics, (4) paradoxical diuresis as in brain tumor patients, and (5) nephrogenic and central diabetes insipidus. Diabetes insipidus is diagnosed intraoperatively by ruling out iatrogenic causes, hyperglycemia, and by demonstrating marked increases in serum sodium and osmolality accompanied by low urine osmolality.

Treatment of diabetes insipidus involves adequate fluid replacement with 5 percent dextrose in water and administration of ADH. Aqueous vasopressin may be given intramuscularly (5–10 U) or as a slow intravenous infusion (3 U/h) for rapid control of intraoperative or postoperative diabetes insipidus.[120] Larger doses may cause hypertension. For less frequent dosage 1 to 2 μg desmopressin (DDAVP) given intravenously or subcuteanously every 6 to 12 h may be administered. DDAVP may be given more frequently if the diabetes insipidus is not controlled. DDAVP has less vasopressor activity than aqueous vasopressin and is preferable to vasopressin in patients with coronary artery disease and hypertension.

OTHER SYSTEMS (see Table 3-5)

Anterior Pituitary Dysfunction

In contrast to posterior pituitary dysfunction (SIADH and diabetes insipidus), anterior pituitary dysfunction is rare in patients who survive head trauma.[119] However, hypothalamic and pituitary damage is common in patients dying of head trauma. Anterior hypothalamic ischemia and hemorrhage

Table 3-5 Other Organ System Effects

Anterior pituitary dysfunction

Metabolic response to head injury

Musculoskeletal
  Cervical spine and maxillofacial injuries
  Succinylcholine-induced hyperkalemia

Disseminated intravascular coagulation (DIC)
  Diffuse intravascular thrombosis
  Consumptive coagulopathy

Gastrointestinal
  Full stomach
  Concurrent intraabdominal injury
  Delayed gastric emptying
  Stress gastritis and ulceration

were observed at autopsy in 40 percent of patients who died of head trauma.[121] Most patients have adequate hormonal reserves so that anterior pituitary dysfunction is not symptomatic for up to several weeks after injury. Adenohypophyseal function may be impaired because of hypothalamic injury, which results in loss of releasing factors, or impairment may be caused by anterior lobe pituitary infarction, due to interruption of the vascular supply. Patients with basal or temporal skull fractures are at higher risk for anterior pituitary dysfunction.[122] Multiple endocrine abnormalities including deficiencies of growth hormone, adrenocorticotropin (ACTH), follicle-stimulating hormone (FSH), luteinizing hormone (LH), prolactin and thyrotropin (TSH) have been reported.[123–126] Abnormalities of thermoregulation may also occur.[119]

Metabolic Response to Head Injury

Severe head traumas, such as burns and other trauma-induced injuries, result in an increased caloric requirement and increased protein catabolism.[127,128] The mean resting metabolic expenditure for head trauma patients was more than twice that expected for uninjured patients.[127] Metabolic demand is further increased by the presence of agitation, fever, secondary infections, and seizures. The increased sympathetic activity causes mobilization of carbohydrate and fat stores and protein catabolism. Protein is broken down to provide alanine and glutamine, required for gluconeogenesis. The most severe protein losses in addition to increased oxygen consumption and carbon dioxide production occur in the more severely injured patients (GCS score <5).[127]

The hypermetabolism resolves in noninfected head trauma patients by the end of the first week after injury.[128] However, nitrogen excretion remains increased, an effect which may reflect equilibration of muscle mass to reduced activity.[128] Head-injured patients had a metabolic response similar to that for patients with burns of 20 to 40 percent of the body surface area.[127]

Musculoskeletal Sequelae

Head trauma patients are at high risk for bone injuries, including maxillofacial, spine, pelvic, and long-bone fractures (Table 3-5). Ten percent of patients with head trauma have a cervical spine injury[129]; therefore, all head-injured patients should be considered to have a cervical spine injury until proved otherwise by x-ray studies or computerized tomography or both. The presence of maxillofacial injuries may also render airway support and endotracheal intubation more difficult. Pneumocephalus, subcutaneous emphysema, intracranial entry of nasogastric tubes,[130] Horner's syndrome, or neck hematomas with airway obstruction may accompany the head injury. Horner's syndrome, diagnosed by a relative miosis, slight ptosis, and preservation of normal light reflex may develop following injury to the facial sympathetic supply.[131] Comparison with the normal pupil may confuse the physical diagnosis of an intracerebral mass lesion.

Head trauma patients with and without paresis may develop hyperkalemia in response to the administration of succinylcholine similar to the time frame and events after a spinal cord injury.[132,133] Hence, succinylcholine should be avoided for 48 to 72 h after severe head trauma.

Coagulopathy

The patient with head trauma is at a high risk for the development of disseminated intravascular coagulation (DIC) (Table 3-5). DIC is a diffuse intravascular thrombosis that arises following the activation of the coagulation cascade (Fig. 3-6).[134] It results in a hemorrhagic diathesis due to the consumption of platelets, fibrinogen, and clotting factors, especially factors V and VIII. The body responds to the intravascular deposition of fibrin by fibrinolysis, in which plasminogen is activated to plasmin. Plasmin degrades fibrin or fibrinogen and destroys factors V and VIII. The fibrin-split products that are formed possess anticoagulant properties that further aggravate the bleeding disorder.

Abnormalities of the standard coagulation tests (fibrinogen, fibrin degradation products, platelet count, prothrombin time, activated partial thromboplastin time, and thrombin clotting time) are extremely common in head trauma patients.[135,136] For instance, 71 percent of children with head injuries had abnormalities of one or more clotting tests and 32 percent of children with head injuries had DIC by laboratory criteria.[137] Even if normal clotting is

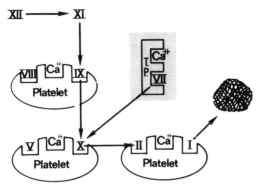

Figure 3-6 Activation of coagulation cascade in DIC. T.P., tissue thromboplastin; Ca^{2+}, calcium; coagulation cascade may be activated by the intrinsic pathway (factors XII, XI, VIII, IX) or by the extrinsic pathway (factor VII). Brain thromboplastin initiates DIC by activating the extrinsic pathway. (*Reprinted by permission of the publisher from Fischbach DP, Fogdall RP.*[134])

found in peripheral blood, jugular vein samples may indicate a localized coagulopathy.[138] Full-blown DIC is particularly common in head trauma patients who have clinical evidence of destruction of brain tissue (e.g., gunshot, massive blunt trauma), whereas it is relatively uncommon in head trauma patients who do not have such clinical evidence (e.g., concussion).[135] Hypofibrinogenemia and low levels of factors V and VIII and platelets were observed in 9 of 13 patients who had direct destruction of brain tissue, but these conditions were not observed in 13 others who had cerebral trauma without obvious brain destruction.[135] Microvascular thrombi, infarction, and secondary hemorrhage were often observed at autopsy in the brain, lungs, liver, pancreas, and kidneys of patients who died of head trauma.[139] This histopathologic evidence of DIC was observed at autopsy in 14 of 16 (88 percent) patients with laboratory evidence of DIC.[139]

The severity of the coagulation abnormalities correlates well with severity of the head injury.[136] Neurologic outcome following head trauma is poorer in patients who develop DIC.[138] An increased level of fibrin degradation products (FDP) is an excellent predictor of a poor outcome from head trauma, being similar to the GCS in prognostic value.[9] Elevation of FDP was a particularly good predictor of poor outcome in patients with moderately severe neurologic injuries, as indicated by GCS scores of 9 to 15.[136] For instance, of the 8 patients who died out of 51 patients with GCS scores of 9 to 12, 7 had severely abnormal levels of FDP. All 25 patients with mildly abnormal FDP levels survived.[136] An increase in FDP levels may also identify patients with head injury who are at high risk for developing ARDS.[9]

The causes of DIC in the head trauma patient are multifactorial.[9,135,140,141] The most significant mechanism of DIC in head trauma is the release of brain thromboplastin into the systemic circulation. The brain contains high concentrations of tissue thromboplastin that is released into the blood stream with destruction of brain tissue. Brain thromboplastin is a potent initiator of the coagulation cascade. Brain thromboplastin causes DIC when it is injected intravenously in dogs.[142] Stagnation of cerebral blood flow, tissue acidosis, hypoxia, and damage to the cerebral endothelium associated with shock, sepsis, and massive transfusions may also contribute to the development of DIC in the head trauma patient.

As the risk of postoperative or recurrent intracranial hemorrhage or both is increased in the presence of abnormalities of coagulation and fibrinolysis, prompt recognition and treatment of the coagulopathy is necessary. Persistent intracranial bleeding may contribute to sudden neurologic deterioration in potentially salvageable patients. Treatment of DIC involves locating and treating the initiating cause, while replacing the consumed clotting factors. Platelets should be replaced to yield a platelet count greater than $100,000/\mu l$. Replacement of factors V and VIII should be accomplished with fresh frozen plasma (or cryoprecipitate for factor VIII), aiming for a normal partial thromboplastin time (PTT). Fibrinogen should be replaced with cryoprecipitate or fresh frozen plasma until the fibrinogen level is greater than 200 mg/dl. Because the risk of bleeding is particularly serious in patients with head injuries, antifibrinolytic therapy (e.g., epsilon aminocaproic acid) and heparin are not advised.

Gastrointestinal System

There are multiple gastrointestinal complications of head trauma, including concurrent intraabdominal injury, delayed gastric emptying, stress gastritis, and ulceration (Table 3-5). Intraabdominal injuries may be present in the patient with an acute head injury. Similar to other trauma patients, all patients with acute head injury should be assumed to have a full stomach. Head trauma patients are at high risk for aspiration of gastric contents, due to the alteration in their mental status. Significant blood alcohol levels have been found in more than 50 percent of head-injured patients.[143] Gastric atony may be present for several weeks following severe head trauma[144] and may adversely affect the outcome from head trauma.

Patients with delayed gastric emptying tolerated enteral feedings at a slower rate compared with patients with normal gastric emptying.[144] There is an association among severity of the head injury, the increase in ICP, and the ability to tolerate enteral feedings.[145] Whereas early nutrition may reduce septic complications after major abdominal trauma,[146] poor nutrition may adversely affect outcome from head trauma. Gastric emptying may be delayed after severe head trauma because of sympathetic nervous system activation associated with stress, elevated ICP, and neurologic damage.

Stress gastritis and ulceration are common after head trauma.[147-150] Gastrointestinal bleeding has been reported in 15 to 20 percent of head trauma patients, with almost half of these occurring within 48 h of injury.[147,148] However, the incidence of severe stress bleeding has decreased within the past 10 years.[151] Currently, a rate of 5 to 8 percent of mild stress-related bleeding is reported.[150]

The prevalence of upper gastrointestinal lesions is much higher than the prevalence of overt gastrointestinal bleeding.[148-150] Over 90 percent of patients with severe head trauma had endoscopic evidence of gastritis less than 12 h after injury.[149] Gastritis after head trauma may result as a physiologic response to severe stress.[152] Because of the concern that hyperacidity may exacerbate the severity of the lesions, prophylactic treatment to raise gastric pH has been advised. However, recent evidence has suggested that prophylactic treatment with antacids or cimetidine may not be effective in reducing stress ulceration,[150] and it may increase the likelihood of nosocomial pneumonia.[16] While histamine receptor type 2 (H_2) blockers and antacids both increase gastric pH, the incidence and severity of stress gastritis were similar in treated and untreated groups,[150] perhaps because the lesions appeared so quickly after injury.[149] Antacids and H_2-blockers may increase the risk of nosocomial pneumonia in critically ill patients.[16] In contrast, prophylactic use of sucralfate, an agent which does not increase gastric pH, may protect against gastric bacterial overgrowth and nosocomial pneumonia.[16]

In summary, there are numerous systemic sequelae of head trauma, both as a direct result of the initial injury as well as an indirect complication from the brain injury. Derangements in the pulmonary, cardiovascular, endocrinologic, musculoskeletal, coagulative, and gastrointestinal systems are common in head trauma patients and contribute to the morbidity and mortality from head trauma.

REFERENCES

1. Katsurada K, Yamada R, Sugimoto T: Respiratory insufficiency in patients with severe head injury. *Surgery* 73:191, 1973.

2. Sinha RP, Ducker TB, Perot PL: Arterial oxygenation: Findings and its significance in central nervous system trauma patients. *JAMA* 224:1258, 1973.

3. Moss IR, Wald A, Ransohoff J: Respiratory functions and chemical regulation of ventilation in head injury. *Am Rev Respir Dis* 109:205, 1974.

4. Frost EAM, Arancibia CU, Shulman K: Pulmonary shunt as a prognostic indicator in head injury. *J Neurosurg* 50:768, 1979

5. Miller JD, Butterworth JF, Gudeman SK, et al: Further experience in the management of severe head injury. *J Neurosurg* 54:289, 1981.

6. Frost EAM: The physiopathology of respiration in neurosurgical patients. *J Neurosurg* 50:699, 1979.

7. Van Besouw JP, Hinds CJ: Fat embolism syndrome. *Br J Hosp Med* 42:304, 1989.

8. Fowler AA, Hamman RF, Good JT, et al: Adult respiratory distress syndrome: Risk with common predispositions. *Am Int Med* 98:593, 1983.

9. Crone KR, Lee KS, Kelley DL: Correlation of admission fibrin degradation products with outcome and respiratory failure in patients with severe head injury. *Neurosurgery* 21:532, 1987.

10. Demling R, Riessen R: Pulmonary dysfunction after cerebral injury. *Crit Care Med* 18:768, 1990.

11. Helling T, Evans L, Fowler D, et al: Infectious complications in patients with severe head injury. *J Trauma* 28:1575, 1988.

12. Braun SR, Levin AB, Clark KL: Role of corticosteroids in the development of pneumonia in mechanically ventilated head-trauma victims. *Crit Care Med* 14:198, 1986.

13. Craven DE, Kunches LM, Kilinsky V, et al: Risk factors for pneumonia and fatality in patients receiving continuous mechanical ventilation. *Am Rev Respir Dis* 133:792, 1986.

14. Luce JM: Medical management of head injury. *Chest* 89:864, 1988.

15. Massei R, Baratta P, Mulazzi D, et al: Impairment of cell-mediated immunity in severe head trauma. *Agressologie* 29:423, 1988.

16. Driks MR, Craven DE, Celli BR, et al: Nosocomial pneumonia in intubated patients given sucralfate as compared to antacids or histamine type 2 blockers: The role of gastric colonization. *N Engl J Med* 317:1376, 1987.

17. Swan K, Black P: Deep vein thromboses and pulmonary emboli in neurosurgical patients: A review. *J Neurosurg* 61:1055, 1984.

18. Kaufman HH, Satterwhite T, McConnell BJ, et al: Deep vein thrombosis and pulmonary embolism in head-injured patients. *Angiology* 34:627, 1983.

19. North BJ, Jennett S: Abnormal breathing patterns associated with acute brain damage. *Arch Neurol* 31:338, 1974.

20. Baigelman W, O'Brien JC: Pulmonary effects of head trauma. *Neurosurgery* 9:729, 1981.

21. Cooper KR, Boswell PA: Reduced functional residual capacity and abnormal oxygenation in patients with severe head injury. *Chest* 84:29, 1983.

22. Berman IR, Ducker TB, Simmons RL: The effects of increased intracranial pressure upon the oxygenation of blood in dogs. *J Neurosurg* 30:532, 1969.

23. Maxwell JA, Goodwin JW: Neurogenic pulmonary shunting. *J Trauma* 13:368, 1973.

24. Pace NL: Fluctuating hypoxemia and pulmonary shunting following fatal head trauma: A case report. *Anesth Analg* 50:129, 1977.

25. Epstein FM, Cooper KR, Ward JD: Profound pulmonary shunting without edema following stereotaxic biopsy of hypothalamic germinoma. *J Neurosurg* 68:303, 1988.

26. Schumacker PT, Rhodes GR, Newell JC, et al: Ventilation-perfusion imbalance after head trauma. *Amer Rev Resp Dis* 119:33, 1979.

27. Popp AJ, Shah DM, Berman RA, et al: Delayed pulmonary dysfunction in head-injured patients. *J Neurosurg* 57:784, 1982.

28. Domino KB, Hlastala MP, Cheney FW: Effect of increased intracranial pressure on regional hypoxic pulmonary vasoconstriction. *Anesthesiology* 72:490, 1990.

29. Cohen HB, Gambill AF, Eggers GWN: Acute pulmonary edema following head injury: Two case reports. *Anesth Analg* 56:136, 1977.

30. Weir BK: Pulmonary edema following fatal aneurysm rupture. *J Neurosurg* 49:502, 1978.

31. Carlson RW, Schaeffer RC, Michaels SG, et al: Pulmonary edema following intracranial hemorrhage. *Chest* 75:731, 1979.

32. Albin MS, Bunegin L, Wolf S: Brain and lungs at risk after cervical spinal cord transection: Intracranial pressure, brain water, blood-brain barrier permeability, cerebral blood flow, and extravascular lung water changes. *Surg Neurol* 24:191, 1985.

33. Braude N, Ludgrove T: Neurogenic pulmonary oedema precipitated by induction of anaesthesia. *Br J Anaesth* 62:101, 1989.

34. Findler G, Cotev S: Neurogenic pulmonary edema associated with a colloid cyst in the third ventricle. *J Neurosurg* 52:395, 1980.

35. Terrence CF, Rao GR, Perper JA: Neurogenic pulmonary edema in unexpected, unexplained death of epileptic patients. *Ann Neurol* 9:458, 1981.

36. Reynolds RW: Pulmonary edema as a consequence of hypothalamic lesions in rats. *Science* 141:930, 1963.

37. Colice GL, Matthay MA, Bass E, et al: Neurogenic pulmonary edema. *Am Rev Respir Dis* 130:941, 1984.

38. Malik AB: Mechanism of neurogenic pulmonary edema. *Circ Res* 57:1, 1985.

39. Ducker TB, Simmons RL: Increased intracranial pressure and pulmonary edema. II. The hemodynamic response of dogs and monkeys to increased intracranial pressure. *J Neurosurg* 28:118, 1968.

40. Maron MB: A canine model of neurogenic pulmonary edema. *J Appl Physiol* 59:1019, 1985.

41. Maron MB: Analysis of airway fluid protein concentration in neurogenic pulmonary edema. *J Appl Physiol* 62:470, 1987.

42. Minnear FL, Kite C, Hill LA, Vander Zee H: Endothelial injury and pulmonary congestion characterize neurogenic pulmonary edema in rabbits. *J Appl Physiol* 63:335, 1987.

43. Maron MB, Dawson CA: Adrenal component to pulmonary hypertension induced by elevated cerebrospinal fluid pressure. *J Appl Physiol* 47:153, 1979.

44. Maron MB, Dawson CA: Pulmonary vasoconstriction caused by elevated cerebrospinal fluid pressure in the dog. *J Appl Physiol* 49:73, 1980.

45. Maron MB: Effect of elevated vascular pressure transients on protein permeability in the lung. *J Appl Physiol* 67:305, 1989.

46. Maron MB: Pulmonary vasoconstriction in a canine model of neurogenic pulmonary edema. *J Appl Physiol* 68:912, 1990.

47. McCellan MD, Dauber IM, Weil JV: Elevated intracranial pressure increases pulmonary vascular permeability to protein. *J Appl Physiol* 67:1185, 1989.

48. Frost EAM: Effects of positive end-expiratory pressure on intracranial pressure and compliance in brain-injured patients. *J Neurosurg* 47:195, 1977.

49. Cooper KR, Boswell PA, Choi SG: Safe use of PEEP in patients with severe head injury. *J Neurosurg* 63:552, 1985.

50. Apuzzo MLJ, Weiss MH, Petersons V, et al: Effect of positive end-expiratory pressure ventilation on intracranial pressure in man. *J Neurosurg* 46:227, 1977.

51. Shapiro HM, Marshall LF: Intracranial pressure responses to PEEP in head-injured patients. *J Trauma* 18:254, 1978.

52. Burchiel K, Steege TD, Wyler AR: Intracranial pressure changes in brain-injured patients requiring positive end-expiratory pressure ventilation. *Neurosurgery* 8:443, 1981.

53. Huseby JS, Pavlin EG, Butler J: Effect of positive end-expiratory pressure on intracranial pressure in dogs. *J App Physiol* 44:25, 1978.

54. Doblar DD, Santiago TV, Kahn AU, et al: The effect of positive end-expiratory pressure ventilation (PEEP) on cerebral blood flow and cerebrospinal fluid pressure in goats. *Anesthesiology* 55:244, 1981.

55. Luce JM, Huseby JS, Kirk W, et al: Mechanism by which positive end-expiratory pressure increases intracranial pressure in dogs. *J Appl Physiol* 52:231, 1982.

56. Cotev S, Paul WL, Ruiz BC, et al: Positive end-expiratory pressure (PEEP) and cerebrospinal fluid pressure during normal and elevated intracranial pressure in dogs. *Intensive Care Med* 7:187, 1981.

57. Aidinis SJ, Lafferty J, Shapiro H: Intracranial responses to PEEP. *Anesthesiology* 45:275, 1976.

58. Clifton GL, Robertson CS, Kyper K, et al: Cardiovascular response to severe head injury. *J Neurosurg* 59:447, 1983.

59. Graff CJ, Rossi NP: Catecholamine response to intracranial hypertension. *J Neurosurg* 49:862, 1968.

60. Clifton GL, Ziegler MG, Grossman RG: Circulatory catecholamines and sympathetic activity after head injury. *Neurosurgery* 8:10, 1981.

61. Brown RS, Mohr PA, Carey JS, et al: Cardiovascular changes after cranial cerebral injury and increased intracranial pressure. *Surg Gynecol Obstet* 125:1205, 1987.

62. Schulte AM, Esch J, Murday H, et al: Haemodynamic changes in patients with severe head injury. *Acta Neurochir* 54:243, 1980.

63. Popp JA, Gottlieb ME, Paloski WH, et al: Cardiopulmonary hemodynamics in patients with serious head injury. *J Surg Res* 32:416, 1982.

64. Cushing H: Concerning a definite regulatory mechanism of the vasomotor center which controls blood pressure during cerebral compression. *Johns Hopkins Hosp Bull* 12:290, 1901.

65. Robard S, Saiki H: Mechanism of the pressure response to increased intracranial pressure. *Am J Physiol* 168:234, 1952.

66. Cushing H: Some experimental and clinical observations concerning states of increased intracranial tension. *Am J Med Sci* 124:375, 1902.

67. Cushing H: The blood-pressure reaction of acute cerebral compression, illustrated by cases of intracranial hemorrhage. *Am J Med Sci* 125:1017, 1903.

68. Kanter RK, Carroll JB, Post EM: Association of arterial hypertension with poor outcome in children with acute brain injury. *Clin Pediatr* 24:320, 1985.

69. Bleyaert AL, Sands PA, Safar P, et al: Augmentation of postischemic brain damage by severe intermittent hypertension. *Crit Care Med* 8:41, 1980.

70. Overgaard J, Christensen S, Hvid-Hansen O, et al: Prognosis after head injury based on early clinical exam. *Lancet* 2:631, 1973.

71. Miner ME, Allen SJ: Cardiovascular effects of severe head injury. In Frost EAM (ed): *Clinical Anesthesia in Neurosurgery*. Boston, Butterworth, 1991:439.

72. Hersch C: Electrocardiographic changes in head injuries. *Circulation* 23:853, 1961.

73. Marshall AJ: Transient atrial fibrillation after minor head injury. *Br Heart J* 38:984, 1976.

74. Di Pasquale G, Pinelli G, Andreoli A, et al: Holter detection of cardiac arrhythmias in intracranial subarachnoid hemorrhage. *Am J Cardiol* 59:596, 1987.

75. Nadas AS, Alimurung MM, Linenthal AJ: Persistent ventricular pacemaker following basal skull fracture; report of case in 5 year old girl. *Am Heart J* 42:888, 1951.

76. McLeod AA, Neil-Dwyer G, Meyer CHA, et al: Cardiac sequelae of acute head injury. *Br Heart J* 47:221, 1982.

77. Rotem M, Constantini S, Shir Y, et al: Life-threatening torsade de pointes arrhythmia associated with head injury. *Neurosurgery* 23:89, 1988.

78. Leipzig TJ, Lowensohn RI: Heart rate variability in neurosurgical patients. *Neurosurgery* 19:356, 1986.

79. Weidler DJ: Myocardial damage and cardiac arrhythmias after intracranial hemorrhage: A critical review. *Stroke* 5:759, 1974.

80. Hersch C: Electrocardiographic changes in subarachnoid haemorrhage, meningitis, and intracranial space-occupying lesions. *Brit Heart J* 26:785, 1964.

81. Rudehill A, Olsson GL, Sundqvist K, et al: ECG abnormalities in patients with subarachnoid haemorhage and intracranial tumours. *J Neurol Neurosurg Psych* 50:1375, 1987.

82. Tobias SL, Bookatz BJ, Diamond TH: Myocardial damage and electrocardiographic changes in acute cerebrovascular hemorrhage: A report of three cases and review. *Heart Lung* 16:521, 1987.

83. Oppenheimer SM, Cechetto DF, Hachinski VC: Cerebrogenic cardiac arrhythmias: Cerebral electrocardiographic influences and their role in sudden death. *Arch Neurol* 47:513, 1990.

84. Yuki K, Kodama Y, Onda J, et al: Coronary vasospasm following subarachnoid hemorrhage as a cause of stunned myocardium. *J Neurosurg* 75:308, 1991.

85. Davies KR, Gelb AW, Manninen PH, et al: Cardiac function in aneurysmal subarachnoid haemorrhage: A study of electrocardiographic and echocardiographic abnormalities. *Brit J Anaesth* 67:58, 1991.

86. Cruickshank JM, Neil-Dwyer G, Hayes Y, et al: Stress/catecholamine induced cardiac necrosis: Reduction by beta 1-selective blockage. *Postgrad Med* 83:140, 1988.

87. Norris JW, Hachinski VC, Myers MG, et al: Serum cardiac enzymes in stroke. *Stroke* 10:548, 1979.

88. Hawkins WE, Clower BR: Myocardial damage after head trauma and simulated intracranial hemorrhage in mice: The role of the autonomic nervous system. *Cardiovasc Res* 5:524, 1971.

89. Uchida M, Saito K, Niitsu T, et al: Model of electrocardiographic changes seen with subarachnoid hemorrhage in rabbits. *Stroke* 20:112, 1989.

90. Abildskov JA: Adrenergic effects on the QT interval of the electrocardiogram. *Am Heart J* 92:210, 1976.

91. Kolin A, Kvasnicka J. Pseudoinfarction pattern of the QRS complex in experimental cardiac hypoxia induced by noradrenalin. *Cardiologia* 43:362, 1963.

92. Hackenberry LE, Miner ME, Rea GL, et al: Biochemical evidence of myocardial injury after severe head trauma. *Crit Care Med* 10:641, 1982.

93. Fabinyi G, Hunt D, McKinley L: Myocardial creatine kinase isoenzyme in serum after subarachnoid hemorrhage. *J Neurol Neurosurg Psychiatry* 40:818, 1977.

94. Kaste M, Somer H, Konttinen A: Heart type creatine kinase isoenzyme (CK MB) in acute cerebral disorders. *Br Heart J* 40:802, 1978.

95. Clifton GL, McCormick WF, Grossman RG: Neuropathology of early and late deaths after head injury. *Neurosurg* 8:309, 1981.

96. Kolin A, Norris JW: Myocardial damage from acute cerebral lesions. *Stroke* 15:990, 1984.

97. Ferrans VJ, Hibbs RG, Weiley HS, et al: A histochemical and electron microscope study of epinephrine-induced myocardial necrosis. *J Mol Cell Cardiol* 1:11, 1970.

98. Hunt D, Gore I: Myocardial lesions following experimental intracranial hemorrhage: Prevention with propranolol. *Am Heart J* 83:232, 1972.

99. Neil-Dwyer G, Cruickshank JM, Doshi R: The stress response in subarachnoid haemorrhage and head injury. *Acta Neurochir* 47(suppl):102, 1990.

100. Marion DW, Segal R, Thompson ME: Subarachnoid hemorrhage and the heart. *Neurosurgery* 18:101, 1986.

101. Grossman MA: Cardiac arrhythmias in acute central nervous system disease: Successful management with stellate ganglion block. *Arch Intern Med* 136:203, 1976.

102. Grad A, Kialeta T, Osredkar J: Effect of elevated plasma norepinephrine on electrocardiographic changes in subarachnoid hemorrhage. *Stroke* 22:746, 1991.

103. De Pasquale G, Pinelli G, Andreoli A, et al: Torsade de pointes and ventricular flutter-fibrillation following spontaneous cerebral subarachnoid hemorrhage. *Int J Cardiol* 18:163, 1988.

104. Andrews BT, Levy ML, Pitts LH: Implications of systemic hypotension for the neurological examination in patients with severe head injury. *Surg Neurol* 28:419, 1987.

105. Shin B, MacKenzie CF, Helrich M: Hypokalemia in trauma patients. *Anesthesiology* 65:90, 1986.

106. Rosa RM, Silva P, Young JB, et al: Adrenergic modulation of extrarenal potassium disposal. *N Engl J Med* 302:431, 1980.

107. Bartter FC, Schwartz WB: The syndrome of inappropriate secretion of antidiuretic hormone. *Am J Med* 42:790, 1967.

108. De Troyer A: Demeclocycline: Treatment for syndrome of inappropriate antidiuretic hormone secretion. *JAMA* 237:2723, 1977.

109. Ayus JC, Krothapali RK, Arieff AI: Treatment of symptomatic hyponatremia and its relation to brain damage. *N Engl J Med* 317:1190, 1987.

110. Nelson PB, Seif S, Gutai J, et al: Hyponatremia and natriuresis following subarachnoid hemorrhage in a monkey model. *J Neurosurg* 60:233, 1984.

111. Diringer MN, Kirsch JR, Ladenson PW, et al: Cerebrospinal fluid atrial natriuretic factor in intracranial disease. *Stroke* 21:1550, 1990.

112. Diringer MN, Lim JS, Kirsch JR, et al: Suprasellar and intra-ventricular blood predict elevated plasma atrial natriuretic factor in subarachnoid hemorrhage. *Stroke* 22:577, 1991.

113. King LR, Knowles HC Jr, McLaurin RL, et al: Glucose tolerance and plasma insulin in cranial trauma. *Ann Surg* 173:337, 1971.

114. Young B, Ott L, Dempsey R, Haack D, et al: Relationship between admission hyperglycemia and neurologic outcome of severely brain-injured patients. *Ann Surg* 210:466, 1989.

115. Lam AM, Winn HR, Cullen BF, et al: Hyperglycemia and neurological outcome in patients with head injury. *J. Neurosurg* 75:545, 1991.

116. King LR, McLaurin RL, Lewis HP, et al: Plasma cortisol levels after head injury. *Ann Surg* 172:975, 1970.

117. Lanier WL, Strangland KJ, Scheithauer BW, et al: The effects of dextrose infusion and head position on neurologic outcome after complete cerebral ischemia in primates. Examination of a model. *Anesthesiology* 66:39, 1987.

118. Shapira Y, Artru AA, Cotev S, et al: Brain edema and neurologic status following head trauma in the rat. *Anesthesiology* 77:79, 1992.

119. Kaufman HH, Timberlake G, Voelker J, et al: Medical complications of head injury. *Med Clin North Am* 77:43, 1993.

120. Harris AS: Clinical experience with desmopressin: Efficacy and safety in central diabetes insipidus and other conditions. *J Pediatr* 114:711, 1989.

121. Crompton MR: Hypothalamic lesions following closed head injury. *Brain* 94:165, 1971.

122. McCullagh EP, Schaffenburg CA: Anterior pituitary insufficiency following skull fracture. *J Clin Endocrinol Metab* 13:1283, 1953.

123. Altman R, Pruzanski W: Postraumatic hypopituitarism: Anterior pituitary insufficiency following skull fracture. *Am Intern Med* 55:149, 1961.

124. Goldman KP, Jacobs A: Anterior and posterior pituitary failure after head injury. *Br Med J* 2:1924, 1960.

125. Paxson CL, Brown DR: Post-traumatic anterior hypopituitarism. *Pediatrics* 57:893, 1976.

126. Weiss SR, Jacobi JD, Fishman LM, et al: Hypopituitarism following head trauma. *Am J Obstet Gynecol* 127:678, 1977.

127. Clifton GL, Robertson CS, Grossman RG, et al: The metabolic response to severe head injury. *J Neurosurg* 60:687, 1984.

128. Deutschman CS, Konstantinides FN, Rupp S, et al: Physiologic and metabolic response to isolated closed-head injury. *J Neurosurg* 64:89, 1986.

129. Shrago GG: Cervical spine injuries; association with head trauma: A review of 50 patients. *Am J Roentgenol Radium Ther Nucl Med* 118:670, 1973.

130. Wyler AR, Reynolds AF: An intracranial complication of nasogastric intubation: Case report. *J Neurosurg* 47:297, 1977.

131. White PR: Horner's syndrome and its significance in the management of head and neck trauma. *Br J Oral Surg* 14:165, 1976.

132. Stevenson PH, Birch AA: Succinylcholine induced hyperkalemia in a patient with a closed head injury. *Anesthesiology* 51:89, 1979.

133. Frankville DD, Drummond JC: Hyperkalemia after succinylcholine administration in a patient with closed-head injury without paresis. *Anesthesiology* 67:264, 1987.

134. Fischbach DP, Fogdall RP: *Coagulation: The Essentials.* Baltimore, Williams & Wilkins, 1981.

135. Goodnight SH, Kenoyer G, Rapaport SI, et al: Defibrination after brain-tissue destruction: A serious complication of head injury. *N Engl J Med* 290:1043, 1974.

136. Olson JD, Kaufman HH, Moake J, et al: The incidence and significance of hemostatic abnormalities in patients with head injuries. *Neurosurgery* 24:825, 1989.

137. Miner ME, Kaufman HH, Graham SH, et al: Disseminated intravascular coagulation fibrinolytic syndrome following head injury in children: Frequency and prognostic implications. *J Pediatr* 100:687, 1982.

138. Kaufman HH, Mattson JC: Coagulopathy in head injury. In Becker DP, Povlishock JT, (eds): *Central Nervous System Trauma Status Report.* Richmond, William Byrd Press, 1985:187.

139. Kaufman HH, Hui KS, Mattson JC, et al: Clinicopathological correlations of disseminated intravascular coagulation in patients with head injury. *Neurosurgery* 15:34, 1984.

140. Clarke JA, Finelli RE, Netsky MG: Disseminated intravascular coagulation following cranial trauma: Case report. *J Neurosurg* 52:266, 1980.

141. Touho H, Hirakawa K, Hiro A, et al: Relationship between abnormalities of coagulation and fibrinolysis and postoperative intracranial hemorrhage in head injury. *Neurosurgery* 19:523, 1986.

142. Cooper HA, Bowie EJW, Owen CA Jr.: Chronic induced intravascular coagulation in dogs. *Am J Physiol* 225:1355, 1973.

143. Kraus JF, Morganstern H, Fife D, et al: Blood alcohol tests: Prevalence of involvement and early outcome following brain injury. *Am J Public Health* 79:294, 1989.

144. Ott L, Young B, Phillips R, et al: Altered gastric emptying in the head-injured patient: Relationship to feeding intolerance. *J Neurosurg* 74:738, 1991.

145. Norton JA, Ott LG, McClain C, et al: Intolerance to enteral feeding in the brain-injured patient. *J Neurosurg* 68:62, 1988.

146. Moore EE, Tones TN: Benefits of immediate jejunostomy feeding after major abdominal trauma: A prospective randomized study. *J Trauma* 26:874, 1986.

147. Kamada T, Fusamoto H, Kawano S, et al: Gastrointestinal bleeding following head injury: A clinical study of 433 cases. *J Trauma* 17:44, 1977.

148. Halloran LG, Zfass AM, Gayle WE, et al: Prevention of acute gastrointestinal complications after severe head injury: A controlled trial of cimetidine prophylaxis. *Am J Surg* 139:44, 1980.

149. Brown TH, Davidson PF, Larson GM: Acute gastritis occurring within 24 hours of severe head injury. *Gastrointest Endosc* 35:37, 1989.

150. Reusser P, Gyr K, Scheidegger D: Prospective endoscopic study of stress erosions and ulcers in critically ill neurosurgical patients: Current incidence and effect of acid-reducing prophylaxis. *Crit Care Med* 18:270, 1990.

151. Groll A, Simon JB, Wigle RD, et al: Cimetidine prophylaxis for gastrointestinal bleeding in an intensive care unit. *Gut* 27:135, 1986.

152. Norton L, Greer T, Eiseman B: Gastric secretary response to head injury. *Arch Surg* 101:200, 1970.

Head Trauma Imaging

Wendy A. Cohen

GENERAL PRINCIPLES OF HEAD TRAUMA IMAGING

Use of CT and MRI in Acute Head Injury

Computerized tomography (CT) has been and remains the radiologic study of choice for the patient with acute cranial trauma.[1] Cranial CT is highly sensitive for diagnosis of acute intracranial hemorrhage and of mass lesions.[2–4] This high sensitivity was shown in early CT studies and remains true despite the development of other imaging techniques. CT continues to be accurate, rapid, easy to perform, and sensitive to the presence of acute intracranial hemorrhage with mass effect that may require neurosurgical intervention.[5–8] CT also shows injury to osseous structures. Subtle parenchymal density differences which, in patients with cranial trauma, may indicate underlying shear injury, are not seen as well with CT.[9] Magnetic resonance imaging (MRI), which measures differences in the behavior of protons in a magnetic field, is more sensitive than CT to parenchymal injury, subacute hemorrhage, and brainstem abnormalities.[9–11] Despite this diagnostic sensitivity, MRI has not become the initial study for traumatic brain injury. Acute hemorrhage, especially subarachnoid hemorrhage, is frequently more difficult to diagnose with MRI than with CT,[12] and osseous injury can be missed because calcified structures do not emit any signal.[7,8] Additionally, the specific requirements of the environment around a high field strength magnet make care of the acutely ill patient difficult. Specialized ventilators and monitoring equipment must be used. Ferromagnetic materials, unidentified intracranial aneurysm clips, metallic foreign bodies in the eye, pacemakers and other electronic medical implants, and Swan-Ganz catheters need to be excluded. Adherence to all of these requirements makes emergent MRI in an unstable trauma patient highly difficult. Currently MRI seems to be best reserved for evaluation of subacute or chronic changes in a patient following cranial trauma.[7] The development of improved medical therapy for the parenchymal components of cranial injury should increase the requirement for early MRI. Other imaging studies, such as single photon emission computed tomography (SPECT) and positron emission tomography (PET) have limited application in patients with cranial injury.

Normal CT and Normal MRI

The basic cranial CT in a head-injured patient consists of a series of 5 to 10-mm-thick axial images. Intravenous iodinated contrast agents, which can obscure the diagnosis of acute hemorrhage, are not used routinely. The usual axial-imaging plane is chosen from frontal and lateral scout projections that have the appearance of anteroposterior (AP) and lateral skull films (Fig. 4-1). These are used to localize the axial image in relation to external landmarks and to display osseous injuries (such as linear skull fractures). We have chosen a scanning plane parallel to a line connecting the orbital floor to the external

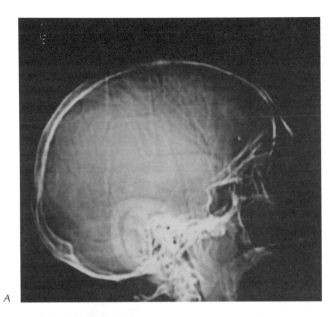

A

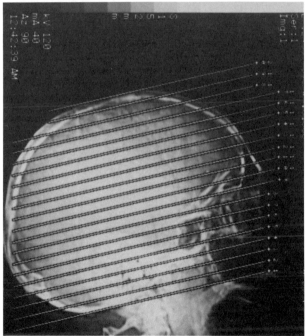

B

Figure 4-1 Lateral scanogram of the head. These digital images, obtained on the CT scanner, are comparable to lateral skull radiographs. *A*. Lateral scanogram shows osseous structures of the skull including sella, calvarium, and vascular grooves. Examination of the scanogram can facilitate the diagnosis of linear skull fractures. *B*. The locations of the CT sections are demonstrated. Notice that the sections pass through the face as well as through the intracranial compartment, allowing survey of facial bones as well as cranial contents for injury in a patient following cranial trauma.

auditory canal. Although this projection increases osseous artifacts within the posterior fossa, it also provides a survey of osseous facial structures, facilitating fracture diagnosis. Each axial section is viewed using three different sets of imaging parameters. *Brain windows,* which are relatively narrow, best display abnormalities within the brain parenchyma. *Subdural (blood) windows,* which are slightly wider and less sensitive to changes in CT density, are used to evaluate collections of blood which lie adjacent to the calvarium and other calcified structures. *Bone windows,* which are very wide and minimally sensitive to changes in CT density, are used to show osseous structures.

A normal CT scan in a young person shows all four ventricles filled with cerebrospinal fluid (CSF). Third and fourth ventricles are midline, and lateral ventricles are symmetrical. The basal cistern (suprasellar cistern, perimesencephalic cisterns, quadrigeminal plate cistern, and cerebellopontine angle cisterns), the Sylvian fissures and the sulci over the convexities can be distinguished, are seen to be symmetrical, and are compatible in size with the age of the patient (Fig. 4-2). In older children, adolescents, and young adults, CSF-containing spaces are normally small. With increasing age, there is an increase in the size of ventricles, sulci, and cisterns. This increase is most noticeable in patients over 60 years of age. On normal scans the gray-white

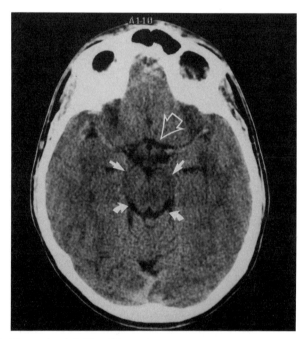

Figure 4-2 Normal axial CT without intravenous contrast administration. This section through the basal cisterns shows the CSF-filled suprasellar cistern (open arrow), quadrigeminal plate cistern (curved arrows), and perimesencephalic cistern (closed arrows).

junction in the cortex and in the basal ganglia can be distinguished. Loss of gray-white differentiation following cranial injury can have multiple causes. In trauma patients, this may reflect ischemic injury or nonhemorrhagic contusion (Fig. 4-3). Sinuses, mastoids, facial bones, and skull should be seen and should be without injury. Neither significant opacification nor air-fluid levels are present in the sinuses or the mastoids in a normal cranial CT.

Similar structures are seen in the normal cranial MRI. Imaging of the head is more complex with MRI because there are a variety of pulse sequences, each with different strengths. The most commonly used sequences produce images with T1-weighted, balanced, and T2-weighted characteristics.[13] For any study, pulse sequences and imaging planes are chosen that best demonstrate anatomic abnormalities and separate different tissue types. For example, CSF (water) is low signal intensity on T1-weighted images, intermediate intensity on balanced images, and increased signal intensity on T2-weighted images. Methemoglobin (subacute blood) is high signal intensity using all standard sequences. Other tissues have other characteristic signal intensity patterns. The rapid development of newer pulse sequences makes any statement about the best sequences to use for imaging of cranial trauma difficult. The best sequence at one point in time may be superseded at another. In general, pulse sequences should be chosen to show anatomical structures and to demonstrate the extent and type of injury. Also, calcium does not emit any signal with MRI. Osseous structures are imaged because of the cellular content of the bones, but the calcified component remains ill-defined.

Important points to remember about cranial MRI are (1) its high sensitivity to nonhemorrhagic parenchymal injury,[9-11] (2) the difficulty in using MRI with identification of acute hemorrhage, (3) the high conspicuity of subacute blood,[7,8] and (4) the problem identifying fractures in calcified bone.[13]

Imaging Characteristics of Hemorrhage

Evaluation of either MRI or CT studies of head-injured patients requires a basic understanding of the imaging characteristics of hemorrhage. The parameters governing the appearance of blood on the two modalities are different. With CT the density of blood reflects the concentration of the protein component of the hemoglobin molecule; thus, the decline in density of clot with time is believed to reflect a decline in protein concentration.[14,15] The more complex MRI appearance of blood is thought to be caused by changes in oxidation state, biochemical form, and location of the hemoglobin molecule.[16,17]

Computerized Tomography

Acute clotted blood of a normal hematocrit, hyperdense to both gray and white matter, measures 50 to 100 Houndsfield units (HU).[14,15] Normal white matter is 25 to 34 HU (mean, 29), gray matter 30 to 40 HU (mean, 35)

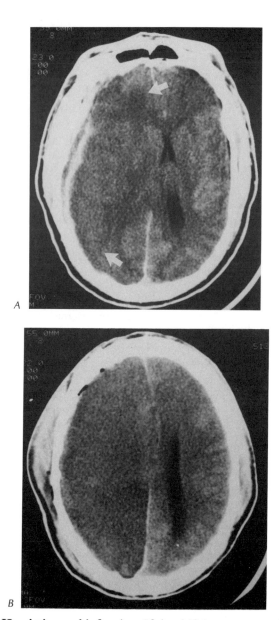

Figure 4-3 Herniation and infarction. If the shift is great enough or if there is direct injury to vessels at the base of the skull or in the neck, there can be secondary infarction within the brain following head trauma. *A.* This axial CT section shows the linear collections of hyperdense and isodense blood-layering within the right subdural space, consistent with a hyperacute SDH. There is subfalcine herniation with flattening of the right lateral ventricle, effacement of the third ventricle, and effacement of sulci in the right hemisphere. On this initial image, there is only a faint suggestion of a loss of differential density between gray and white matter in the inferior frontal and superior temporal

and CSF 0 to 5 HU (mean, 3).[18] Unclotted blood, either recent hemorrhage or flowing blood, is similar in density to brain at 25 to 30 HU.[15] Thus, on CT a hyperacute hemorrhage, a hemorrhage with ongoing extravasation at the time of the scan, a bleed without significant clot formation because the patient has been anticoagulated, or an acute hemorrhage in a patient with a low hematocrit, may not be hyperdense to brain parenchyma. This is the least common case, however. Most acute clots are hyperdense to brain on noncontrast CT.

With resolution of the hemorrhage (subacute), the density of an intraparenchymal clot decreases 1.5 HU per day.[19] This process starts peripherally and progresses centrally. The mass effect of the clot resolves at a slower rate than its density[20,21] and may still be present when the clot is hypodense to brain. Thus, with CT a subacute hemorrhage in the brain 4 to 21 days after injury may be seen as an isodense region of focal mass effect. The exact length of time for a clot to demonstrate this appearance depends upon the initial size of the hemorrhage. The time frame of clot resolution is similar in both the subdural and epidural spaces.[22] In the subarachnoid space the blood is cleared as well as metabolized; therefore, the time to resolution may be faster. Chronic hemorrhage appears hypodense to brain on CT.

Magnetic Resonance Imaging

As with CT, the imaging characteristics and the time frame to resolution of intracranial hemorrhage has been best described for intraparenchymal bleeds. Acute hemorrhage, which commonly consists of intracellular oxyhemoglobin, is essentially isointense to surrounding brain on T1-weighted, proton density, and T2-weighted sequences.[7,16,17] With the change in oxidation state to intracellular deoxyhemoglobin, the signal becomes hypointense to brain using these same sequences. With continuing degradation, intracellular deoxyhemoglobin changes to intracellular methemoglobin, then to extracellular methemoglobin. The corresponding signal intensity passes from hypo- to iso- to hyperintense to brain (Fig. 4-4). This change tends to occur earlier on T1- than on T2-weighted images. As a rule of thumb, using a high field-strength system (1 to 1.5 Tesla), the signal from a clot will be hyperintense to brain

---

lobes (arrows). This subtle loss of gray-white differentiation is a sign of early infarction. *B.* Axial CT obtained 24 h later, following evacuation of the subdural hematoma. There is generalized loss of gray-white differentiation throughout the right hemisphere, most noted when right and left hemispheres are compared. The right-sided ventricular structures and the right-sided sulci are totally compressed. The entire right hemisphere has infarcted with compression of the right internal carotid artery secondary to herniation.

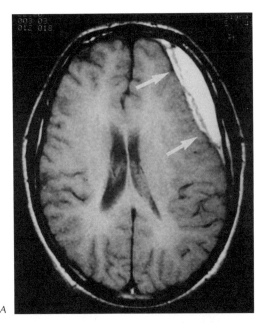

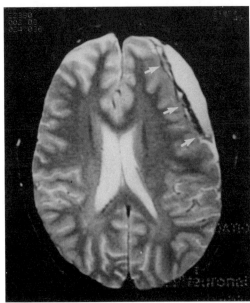

Figure 4-4 Subacute subdural hematoma. These always show the signal characteristics of subacute hemorrhage collections. *A.* T1-weighted image (TR 600, TE 11) shows a hyperintense subdural collection in the left frontal region (arrows) that flattens sulci and causes a mild subfalcine herniation. The bulk of this collection is of markedly increased signal intensity compared to brain. *B.* T2-weighted image (TR 2700, TE 80) at the same level again shows the subdural collection in the left frontal region. This collection is also of high signal intensity on this image. The medial border of the collection (arrows) is hypointense to brain and more apparent than on the corresponding T1-weighted image. This appearance (in *A* and *B*) suggests the presence of extracellular methemoglobin within the subdural space. This is of high signal intensity on both T1- and T2-weighted images. The markedly hypointense medial margin suggests the presence of hemosiderin.

by 1 week on T1-weighted images and by approximately 2 weeks on T2-weighted images. Similar to the CT appearance of resolving intracranial hemorrhage, the process of clot resorption and corresponding signal changes begins peripherally and moves centrally.[16] The chronic residual of an intraparenchymal hemorrhage, hemosiderin, is hypointense to brain on all imaging sequences. The area of signal dropout (blooming) is more apparent on T2- than on T1-weighted images (Fig. 4-5). This appearance is due to a local inhomogeneity of the magnetic field caused by the presence of hemosiderin. In summary, CT is sensitive to acute blood, to osseous injury, and is easy to obtain in the acute trauma setting; MRI is more sensitive than CT to both subacute and chronic hemorrhage and to all forms of parenchymal injury.

CT Classification of Head Injury/CT Signs of Increased ICP

Cranial injury can occur as a focal process, a diffuse process, or a combination of both.[23] As previously mentioned, the early reports of CT use for traumatic head injury stressed identification of focal lesions, such as subdural hematoma, epidural hematoma, intraparenchymal hemorrhage, and infarct.[2,3] Diagnosis of diffuse shear injury by CT was possible only in severely injured individuals. The CT diagnosis required demonstration of punctate hemorrhages in the corpus callosum and brainstem.[24] More recent observations based upon MRI of head-injured patients and upon animal research suggest that there is a wider range of severity of diffuse cranial injury (diffuse shear injury) than that suggested by early CT. Patients with nonhemorrhagic punctate lesions in the white matter and at the gray-white junction on MRI are also a part of the spectrum of diffuse shear injury. Gentry and Kelly and coworkers have related this appearance to acceleration/deceleration injury.[9,10,25,26]

Another classification of cranial injury, derived from information from the Traumatic Coma Data Bank, extrapolates physiologic dysfunction from the anatomic changes visible with cranial CT. In this study all patients had a Glasgow Coma Scale (GCS) score ≤ 8. Four grades of diffuse injury were defined[27]: *Diffuse injury I*-normal CT; *diffuse injury II*-basal cisterns open, midline shift ≤ 5 mm and no parenchymal lesion > 25 cc; *diffuse injury III*-basal cisterns compressed or absent, midline shift ≤ 5 mm and no parenchymal lesion > 25 cc; *diffuse injury IV*-midline shift > 5 mm and a focal lesion > 25 cc. Although this classification was first proposed as a method for predicting outcome, the obscuration of basal cisterns on an initial CT is found to be a predictor of increased intracranial pressure (ICP). Patients with compressed or absent mesencephalic cisterns are 3 times more likely to have increased ICP than are patients with visible cisterns. Similarly significant are the presence of midline shift and a mass lesion greater than 25 cc, even if the lesion is evacuated.[28]

Other researchers have used basal cistern compression alone,[29] basal cistern compression combined with third ventricular compression,[30] size of subdural

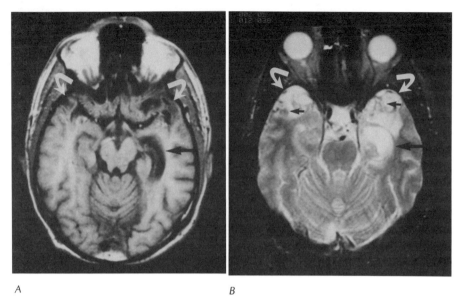

A   B

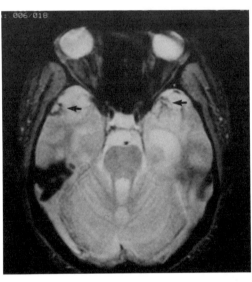

C

Figure 4-5 Old injury. Three axial MRI sequences demonstrating the appearance of old traumatic injury of the brain. *A.* T1-weighted sequence (TR 600, TE 11) shows enlargement of the left temporal horn (straight arrow) and areas of lower signal intensity within both anterior temporal lobes (curved arrows). These intraaxial areas of intermediate to very low signal intensity suggest gliosis combined with focal cystic change. The bitemporal distribution of injury is common following head trauma. *B.* On the T2-weighted sequence (TR 2700,TE 80) CSF is of high signal intensity. Seen again is the dilated temporal horn (large arrow) and bilateral contusions of the anterior temporal tips (curved arrows). Areas of gliosis and cystic change are increased in signal intensity on T2-weighted images. Areas of lower signal

hematoma (SDH), size of ventricles, status of cerebral contusion, and midline shift in descending order of importance as predictors of increased ICP.[31] A less commonly reported sign of increased ICP is the trapping of a ventricle on the side opposite the mass lesion, thereby causing focal ventricular enlargement.[32] Medial displacement of the uncus with deformity of the midbrain is a direct indicator of uncal herniation (Fig. 4-6). This displacement may be unilateral or bilateral and is separate from midline shift of the third ventricle. The presence of traumatically elicited subarachnoid blood does not correlate with the development of increased ICP (Fig. 4-7). Although the diagnosis of diffuse injury is best made with MRI, the clinical diagnosis is commonly based upon the patient's poor clinical grade at presentation in association with a CT scan without large focal lesions.

In summary, in any patient, the severity of a cranial injury, as demonstrated by CT, depends upon the size of the clot, the location of the clot (such as frontal versus brainstem), the extent of midline shift, the severity of the sulcal compression, the presence of medial displacement of the uncus with deformity of the midbrain, and the size and configuration of the basal cisterns. For example, a 10-mm-thick subdural hematoma in an 18-year-old patient usually would result in significant midline shift, uncal herniation and sulcal effacement. The same size SDH in a 75-year-old patient might merely flatten the sulci without significant shift of midline because of the presence of prior parenchymal volume loss.

Other Injuries Associated with Cranial Trauma

Spinal and facial injuries are frequently associated with traumatic brain injury. Michael and coworkers in a single trauma center found 22 of 451 patients with both head and cervical spine injuries.[33] In their series, 24 percent of patients with cervical spine injuries had cranial injury while 6 percent of head-injured patients had a cervical spine injury. Cervical spine injury was present

---

intensity within both contusions (small arrows) suggest the presence of hemosiderin. Hemosiderin causes local inhomogeneity of the magnetic field resulting in a much lower signal intensity on T2 and gradient echo images than on T1-weighted images (blooming). *C.* Gradient echo sequence (TR 650; TE 30; flip angle, 15°) again shows high signal intensity CSF in the dilated left temporal horn and contusions in both anterior temporal lobes. Better seen than on the T2-weighted image are the areas of low signal intensity (arrows) reflecting local changes in the magentic field caused by hemosiderin. The more posterior areas of low signal intensity are caused by the petrous ridges.

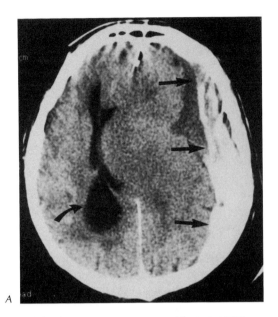

A

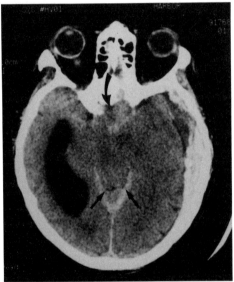

B

Figure 4-6 Subfalcine and uncal herniation. *A.* Axial CT shows a large, hyperacute SDH on the left (straight arrows). The lateral ventricles have been shifted across midline and there is dilation of the right atrium (curved arrow). *B.* The marked dilatation of the right temporal horn is better seen on the CT section immediately caudal to the section in *A.* Basal cisterns are totally effaced and the margins of the brainstem are difficult to discern. The quadrigeminal plate cistern is small (straight arrows) and the left uncus is displaced medially (curved arrow). The subdural hematoma extends into the floor of the middle cranial fossa under the temporal lobe. This large SDH has caused uncal and subfalcine herniation.

in 2.4 percent of comatose patients (GCS score < 8). Other researchers report rates of 1.2 to 1.7 percent for cervical spine injury associated with head injury.[34] Similar to Michael's findings, 19 to 21 percent of patients with cervical spine injury have associated cranial injury.[35,36] A high index of suspicion of cervical spine injury has to be considered in the patient with cervical spine or cranial trauma.

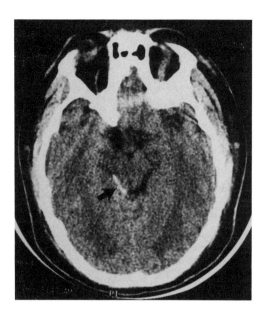

Figure 4-7 Subarachnoid hemorrhage. At times posttraumatic SAH is small and there are few other signs of intracranial injury. This axial CT section shows a small amount of blood in the quadrigeminal plate cistern (arrow). There are no other abnormalities noted on the scan at any level.

Injury to the face with concomitant intracranial injury is also frequent. As in the cervical spine, recognition of the patient with cranial and facial injuries depends upon the screening mechanism chosen. Lee and coworkers evaluated cranial CT in patients with facial fractures: Fifty-six percent of those with injuries to the upper face had moderate or severe cranial injury. The prevalence was only 14 percent in those with mandibular or midface injuries.[37] Davidoff and coworkers, using loss of consciousness or posttraumatic amnesia as an indicator of cranial injury, found associated mild cranial injury in 55 percent of patients admitted for facial injury. Vehicular trauma was more likely than other types of trauma to cause facial and cranial injury (68 percent versus 43 percent).[38] Injury to the upper face should raise concern about concomitant intracranial injury.

PATTERNS OF CRANIAL INJURY

Fracture-Osseous Injury

The presence of a linear skull fracture is of little import when attempting to recognize the patient with an intracranial injury. Masters and coworkers evaluated head trauma in 7035 patients and looked at multi-institutional data for 22,058 patients. In adults, 91 percent of patients with intracranial injury did not have skull fractures. This fact led these authors to suggest that radiographs of the skull in those patients at moderate and high risk for cranial injury[1] were less useful than neurologic examination and CT. Controversy continues over the need for skull films in patients with minor head injuries,[39-42] and some authors still propose the use of screening radiographs. Nevertheless, radiographs of the skull remain useful if the condition of the osseous structures is important. This concern might occur in a patient with cervical and cranial injury who requires placement of Gardner-Wells tongs.

Skull fractures, in particular, those fractures parallel to the CT plane of section, may be difficult to diagnose from the axial images, however frequently these parallel fractures may be diagnosed from the CT scout, which is equivalent to a skull radiograph (Fig. 4-1). Using early scanners, only 20 percent of fractures seen with plain radiographs were diagnosed with CT.[2] In view of the greater interest in the status of the brain parenchyma, these fracture studies have not been repeated with current high-resolution scanners. In contrast, depressed skull fractures, which deform the calvarium, are well seen on axial-imaging planes. The deformity of the calvarium can be assessed in terms of the severity of displacement of fracture fragments in relation to the remainder of the skull or in relation to underlying parenchymal injury.

Elevation of the depressed fracture fragments may need to be performed if the wound is open or if there is cosmetic deformity; elevation for other reasons is more controversial.[43] Fractures through the temporal bones and skull base are more difficult to diagnose with CT, requiring thin-section axial and coronal-imaging techniques to demonstrate them in detail.[44,45] If these fractures pass through foramina for vascular structures, such as the carotid canal, early diagnosis may help identify potential vascular injuries in patients. Often, other acute management issues associated with basilar skull fractures, such as the presence of a CSF leak or a cranial nerve dysfunction, may resolve spontaneously. Therefore, high-resolution imaging of a skull-base fracture is often postponed until the subacute period when persistence of meningitis or cranial nerve deficit makes detailed diagnosis necessary.[46] For example, a fracture through the carotid canal, injuring the carotid artery may cause distal ischemia, a carotid-cavernous fistula, or may be the source of emboli. Catheter angiography is currently the study of choice to clarify this diagnosis. Although the increasing resolution of magnetic resonance angiography (MRA) may soon make this method the preferred imaging in these patients, as yet there are few studies comparing the sensitivity of MRA versus angiography for traumatic injuries, such as carotid dissections.

Epidural Hematoma

Epidural hematomas (EDH) are seen on either CT or MRI as a focal, lens-shaped (biconvex) collection with its inner surface curved away from the skull[2] (Fig. 4-8). Associated skull fractures are found in up to 80 to 90 percent of patients.[22] Most EDH are acute (hyperdense to brain on CT) or hyperacute

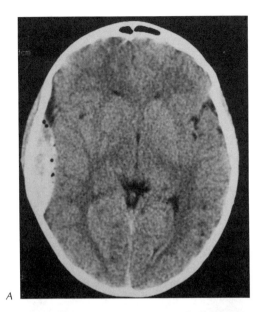

A

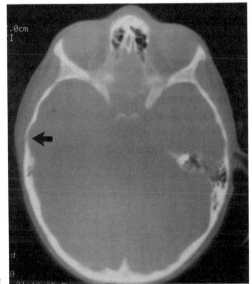

B

Figure 4-8 Epidural hematoma. Epidural hematomas are commonly associated with skull fracture and are seen as biconvex or lenticular collections of blood lying superficial to the brain. The presence of intracranial air in a patient with a closed head injury leads to a presumptive diagnosis of a fracture into an air-containing space, such as the mastoid air cells or the sinuses. *A.* Axial CT showing mixed iso- to-hyperdense collection in the epidural space of the right middle cranial fossa. Several small low attenuation foci caused by intracranial air are seen at the margin of the collection. The medial surface of the collection is bowed away from the skull. The mixture of iso- to-hyperdensity within the EDH suggests that the injury is active and that clot formation is incomplete. *B.* Axial CT section obtained more inferiorly in the same patient. The section, displayed using bone windows, shows a linear fracture in the right temporal bone (arrow). The EDH was immediately adjacent to the fracture.

lesions (mixed isodensity/hyperdensity to brain).[47] These latter may occur with an arterial bleeding point.[22,47] EDH may cross points of attachment of the dural sinuses, such as the midline at the vertex. The brain under the epidural collection is frequently uninjured or has minimal injury. Delayed EDH have been reported, usually in younger patients and commonly with a fracture. Sakai and coworkers followed up patients with EDH by CT if early evacuation did not occur; the EDH enlarged in 19 of 28 patients.[48] Notably in this group, the final size of the EDH could not be correlated with increased ICP.

Subdural Hematoma

Subdural hematoma (SDH) forms in the potential space between the dura and the arachnoid. Associated injury to the brain parenchyma is common. Selig and coworkers found 65 percent of 82 patients with acute SDH had an accompanying contusion or hematoma.[49] On sectional-imaging studies, the margin of an SDH tends to parallel the calvarium, and the SDH, although thin, may be quite extensive and may track caudad to the brain, particularly in the middle fossa (Fig. 4-6). Using CT, both brain windows and subdural windows should be evaluated in order to recognize a thin, acute SDH lying adjacent to the calvarium. An acute SDH is most commonly hyperdense, although acute isodense SDH has been reported from hemorrhage in anemic patients or as part of hyperacute collections in which the extravasated blood has not yet clotted.[50–52]

Chronic SDH tend to occur after minor trauma in older patients with underlying cerebral volume loss. Bridging veins that cross the subdural space are commonly stretched in these individuals and can tear with minor trauma.[53] Repeated tearing with repeated small hemorrhages from these bridging veins results in a mixed density collection in the subdural space. The presence of both acute and chronic hemorrhage is suggested by the presence of hyperdense blood layering in a dependent relationship to the older, iso- to hypodense portions of the clot. Occasionally an acute rebleed into a chronic SDH can result in an isodense SDH (Fig. 4-8) or layering with hypodense collection[54] (Figs. 4-9, 4-10).

Subarachnoid Hemorrhage

As an isolated entity, subarachnoid hemorrhage (SAH) is less commonly associated with trauma than with rupture of intracranial aneurysms. However, blood within the subarachnoid space is not unusual following cranial trauma, particularly if there is a hemorrhagic parenchymal injury. Rarely, head trauma will present as subarachnoid hemorrhage without other injuries seen with CT.

On CT the appearance of posttraumatic SAH is similar to aneurysmal-type bleeds. The basal cisterns are of increased density, frequently filled with clot, and without a distortion of the normal parenchymal or cisternal architecture. One complication of SAH, vascular spasm, can occur following posttraumatic subarachnoid hemorrhage, although the incidence is not well defined. This is radiographically similar to spasm occurring subsequent to aneurysmal hemorrhage (Fig. 4-11).

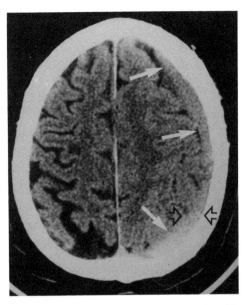

Figure 4-9 Isodense subdural hematoma. Isodense subdural hematoma frequently occurs when there is rebleeding into a chronic subdural collection. Uniform mixing of denser acute blood cells with hypodense chronic SDH results in an isodense collection on CT. Other causes of isodense SDH on CT are subacute SDH imaged at the point when the blood, passing from hyperdensity through to hypodensity is isodense, and acute hemorrhage in an anemic patient. In this patient of 60 years of age, there is a 1-cm-thick isodense SDH on the left (closed arrows). There is also moderate enlargement of sulcal structures in the uninvolved right hemisphere. The SDH is likely to have been caused by minor, repeated trauma to stretched draining veins. The presence of a region of relative hyperdensity in the inferior portion of the SDH suggests the presence of acute blood cells layered in a dependent position (open arrows).

Intraparenchymal Injury/Coup-Contrecoup Injury

Intraparenchymal brain injury (contusion) has a range of severity. In its mild form there may be edema without hemorrhage. When severe, a large clot may be present within the bed of contused brain. There are gradations of severity between these two extremes.[3] The CT appearance of the intermediate form is one of multiple punctate areas of hemorrhage within a region of lower attenuation. These correspond to petechial hemorrhages. Small, subtle contusions may be seen as areas of lower density without hemorrhage while other areas of contusion with a large component of vascular injury may appear predominantly hemorrhagic.[2] In some cases the initial, minimally hemorrhagic contusion may progress to larger clots (delayed hemorrhage).[55,56] Contusions tend to be found at the edges of the brain, such as the anterior and posterior temporal tips, the inferior frontal lobes or the

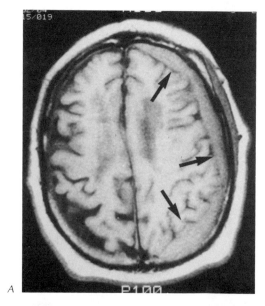

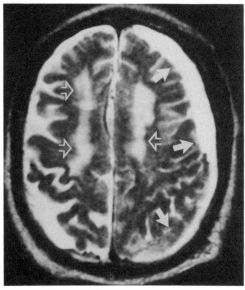

Figure 4-10 Chronic subdural hematomas. As collections of blood break down on MRI they diminish in signal intensity until only proteinaceous fluid remains. This is then cleared by normal physiologic mechanisms. *A.* Axial T1-weighted image (TR 600, TE 11) at the level of centrum semiovale in this elderly patient. The marked degree of cerebral volume loss is visible in the right hemisphere. On the left there is a relatively isointense subdural hematoma (arrows). *B.* T2-weighted sequence (TR 2500, TE 80). This axial image at the same level again shows cerebral volume loss in the right hemisphere and a high signal intensity subdural collection (closed arrows) on

occipital poles, and all areas where soft brain comes in contact with the irregular inner surface of the skull.[4] These contusions may be either the result of the direct blow or part of a *coup-contrecoup*-type injury. This latter term describes the injuries that occur due to differences in the rate of acceleration and deceleration of the brain compared with the skull in response to the same force. Following a blow to the head, the brain can rebound at a rate that differs from that of the skull. Injured brain is often present on the side of the head opposite the initial, direct blow, and the more severe parenchymal lesion may be either the direct coup or the indirect contrecoup injury (Fig. 4-12). In many cases, only an examination of the patient for signs of external injury or fracture can identify the point of direct cranial trauma.

Similar to other cranial processes, for an individual patient the clinical concerns following contusion reflect the size of the injury, its location, other associated cranial injuries, the extent of the midline shift, the extent of cisternal compression, and the associated neurologic deficit. For example, a 2-cm contusion in the inferior right frontal pole would be expected to cause a less severe functional deficit than the deficit caused by the same size contusion in the left posterior temporal lobe near the primary speech cortex.

Intraparenchymal Hemorrhage

Intraparenchymal hematomas are found in the same anatomic regions as contusions and coup-contrecoup injuries. Intraparenchymal hematoma may not be apparent on an initial CT scan. However, sequential CT studies have shown the development of an intra-parenchymal clot in 1 to 9 percent of patients[56,57] while others noted that over half of patients with a GCS score of 12 developed these lesions on CT[55,56] (Fig. 4-10). Delayed hemorrhage may develop in already injured brain parenchyma.[58,59] In imaging appearance, delayed hematoma is no different from any other intraparenchymal clot except in the time course of its appearance (Fig. 4-13).

the left. This appearance can occur when extracellular methemoglobin is in the process of further degrading into its proteinaceous components. This chronic subdural hematoma is presumed to have occurred when bridging veins were torn following minor trauma. The dependent portion is of lower signal intensity than the remainder of the SDH. This may be a loculated portion of the SDH, which continues to be predominantly intracellular methemoglobin (isointense on T1-weighted images and hypointense on T2-weighted images.) Incidentally seen are areas of increased signal intensity in the white matter of the centrum semiovale (open arrows). This represents parenchymal changes secondary to small vessel occlusive disease, possibly hypertensive or atherosclerotic in origin, in this elderly patient.

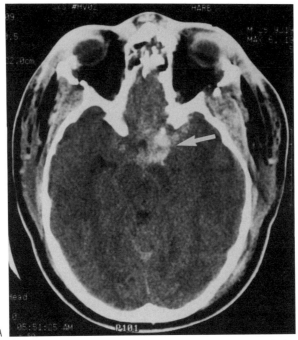

Figure 4-11 Subarachnoid hemorrhage and spasm. Although subarachnoid blood is frequently reported in conjunction with other cranial injuries, a large volume of subarachnoid blood and subsequent clinically apparent spasm is uncommon. *A.* This patient presented with a large amount of subarachnoid blood and no focal parenchymal lesions following a motor vehicle accident. Blood is seen within the suprasellar cistern on the axial CT section (arrow). The perimesencephalic cisterns are obscured. There is no midline shift. *B.* Axial CT section obtained 8 days later shows an acute infarct in the head of the left caudate nucleus (arrow). *C.* Subsequent left internal carotid arteriogram demonstrates marked narrowing of the supraclinoid carotid (arrows) and relatively poor filling of distal middle cerebral artery branches. This is consistent with marked vasospasm of the supraclinoid carotid artery. Again, although not commonly seen in the setting of trauma, subarachnoid hemorrhage and vasospasm can be components of traumatic cranial injury.

Diffuse Cerebral Injury

Diffuse intracranial injury, commonly also called diffuse shear injury, has been previously mentioned in the section discussing signs of increased intracranial pressure. As noted, diffuse shear injury often is the result of an acceleration/deceleration injury of the brain. The injury is postulated to occur when axons slide past each other during rapid changes in the rate of motion of the head

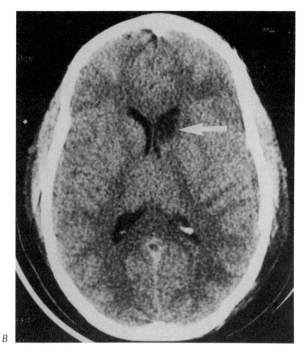

B

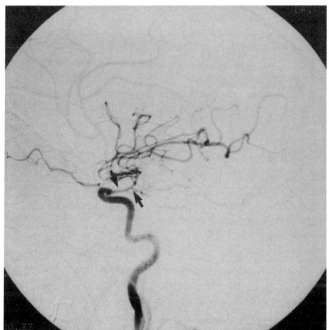

C

Figure 4-11 *(Continued)*

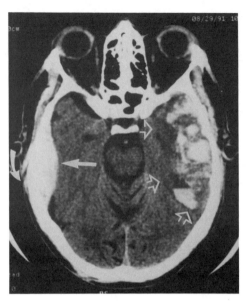

Figure 4-12 Coup-contrecoup injuries. Coup-contrecoup injuries are common in patients with cranial trauma. In this patient there is an epidural hematoma on the left (closed arrow). On the right there is a large hemorrhagic contusion in the temporal lobe (open arrows). Although the exact site of impact is difficult to confirm, on CT there is a suggestion of soft tissue swelling external to the epidural hematoma (curved arrow). This places the primary injury on the right resulting in an epidural hematoma with its underlying fracture. The contrecoup injury on the left is the result of differences in the rate of acceleration/deceleration between brain and skull.

associated with rotational forces. The imaging appearance depends upon the severity; milder injury consists of punctate areas of edema (punctate areas of increased T2 signal on MRI with minimal to no CT changes) while severe injury may present as punctate hemorrhages found particularly in the corpus callosum, small intraventricular hemorrhages, or, as described by Marshall,[27] effacement of basal cisternal structures without significant midline shift or focal mass lesions. MRI is more sensitive than CT for making this diagnosis; however, in most patients with traumatic brain injury, the diagnosis needs to be suggested acutely from the CT scan. The significance of this diagnosis, particularly in patients without surgical lesions, lies in the risk that these patients may develop increased intracranial pressure. Thus the importance is in identifying ICP problems in patients at risk who can often be treated with close monitoring techniques and aggressive medical management.

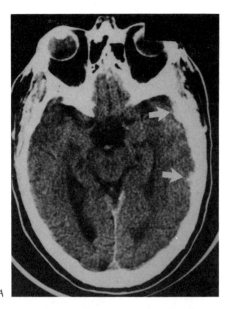

A

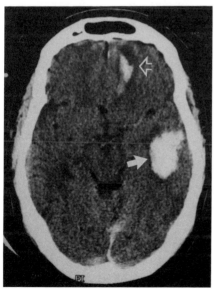

B

Figure 4-13 Delayed hemorrhage. Delayed hemorrhage which occurs 12 to 24 h following injury can cause deterioration in the patient's clinical status. *A*. The initial axial imaging section in this 42-year-old male shows small superficial contusions (arrows) in the left temporal lobe. These are accompanied by generalized effacement of sulci, flattening of the Sylvian cistern and medial displacement of the temporal horn. Basal cisterns remain open. Sections through the frontal lobe do not show any hemorrhage. *B*. Two areas of frank hemorrhage are present on a scan performed 18 h later. One is within the left temporal lobe deep to the previously seen superficial hemorrhage (closed arrow). The second is in the inferior left frontal lobe (open arrow). Delayed hemorrhage tends to occur in brain that has a nonhemorrhage injury.

SUMMARY

This short description of imaging concerns in patients with cranial injury should serve as an initial guide to the areas in which imaging can be of aid in diagnosis and patient management. It is intended to demonstrate the major areas in which imaging can help management; it is not meant to be a comprehensive discussion of all of the concerns in imaging traumatic brain injury.

REFERENCES

1. Masters SJ, McClean PM, Arcarese MS, et al: Skull X-ray examinations after head trauma. *N Engl J Med* 316:84, 1987.

2. Dublin AB, French BN, Rennick JM: Computed tomography in head trauma. *Radiology* 122:365, 1977.

3. French BN, Dublin AB: The value of computerized tomography in the management of 1000 consecutive head injuries. *Surg Neurol* 7:171, 1977.

4. Koo HA, LaRoque RL: Evaluation of head trauma by computed tomography. *Radiology* 123:345, 1977.

5. Johnson MH, Lee HS: Computed tomography of acute cerebral trauma. *Radiol Clin North Am* 30:325, 1992.

6. Stein S, Young G, Talucci R, et al: Delayed brain injury after head trauma: Significance of coagulopathy. *Neurosurg* 30:160, 1992.

7. Zimmerman RA, Bilaniuk LT, Hackney DG, et al: Head injury: Early results of comparing CT and high-field MR. *Am J Neuroradiol* 7:757, 1986.

8. Snow RB, Zimmerman RD, Gandy SE, et al: Comparison of magnetic resonance imaging and computed tomography in the evaluation of head injury. *Neurosurg* 18:45, 1986.

9. Kelly AB, Zimmerman RD, Snow RB, et al: Head trauma: Comparison of MR and CT experience in 100 patients. *Am J Neuroradiol* 9:699, 1988.

10. Gentry LR, Godersky JC, Thompson B, et al: Prospective comparative study of intermediate-field MR and CT in the evaluation of closed head trauma. *Am J Neuroradiol* 9:91, 1988.

11. Han JS, Kaufman B, Alfidi RJ, et al: Head trauma evaluated by magnetic resonance and computed tomography: A comparison. *Radiology* 150:71, 1984.

12. Bradley WJ, Schmidt P: Effect of methemoglobin formation on the MR appearance of subarachnoid hemorrhage. *Radiology* 156:99, 1985.

13. Pykett IL, Newhouse JH, Buonanno FS, et al: Principles of nuclear magnetic resonance imaging. *Radiology* 143:157, 1982.

14. New P, Aronow S: Attenuation measurements of whole blood and blood fractions in computed tomography. *Radiology* 121:635, 1976.

15. Norman D, Price D, Boyd D, et al: Quantitative aspects of computed tomography of the blood and cerebrospinal fluid. *Radiology* 123:335, 1977.

16. Gomori J, Grossman R, Goldberg H, et al: Intracranial hematomas: Imaging by high-field MR. *Radiology* 157:87, 1985.

17. Gomori J, Grossman R, Hackney D, et al: Variable appearances of subacute intracranial hematomas on high-field spin-echo MR. *Am J Neuroradiol* 8:1019, 1987.

18. Weinstein MA, Duchesneau PM, MacIntyre WJ: White and gray matter of the brain differentiated by computed tomography. *Radiology* 122:699, 1977.

19. Scotti G, Terbrugge K, Melancon D, et al: Evaluation of the age of subdural hematomas by computerized tomography. *J Neurosurg* 47:311, 1977.

20. Dolinskas C, Bilaniuk L, Zimmerman R, et al: Computed tomography of intracerebral hematomas: I. Transmission CT observations on hematoma resolution. *Am J Roentgenol* 129:681, 1977.

21. Messina V, Chernik N: Computed tomography: The "resolving" intracerebral hemorrhage. *Radiology* 18:609, 1975.

22. Zimmerman RA, Bilaniuk LT: Computed tomographic staging of traumatic epidural bleeding. *Radiology* 144:809, 1982.

23. Hume J, Graham D, Murray LS, et al: Diffuse axonal injury due to nonmissile head injury in humans: An analysis of 45 cases. *Ann Neurol* 12:557, 1982.

24. Zimmerman RA, Bilaniuk LT, Gennarelli T: Computed tomography of shearing injuries of the cerebral white matter. *Radiology* 127:393, 1978.

25. Gennarelli TA, Adams J, Graham D: Acceleration-induced head injury in the monkey: I. The model, its mechanical and physiologic correlates. *Acta Neuropathol* 7(suppl):23, 1981.

26. Adams H, Mitchell DE, Graham DI, et al: Diffuse brain damage of the immediate impact type: Its relationship to primary brain stem damage in head injury. *Brain* 100:489, 1977.

27. Marshall LF, Marshall SB, Klauber MR, et al: A new classification of head injury based on computerized tomography. *J Neurosurg* 75:S14, 1991.

28. Eisenberg HM, Gary HE Jr, Aldrich EF, et al: Initial CT findings in 753 patients with severe head injury: A report from the NIH Traumatic Coma Data Bank. *J Neurosurg* 73:688, 1990.

29. Toutant S, Klauber M, Marshall L: Absent or compressed basal cisterns on first CT scan: Ominous predictors of outcome in severe head injury. *J Neurosurg* 61:691, 1984.

30. Colquhoun IR, Burrows EH: The prognostic significance of the third ventricle and basal cisterns in severe closed head injury. *Clin Radiol* 40:13, 1989.

31. Mizutani T, Manaka S, Tsutsumi H: Estimation of intracranial pressure using computed tomography scan findings in patients with severe head injury. *Surg Neurol* 33:178, 1990.

32. Sadhu V, Sampson J, Haar F, et al: Correlation between computed tomography and intracranial pressure monitoring in acute head trauma patients. *Radiology* 133:507, 1979.

33. Michael DB, Guyot DR, Darmody WR: Coincidence of head and cervical spine injury. *J Neurotrauma* 6:177, 1989.

34. Gbaanador GBM, Fruin A, Taylor C: The role of routine emergency cervical radiography in head trauma. *Am J Surg* 152:643, 1986.

35. Bohlman HH: Acute fractures and dislocations of the spine. *J Bone Joint Surg* 61A:1119, 1979.

36. Bachulis BL, Long WL, Hynes SG, et al: Clinical indications for cervical spine radiographs in the traumatized patient. *Am J Surg* 153:473, 1987.

37. Lee KF, Wagner LK, Lee YE, et al: The impact-absorbing effects of facial fractures in closed-head injuries. *J Neurosurg* 66:542, 1987.

38. Davidoff G, Jakubowski M, Thomas D, et al: The spectrum of closed-head injuries in facial trauma victims: Incidence and impact. *Ann Emerg Med* 17:6, 1988.

39. Macpherson P, Jennett B, Anderson E: CT scanning and surgical treatment of 1551 head-injured patients admitted to a regional neurosurgical unit. *Clin Radiol* 42:85, 1990.

40. Servadei F, Ciucci G, Papago F, et al: Skull fracture as a risk factor of intracranial complications in minor head injuries: A prospective CT study in a series of 98 adult patients. *J Neurol Neurosurg Psychiatry* 51:526, 1988.

41. Hackney DB: Skull radiography in the evaluation of acute head trauma: A survey of current practice. *Radiology* 181:711, 1991.

42. Rosenorn J, Duus B, Nielsen K, et al: Is a skull X-ray necessary after milder head trauma? *Br J Neurosurg* 5:135, 1991.

43. Cooper PR: Skull fracture and traumatic cerebrospinal fluid fistulas, in Cooper PR (ed): *Head Injury,* 2d ed. Baltimore, Williams and Wilkins, 1993.

44. Johnson MH, Hasso A, Stewart CI, et al: Temporal bone trauma: High resolution computed tomographic evaluation. *Radiology* 151:411, 1984.

45. Holland B, Braut-Zawadski M: High-resolution CT of temporal bone trauma. *Am J Neuroradiol* 5:291, 1984.

46. Guha A, Fazl M, Cooper PW: Isolated basilar artery occlusion associated with a clivus fracture. *Can J Neurol Sci* 16:81, 1989.

47. Tapiero B, Richer E, Laurent F, et al: Posttraumatic extradural hematomas. *J Neuroradiol* 11:213, 1984.

48. Sakai H, Takago H, Ohtaka H, et al: Serial changes in acute extradural hematoma

size and associated changes in level of consciousness and intracranial pressure. *J Neurosurg* 68:566, 1988.

49. Seelig JM, Becker DP, Miller JD, et al: Traumatic acute subdural hematoma: Major mortality reduction in patients treated within four hours. *N Engl J Med* 304:1511, 1981.

50. Kaufman H, Singer J, Sadju V, et al: Isodense acute subdural hematoma. *J Comput Assist Tomogr* 4:557, 1980.

51. Smith WJ, Batnitzky S, Rengachary S: Acute isodense subdural hematomas: A problem in anemic patients. *Am J Roentgenol* 136:543, 1981.

52. Greenberg J, Cohen WA, Cooper P: The "hyperacute" extra-axial intracranial hematoma: Computed tomographic findings and clinical significance. *Neurosurgery* 17:48, 1985.

53. Yashima T, Friede RL: Why do bridging veins rupture into vertical subdural space? *J Neurol Neurosurg Psychiatry* 47:121, 1984.

54. Kao M: Sedimentation level in chronic subdural hematoma visible on computerized tomography. *J Neurosurg* 58:246, 1983.

55. Cooper P, Maravilla K, Moody S, et al: Serial computerized tomographic scanning and the prognosis of severe head injury. *Neurosurgery* 5:566, 1979.

56. Diaz F, Yock DJ, Larson D, et al: Early diagnosis of delayed posttraumatic intracerebral hematomas. *J Neurosurg* 50:217, 1979.

57. Lipper M, Kishore P, Girevendulis A, et al: Delayed intracranial hematoma in patients with severe head injury. *Radiology* 133:635, 1979.

58. Gudeman S, Kismore P, Miller J, et al: The genesis and significance of delayed traumatic intracerebral hematoma. *Neurosurgery* 5:309, 1979.

59. Taneda M, Irino T: Enlargement of intracerebral hematomas following surgical removal of epidural hematomas. *Acta Neurosurg* 51:73, 1979.

CHAPTER 5

Management of Acute Head Injury: Initial Resuscitation

M. Sean Grady and Arthur M. Lam

INITIAL RESUSCITATION
  Pre-Hospital Care
  Emergency Department Management

Comprehensive management of traumatic brain injury (TBI) begins at the site of injury, continues through transport and hands off to definitive neurosurgical management at the treatment facility. This chapter is divided into two segments: initial resuscitation and surgical management. Initial resuscitation starts at the injury site and continues to the point of definitive surgical care. Resuscitation includes care in the emergency department and diagnostic evaluation. A few basic principles must be adhered to in order to optimize outcome from TBI. Simply, the brain must receive adequate oxygen and glucose to continue normal metabolism.[1,2] This fact translates into the ABCs of trauma resuscitation: Airway, Breathing, and Circulation.[3] Ensuring that these needs are met will be the focus of the first half of this chapter.

INITIAL RESUSCITATION

Prehospital Care

Outcome from TBI is directly influenced by the early care of these patients. Hypotension and hypoxia are associated with severe TBI in almost 50 percent of cases[4,5] (see also Chap. 3). Hypotension is almost always due to systemic injuries, rather than hemorrhage or loss of vascular tone due to the brain injury.[6] The rare exceptions to this statement may be found in children under the age of 4, where blood loss from scalp lacerations can cause hemorrhagic shock, or, in cases of lethal TBI, with medullary brainstem failure. Hypoxia, on the other hand, may be caused by systemic injuries (pneumothorax, hemothorax) or may be due to airway obstruction because of coma or trauma. No matter what the cause, hypoxia and hypotension should be addressed in the field by trained personnel through intubation and fluid resuscitation.

Hypoxemia is frequently found in patients transported to the hospital by emergency personnel. In 1978, Miller et al. reported that 30 percent of severely head-injured patients had an initial arterial P_{O_2} <65 mmHg.[7] Even with recognition of the adverse consequences of hypoxemia, pilot data from the National Coma Data Bank showed that 20 percent of patients with severe brain injury had an initial arterial P_{O_2} <60 mmHg.[8] Eisenberg et al. identified a relationship between outcome and hypoxemia: vegetative or severely disabled patients were more likely to be hypoxemic in the emergency department (45 percent) than patients with a good outcome (20 percent).[4] Improvement in incidence of mortality after severe TBI has been associated with in-field intubation.[9]

Airway control for the purpose of avoiding hypoxemia has the added benefit of directly controlling events within the cranial cavity and avoiding hypercarbia. Intracranial blood volume is exquisitely sensitive to CO_2 tension in the blood.[10] Each mmHg change in P_{CO_2} results in approximately 3 to 4 percent change in cerebral blood flow. Cerebral blood vessel tone responds to hypercarbia by dilating and, conversely, by constricting in response to hypocarbia. In a poorly ventilated state, the cerebral vessels dilate, increasing flow to the brain but having the negative consequence of increasing intracranial pressure (ICP) because of increased blood volume. As a result, cerebral perfusion may be compromised by the increase in ICP due both to mass lesions or cerebral edema as well as the increased blood volume resulting from hypercarbia. On the other hand, ICP can be decreased by hyperventilation to mild levels of hypocarbia (P_{CO_2} = 30 to 35 mmHg).

Airway control and ventilation may be achieved through a variety of means, including endotracheal intubation, or if there are multiple facial fractures or swelling, through cricothyroidotomy or tracheotomy. Injuries to the cervical spine are present in 10 percent of high-speed trauma victims, and caution should be exercised during intubation.[1] Concerns about extending the cervical spine during intubation in the multi-injured patient have led some researchers to advocate nasotracheal intubation with the head held in a neutral position, but currently there are no data to support either the oral or the nasal route. Paramedics associated with our trauma center are trained to perform oral endotracheal intubation facilitated by the administration of 1 mg/kg succinylcholine and 1.5 mg/kg lidocaine. One hundred percent oxygen and appropriate rates of ventilation should be administered during transport to the emergency facility.

As with hypoxia, there is a significant incidence of hypotension with severe TBI.[11,12] The National Coma Data Bank documented a 35 percent incidence of hypotension (<90 mmHg) as the first-recorded blood pressure determination in the emergency department in patients with severe TBI. The presence of hypotension was associated with a general increase in mortality from 27 to 50 percent.[12] Hypotension is usually caused by systemic injury, rather than loss of autonomic-controlled vascular tone. Cervical or high thoracic spinal cord injury may cause hypotension as a result of autonomic pathway interruption, but the patient is usually bradycardic, compared with the tachycardic patient, as in hypovolemic shock.

In-field resuscitation of hypovolemic shock consists of intravenous administration of crystalloid solutions such as Ringer's lactate. Glucose-containing solutions may have an adverse impact on the brain during periods of ischemia, based on data derived from patients with diabetes who suffer stroke.[13] Experimental studies have shown that the brain continues to metabolize glucose during periods of oxygen deprivation, leading to excessive lactate production.[14-17] The relative acidosis induced by lactic acid may account for the worse outcome after stroke in diabetic patients with poor blood glucose control when compared with diabetics with good blood glucose control. In patients with TBI, hyperglycemia has also been shown to be associated with poor prognosis.[18-20] Glucose-containing solutions should not be administered unless the presence of hypoglycemia is suspected or established. Regardless of the components of the crystalloid solution used, the clinical consequences of hypovolemic shock are so definitive that every attempt should be made to obtain a normal blood pressure during prehospital care.[21] Once the patient is normotensive, fluid administration should be regulated to avoid fluid over-load, a situation that can exacerbate pulmonary problems or adversely affect ICP by worsening cerebral edema.

Hypertonic saline (3 to 6 percent) may prove to be an even better intrave-nous solution for the purpose of fluid resuscitation. A number of experimental studies have demonstrated that hypertonic saline in very small quantities (about 10 percent of the resuscitation volume of isotonic solutions) can markedly increase blood pressure and cardiac index.[22,23] Such small quantities are rapidly infused and have a negligible effect on ICP.[24] Hypertonic saline pulls fluid from the large reservoir of fluid in the extravascular space, and the effect, therefore, is limited by that volume. The intravascular expansion effect is short-lived, about 15 to 30 min, and other fluids must be administered intravenously. However, because such a small bolus is needed, it can be given rapidly while large venous catheters are established and large volumes of isotonic fluids infused.

Hypertonic solutions commonly used in treatment of elevated ICP, such as mannitol, do not have the same profound cardiovascular effect as hypertonic saline. Generally, if the patient has a stable or improving neurologic status, mannitol is not used in prehospital management. Mannitol, because it is an osmotic diuretic, can have the negative systemic effect of dehydrating the patient at the time when maintenance of an adequate intravascular volume is critical. Whether mannitol exacerbates intracranial hemorrhage is unclear.

Steroids such as dexamethasone or methylprednisolone given early in the course of TBI do not improve clinical outcome, based on double blind, randomized placebo-controlled trials.[25,26] Likewise, steroids do not affect cerebral edema from trauma, compared with their clear effect on tumor-induced cerebral edema. However, the dosages of steroids used in these trials may have been insufficient. Methylprednisolone at extremely high doses does improve outcome from spinal cord injury and must be given within 8 h of injury.[27] Since patients with serious brain injury may be unable to communi-cate, spinal cord injury must be diagnosed by spine radiographs (see Chap. 4). In those patients with TBI and suspected spinal cord injury, methylprednis-olone should be administered at the recommended dose of 30 mg/kg intrave-nous bolus, followed by a 5.4 mg/kg per h intravenous infusion. Steroid drug trials at these dosages for treatment of TBI have not been initiated for a number of reasons, not the least of which is the difficulty in quantifying meaningful clinical outcome measures. Furthermore, a number of related compounds that can prevent neuronal death without glucocorticoid side effects have been developed and are presently in clinical trials.[28]

Clinical classification of the brain injury occurs in the field, generally by paramedics. The Glasgow Coma Scale (GCS) is a simple, rapid scoring system that has high interobserver reliability and has proven extremely useful in grading the severity of the TBI. The GCS is based on neurologic tests involv-ing motor, verbal, and eye responses to verbal command or painful stimulus.[29] The score ranges from 3, a very severe brain injury, to 15, which is normal.

Operational definitions of the severity of TBI have been developed using the GCS, and are widely accepted.[3] A severe TBI is defined as a GCS of 3 through 8; a moderate TBI, a GCS of 9 through 12; and a mild TBI, a GCS of 13 through 15. Reappraisal of the patient's neurologic status every 15 min using the GCS permits a continual monitor of neurologic function and helps detect neurologic decline that otherwise might be overlooked in the complex, multi-injured patient.

The final critical point in prehospital care of the head-injured patient involves transport.[9] Patients with TBI should have spinal column immobilization. At least 10 percent of severely head-injured patients have an associated spinal column or spinal cord injury. Unless the patient is firmly secured to a backboard, movement of the patient's spine during extraction or transport may create or worsen a spinal cord injury. The patient should stay restrained to the backboard until cleared by clinical exam, using radiographs as needed. Use of aircraft as opposed to land transport may be useful when travelling long distances or through heavy traffic. Resuscitation of a patient during transport is difficult at best, and travel time should be minimized.

Emergency Department Management

Resuscitation efforts targeted toward airway, breathing and circulation continue in the emergency department. If an airway has not been secured in the field, or there is a decline in the patient's ventilatory status, intubation can occur in the slightly more controlled environment of the emergency department. Assessment of neurologic function continues, using a simple neurologic examination consisting of the GCS, pupillary reaction to light, and determination of power and sensation in the extremities. Pupillary light responses are not affected if the patient is pharmacologically paralyzed for the purposes of airway or ventilatory control. Other systemic injuries are identified and triaged for treatment according to their potential impact on morbidity or mortality. Efficient trauma management in the emergency department is critical for patients with intracranial mass lesions that require evacuation.[30] The length of time to definitive surgical evacuation of traumatic subdural hematomas had a significant impact on outcome in a series of patients reported by Seelig et al.[31] Those patients who underwent craniotomy for subdural hematoma within 4 h of the time of injury were much more likely to have a good outcome than those operated on after this interval.

Airway Management

Because of the potential spinal column/cord injury, management of the airway in a patient with TBI can be a very challenging problem. The goal is to establish a definitive airway allowing improved oxygenation and ventilation without aggravating any potential injury to the spinal cord. The optimal method of tracheal intubation depends on the patient's condition, the level of cooperation, and the skill and experience of the anesthesiologist. The difficulty can be highlighted by the following facts:

1. A patient with mild to moderate TBI may require tracheal intubation, but may be strong or alert enough to resist an intubation attempt without pharmacologic restraints in the form of hypnotic and neuromuscular blockers.
2. Collars, whether soft or rigid, do not completely eliminate movement of the neck during intubation. Although the rigid collar is more effective,[32] it may hinder tracheal intubation.
3. The patient's condition may not allow postponement of intubation until a radiograph of C-spine is taken.
4. A negative cross-table lateral x-ray does not rule out all cervical spinal injuries; Woodring and Lee reported that 30 percent of patients with cervical spinal injuries may be missed.[33] However, this is frequently used as the criterion to "clear" the spine in many centers.[34] A CT scan is therefore often required to rule out cervical spine injuries.
5. Nasotracheal intubation is contraindicated in patients with basal skull fractures; not only can infection be introduced into the brain, but the endotracheal tube has also been reported to enter the brain through the site of fracture.
6. Manual in-line traction (MILT), although effective in immobilizing the neck during tracheal intubation, does not eliminate movement completely and may cause increased distraction in patients with fracture-dislocations.[35]
7. In patients with associated facial trauma, conventional tracheal intubation may be impossible, and transtracheal jet ventilation or surgical airway (cricothyroidotomy or tracheotomy) may be required.
8. Fiberoptic bronchoscopic intubation is generally not applicable in patients with TBI because of the urgent nature.

In the final analysis, the skill and clinical experience of the anesthesiologist is as important as these eight considerations.[36,37]

To provide a frame of reference, the airway management protocol of Advanced Trauma Life Support (ATLS) advocated by the American College of Surgeons is shown in Fig. 5-1.[38] This protocol, however, does not assume the presence of a skilled anesthesiologist and therefore makes no provision for the use of hypnotics and muscle relaxants. In general, oral tracheal intubation under MILT is the preferred method of choice, and has an excellent safety record[39,40] that is comparable to that of awake intubation.[41,42] Although patients with low GCS score are generally intubated in the field by paramedics with or without the use of neuromuscular blocking agents, patients with mild to moderate TBI will require a hypnotic either in addition to or without a neuromuscular blocking agent in order to facilitate tracheal intubation. Endotracheal intubation elicits an intense sympathetic response, and the associ-

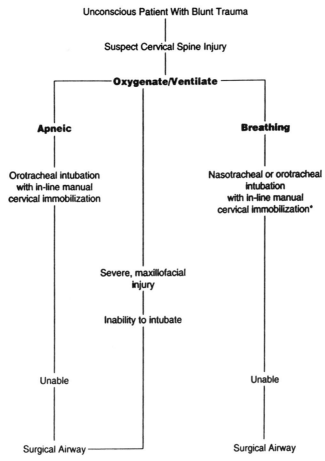

Figure 5-1 Immediate need for definitive airway. Airway algorithm for patients suffering from traumatic injury. *Proceed according to clinical judgment and skill/experience level. (*Reproduced from Advanced Trauma Life Support Course, with permission from the American College of Surgeons.*)

ated increase in intracranial pressure (ICP) may be detrimental. Moreover, coughing or bucking during tracheal intubation can trigger an even larger increase in ICP. It is therefore prudent to administer both a hypnotic agent as well as a neuromuscular blocker in these patients. The choice of agents is dependent on the patient's hemodynamic stability and the anesthesiologist's preference. Thiopental, propofol and etomidate are all cerebral vasoconstrictors and will reduce ICP. All are capable of causing systemic hypotension although etomidate is the least likely agent to do so. Because all patients with TBI are at risk of gastric aspiration and many are intoxicated from recent alcohol consumption, a rapid sequence technique with cricoid pressure should be followed. Although the use of cricoid pressure in a patient with potential cervical spinal cord injury is controversial, it has been used successfully[43,44] and should only be withheld in patients with established disruption of the cervical spinal column. Although not directly relevant, the American Society of Anesthesiologists has recently published *Practice Guidelines for Management of the Difficult Airway,* which should also be consulted (*Anesthesiology* 78:597–602, 1993).

The choice of neuromuscular blockers is equally controversial. Succinylcholine remains the muscle relaxant with the quickest onset and shortest duration. It would allow immediate establishment of a protected airway in a patient with TBI and assessment of neurologic function shortly after if deemed necessary. However, it has been reported to result in increase in ICP in several studies.[45–48] Experimental study in canines has identified that the increase in ICP is a result of increase in cerebral blood flow secondary to stimulation of the gamma motor neurons.[45] However, animals suffering from cerebral ischemia do not mount this response,[49] and a similar lack of response has been reported in patients with neurologic injury or in deeply anesthetized patients.[50–52] Thus, it would appear that succinylcholine remains the muscle relaxant of choice when an airway needs to be established expeditiously in a patient with TBI. In nonemergent situations, the use of a slower onset nondepolarizing blocker, such as vecuronium, is appropriate although succinylcholine can still be used. In patients with focal neurologic deficits, hyperkalemia from denervation sensitivity may occur with the administration of succinylcholine. Similar response has also been reported in patients with closed head injury but without focal neurologic signs.[53] However, this hyperkalemic response does not occur acutely and succinylcholine is safe to use within the first 24 to 48 h of the initial injury. A recommended algorithm for the choice of hypnotics and neuromuscular blockers is shown in Table 5-1.

Radiologic and Laboratory Investigations

Initial radiologic diagnostic tests obtained on the multiply injured patient include chest, abdomen, and lateral cervical spine radiographs. Other radiologic tests can be delayed until a determination is made whether the patient will need to be taken to surgery immediately. Skull radiographs are of insufficient value in patients with moderate or severe TBI to warrant their use.[54] Instead, a CT scan is a much better tool for diagnostic purposes and should be obtained when the patient has a secure airway and is hemodynamically stable. The use of exploratory burr holes in the emergency department is not recommended as a substitute for a CT scan. Andrews et al. have described the use of exploratory burr holes placed in the operating room in order to

Table 5-1 Suggested Choice

GCS Score	Hemodynamic Stability	Hypnotic	Urgency	Neuromuscular Blocker
3–8	Yes	Lidocaine 1.5 mg/kg	Yes ↑	Sux 1.0 mg/kg
	No			
9–12	Yes	Thiopental 2–3 mg/kg or propofol 1–2 mg/kg ±lidocaine 1.5 mg/kg	Yes ↑ / No ↑	Sux 1.0 mg/kg / Vec 0.02 mg/kg
	No	Etomidate 1–2 mg/kg	Yes ↑	Sux 1.0 mg/kg
13–15	Yes	Thiopental 3–4 mg/kg or propofol 1.5–2.0 mg/kg ±lidocaine 1.5 mg/kg	Yes ↑ / No ↑	Sux 1.0 mg/kg / Vec 0.02 mg/kg
	No	Etomidate 1–2 mg/kg	Yes ↑	Sux 1.0 mg/kg

Sux = succinylcholine; Vec = vecuronium; GCS = Glasgow Coma Scale

avoid the sometimes lengthy wait needed to obtain a CT scan, but a timely CT is a better diagnostic tool than burr holes.[55] Laboratory investigations should include a baseline hemogram, in addition to tests for coagulation, glucose, electrolytes, and arterial blood gases, as well as a toxicology screen. Blood should also be typed and reserved.

Monitoring

Certain monitoring tools are available in the emergency department. It is time consuming and difficult to place arterial catheters in the emergency department for hemodynamic measurement; automatic noninvasive blood pressure monitoring through self inflating cuffs is a better alternative. Arterial oxygenation and end tidal CO_2 can be monitored continuously with pulse oximetry and capnometer, along with standard arterial blood gas measurement. Close clinical observation remains the best tool for neurologic monitoring in the emergency dept. A fiberoptic intracranial pressure monitor can be easily and rapidly inserted in those patients with moderate or severe TBI, but ICP measurement should not take the place of frequent (every 15 min or less) neurologic checks using the GCS and pupillary examination.

A coordinated medical approach to the trauma patient with brain injury is critical to outcome. Several key physicians play central roles in the immediate evaluation and treatment of these patients. These include an emergency department physician, anesthesiologist and a trauma surgeon.[56] There should be immediate availability of a neurological surgeon for care of the patient with a brain or spinal cord injury. Delay in consultation should be avoided, and if a neurological surgeon is not available at the treatment facility, strong consideration should be given to transfer to an institution where such consultation is provided.

REFERENCES

1. Mahoney BD, Ruiz E: Acute resuscitation of the patient with head and spinal cord injuries. *Emerg Med Clin North Amer* 1:583, 1983.

2. Miller JD, Becker DP: Secondary insults to the injured brain. *J R Coll Surg Edinb* Sept.: 292, 1982.

3. Levison M, Trunkey DD: Initial assessment and resuscitation. *Surg Clin North Am* 62:9, 1982.

4. Eisenberg HM, Cayard C, Papanicolaou FF, et al: The effects of three potentially preventable complications on outcome after severe closed head injury. In Ishal S, Nagai H, Brock M (eds): *Intracranial Pressure V*. Tokyo, Springer Verlag, 1983: 549–553.

5. Jennett B, Carlin J: Preventable mortality and morbidity after head injury. *Injury* 10:31, 1978.

6. Youmans JR: Causes of shock with injury. *J Trauma* 4:204, 1964.

7. Miller JD, Sweet RC, Narayan R, et al: Early insults to the injured brain. *JAMA* 240:439, 1978.

8. Marshall LF, Becker DP, Bowers SA, et al: The National Traumatic Coma Data Bank. I: Design, purpose, goals, and results. *J Neurosurg* 59:276, 1983.

9. Gildenberg PL, Maleka M: Effect of early intubation and ventilation on outcome following head trauma. In Dacey RG Jr, et al (eds): *Trauma of the Central Nervous System*. New York, Raven Press, 79–90, 1985.

10. Symon L: Flow thresholds in brain ischaemia and the effects of drugs. *Br J Anaesth* 57:34, 1985.

11. Cooper PR: Delayed brain injury: Secondary issues. In Becker DP, Povlishock JT (eds): *Central Nervous System Trauma Status Report*. Washington, D.C., National Institute of Neurological and Communicative Disorders and Stroke, National Institutes of Health, 1985:217–228.

12. Marmarou A, Anderson RL, Ward JD: Impact of ICP instability and hypotension on outcome in patients with severe head trauma. *J Neurosurg* 75:S59, 1991.

13. Pulsinelli WA, Levy DE, Sigsbee B, et al: Increased damage after ischemic stroke in patients with hyperglycemia with or without established diabetes mellitus. *Am J Med* 74:540, 1983.

14. Kalimo H, Rehncrona S, Soderfelt B: The role of lactic acidosis in the ischemic nerve cell injury. *Acta Neuropathol* 7(Suppl):20, 1981.

15. Marsh WR, Anderson RE, Sundt TM Jr: Effect of hyperglycemia on brain pH levels in areas of focal incomplete cerebral ischemia in monkeys. *J Neurosurg* 65:693, 1986.

16. Rehncrona S, Rosen I, Siesjo BK: Brain lactic acidosis and ischemic cell damage: I. Biochemistry and neurophysiology. *J Cereb Blood Flow Metab* 1:297, 1981.

17. Siemkowicz E: Hyperglycemia in the reperfusion period hampers recovery from cerebral ischemia. *Acta Neurol Scand* 64:207, 1981.

18. Young B, Ott L, Dempsey R, et al: Relationship between admission hyperglycemia and neurologic outcome of severely brain-injured patients. *Ann Surg* 210:466, 1989.

19. Lam AM, Winn HR, Cullen BF, et al: Hyperglycemia and neurological outcome in patients with head injury. *J Neurosurg* 75:545, 1991.

20. Michaud LJ, Rivara FP, Longstreth WT Jr, et al: Elevated initial blood glucose levels and poor outcome following severe brain injuries in children. *J Trauma* 31:1356, 1991.

21. Miller JD: Head injury and brain ischaemia—implications for therapy. *Br J Anaesth* 57:120, 1985.

22. Nakayama S, Sibley L, Gunther RA, et al: Small volume resuscitation with hypertonic saline (2,400 mosm/liter) during hemorrhagic shock. *Circ Shock* 13:149, 1984.

23. Wisner DH, Schuster L, Quinn C: Hypertonic saline resuscitation of head injury: Effects on cerebral water content. *J Trauma* 30:75, 1990.

24. Gunnar W, Jonasson O, Merlotti G, et al: Head injury and hemorrhagic shock: Studies of the blood brain barrier and intracranial pressure after resuscitation with normal saline solution, 3% saline solution, and dextran-40. *Surgery* 103:398, 1988.

25. Cooper PR, Moody S, Clark WK, et al: Dexamethasone and severe head injury: A prospective double-blind study. *J Neurosurg* 51:307, 1979.

26. Giannotta SL, Weiss MH, Apuzzo MLJ, et al: High dose glucocorticoids in the management of severe head injury. *Neurosurgery* 15:497, 1984.

27. Bracken MB, Shepard MJ, Collins WF, et al: A randomized, controlled trial of methylprednisolone or naloxone in the treatment of acute spinal-cord injury. *N Engl J Med* 322:1405, 1990.

28. Hall ED, Yonders PA, Andrus PK, et al: Biochemistry and pharmacology of lipid antioxidants in acute brain and spinal cord injury. *J Neurotrauma* 9:S425, 1992.

29. Teasdale G, Jennett B: Assessment of coma and impaired consciousness. A practical scale. *Lancet* 2:81, 1974.

30. Becker DF, Miller JD, Ward JD, et al: The outcome from severe head injury with early diagnosis and intensive management. *J Neurosurg* 47:491, 1977.

31. Seelig JM, Becker DP, Miller JD, et al: Traumatic acute subdural hematoma: Major mortality reduction in comatose patients treated within four hours. *N Engl J Med* 304:1511, 1981.

32. Majernick TG, Bieniek R, Houston JB, et al: Cervical spine movement during orotracheal intubation. *Ann Emerg Med* 15:417, 1986.

33. Woodring JH, Lee C: Limitations of cervical radiography in the evaluation of acute cervical trauma. *J Trauma* 34:32, 1993.

34. Mirvis SE, Diaconis JN, Chirico PA, et al: Protocol-driven radiologic evaluation of suspected cervical spine injury: Efficacy study. *Radiology* 170:831, 1989.

35. Bivins HG, Ford S, Bezmalinovic Z, et al: The effect of axial traction during orotracheal intubation of the trauma victim with an unstable cervical spine. *Ann Emerg Med* 17:25, 1988.

36. Crosby ET, Lui A: The adult cervical spine: Implications for airway management. *Can J Anaesth* 37:77, 1990.

37. Hastings RH, Marks JD: Airway management of trauma patients with potential cervical spine injuries. *Anesth Analg* 73:471, 1991.

38. Advanced Trauma Life Support Course for Physicians Manual. American Coll Surgeons. 1993; 57.

39. Grande CM, Barton CR, Stene JK: Appropriate techniques for airway management of emergency patients with suspected spinal cord injury. *Anesth Analg* 67:714, 1988.

40. Rhee KJ, Green W, Holcroft JW, et al: Oral intubation in the multiply injured patient: The risk of exacerbating spinal cord damage. *Ann Emerg Med* 19:511, 1990.

41. Suderam VS, Crosby ET, Lui A: Elective oral tracheal intubation in cervical spin-injured adults. *Can J Anaesth* 38:785, 1991.

42. Meschino A, Devitt JH, Szalai JP, et al: The safety of awake tracheal intubation in cervical spin injury. *Can J Anaesth* 39:114, 1992.

43. Talucci RC, Shaikh KA, Schwab CW: Rapid sequence induction with oral endotracheal intubation in the multiply injured patient. *Am Surg* 54:185, 1988.

44. Doolan LA, O'Brien JF. Safe intubation in cervical spine injury. *Anaesth Intensive Care* 13:319, 1985.

45. Lanier WL, Iaizzo PA, Milde JH: Cerebral function and muscle afferent activity following intravenous succinylcholine in dogs anesthetized with halothane: The effects of pretreatment with a defasciculating dose of pancuronium. *Anesthesiology* 71:87, 1989.

46. Minton MD, Grosslight F, Stirt JA, et al: Increases in intracranial pressure from succinylcholine: Prevention by prior nondepolarizing blockade. *Anesthesiology* 65:195, 1986.

47. Cottrell JE, Hartung J, Griffin JP, et al: Intracranial and hemodynamic changes after succinylcholine administration in cats. *Anesth Analg* 62:1006, 1983.

48. Atru AA. Succinylcholine-induced increases in CSF pressure are not affected by $Paco_2$ oar mean arterial pressure in dogs. *J Neurosurg Anesth* 2:4, 1990.

49. Lanier WL, Iaizzo PA, Milde JH: The effects of intravenous succinylcholine on cerebral function and muscle afferent activity following complete ischemia in halothane-anesthetized dogs. *Anesthesiology* 73:485, 1990.

50. White PF, Schlobohm RM, Pitts LH, et al: A randomized study of drugs for preventing increases in intracranial pressure during endotracheal suctioning. *Anesthesiology* 57:242, 1982.

51. Kovarik WD, Mayberg TS, Lam AM, et al: Succinylcholine does not change intracranial pressure, cerebral blood flow velocity, or the electroencephalogram in patients with neurologic injury. *Anesth Analg* 78:469, 1994.

52. Lam AM, Nicholas JF, Manninen PH. Influence of succinylcholine on lumbar cerebral spinal pressure in man. *Anesth Analg* 63:240, 1984.

53. Frankville DD, Drummond JC: Hyperkalemia after succinylcholine administration in a patient with closed head injury without paresis. *Anesthesiology* 67:264, 1987.

54. Cooper PR, Ho V: The role of emergency skull x-ray films in the evaluation of the head-injured patient: A retrospective study. *Neurosurgery* 13:136, 1983.

55. Andrews BT, Pitts LH, Lovely MP, et al: Is computed tomographic scanning necessary in patients with tentorial herniation? Results of immediate surgical

exploration without computed tomography in 100 patients. *Neurosurgery* 19:408, 1986.

56. Trunkey DD: Neural trauma: From the point of view of the general surgeon. In Dacey RG Jr, Winn HR, Rimel R, et al. (eds): *Trauma of the Central Nervous System* (Seminars in Neurological Surgery Series). New York, Raven Press, 1985: 2–17.

CHAPTER 6

Surgical Management of Acute Head Injury

Peter D. Le Roux and H. Richard Winn

Although the initial management of head injury is multidimensional, it is centered on identifying and surgically evacuating intracranial mass lesions as quickly as possible to prevent permanent neurologic dysfunction. In addition to causing injury to the brain, such lesions can disrupt the integrity of the skull and meninges. Early surgical restoration of normal anatomy can prevent deleterious long term sequelae such as infection. Although the benefits of surgery are well documented, its success is critically dependent on the careful attention to the systemic effects of trauma, as the injured brain does not withstand secondary insults.[1]

Intracranial pressure monitoring is discussed elsewhere in the book; this chapter will review surgical pathology, indications for acute surgery, and outcome after head trauma. Although injuries of the skull and meninges are often associated with injuries to the brain, the principles of employing craniotomy for mass lesions and craniectomy for skull fractures and open wounds will be discussed separately. The underlying principle behind both operations is to prevent neurologic compromise in both the short and long term.

CRANIOTOMY FOR MASS LESIONS

Evaluation and Indications for Surgery

There is considerable evidence that early evacuation of traumatic intracranial hemorrhage can improve outcome. Operative indications are defined by both clinical evaluation and radiologic investigations. Clinical evaluation allows an assessment of the severity of the injury and provides information to predict prognosis. The clinical triad of depressed consciousness, pupillary anisocoria, and hemiparesis, often secondary to brainstem compression, is the classic presentation of a traumatic mass lesion. However, even without the presence of these findings the presence of a mass lesion cannot be discounted even in the fully conscious person.[2] Traumatic mass lesions are more likely to occur in older patients, alcoholics, persons injured in falls and persons presenting with a skull fracture, particularly if the fracture crosses the middle meningeal artery or a major venous sinus.[3] Subtle signs, such as restlessness and disorientation, may indicate the presence of a mass lesion. However, stable patients may suddenly deteriorate as intracranial compensatory mechanisms are exhausted. To prevent permanent neurologic damage, recognition of a mass and its decompression should occur before clinical deterioration develops. Repeated neurologic evaluation may be necessary as assessed by the Glasgow Coma Scale.[4] The Glasgow Coma Scale (GCS) allows different observers to consistently evaluate neurologic function.

Although a depressed GCS score is a very reliable indicator of a mass lesion, nearly 20 percent of patients with traumatic intracranial hemorrhage can have an initial GCS score that is normal.[2,3] Investigative techniques are thus essential to define traumatic mass lesions (Fig. 6-1). The development of computed tomography (CT), which has revolutionized the management of head injury, allows early identification of mass lesions and may also predict clinical deterioration. All patients with altered consciousness, even transient, and those at risk for mass lesions should have an admission CT scan. The utility of magnetic resonance imaging (MRI) remains to be determined in patients with acute head trauma. The radiologic features of head injury are discussed in Chap. 4, but certain CT findings are important guidelines for surgical intervention. One of the primary goals of surgery is to relieve increased intracranial pressure (ICP). Intracranial hypertension can be suspected from several CT features: effacement of cerebrospinal fluid (CSF) spaces, particularly the perimesencephalic cisterns, hematoma size, and midline shift.[5] In the fully conscious patient an extraaxial hematoma >1 cm thick or an intracranial hematoma (ICH) >3 cm in diameter should be considered for surgical removal, if accessible, because intracranial hypertension invariably

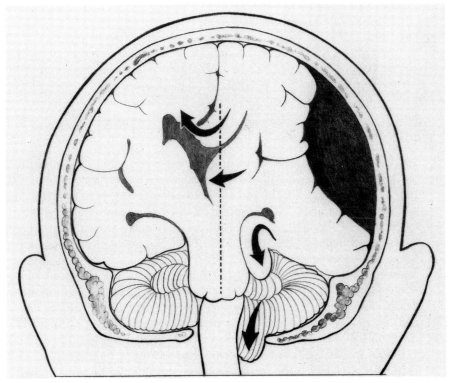

Figure 6-1 The presence of an extradural hematoma, subdural hematoma, or intracerebral hematoma may contribute to uncal, transtentorial or tonsillar herniation following head injury. The goal of surgery is to evacuate the space-occupying lesion before herniation occurs.

develops. Midline shift may be a more reliable indicator for surgery than hematoma size alone. Ropper[6] has established that 8 mm of shift is associated with coma and 6 mm with stupor; therefore, any lesion causing >5 mm shift should be considered for evacuation irrespective of the hematoma's size and patient's clinical condition. Just as repeat clinical evaluation is necessary, so also is a follow-up CT scan. Admission CT scan can often miss a developing lesion if the patient is evaluated between 1 or 2 h after injury.[10,11] Significant swelling, delayed extraaxial or intracerebral hematomas or both may be found on follow-up CT scan within 24 to 48 h of trauma. A repeat CT is warranted in all patients whose initial CT demonstrates an abnormality, or whose GCS score is less than 10 or whose condition deteriorates.

In the conscious patient, whose lesions do not meet the CT criteria described previously, inserting an ICP monitor may be useful. Surgery is indicated if pressure is >25 mm Hg.[7-9] However, standard ICP monitoring may not reflect local pressure changes in the presence of temporal or cerebellar lesions, and the ICP may be misleadingly low. Moreover, these locations, because of their proximity to the brainstem, can cause rapid deterioration and are particularly dangerous as ICP changes may not predict their evolution.

The combination of neurologic and radiologic evaluation is necessary to determine which patients require craniotomy. Neither poor neurologic condition nor normal neurologic function in the presence of a significant mass lesion are contraindications to surgery. Once identified, mass lesions should be evacuated as quickly as possible.

Preparation for Surgery

Despite the required urgency of diagnosis and treatment of patients with head injury, the physician should not forget the simple ABCs of trauma care. Initial resuscitation has been discussed in detail in the first part of this chapter and anesthetic care in Chap. 7, but certain important points require emphasis. Other injuries are often superimposed on head injury and can contribute to hypoxia and hypotension, both of which will adversely affect outcome.[12,13] Respiratory insufficiency, manifested by poor airway control, hypoxemia, decreased functional reserve and compliance, is common after head injury[14] (see Chap. 3). On arrival in the OR, airway and respiratory function are the first priority of care. Hyperventilation may provide a protective effect on ICP and intracranial compliance in the short term and should be instituted to maintain Pa_{O_2} >100 mmHg and Pa_{CO_2} of 25 to 30 mmHg.[15]

Blood pressure (BP) is frequently elevated in the face of a mass lesion as part of a vasopressor response to maintain cerebral perfusion pressure (CPP). The relief of systemic hypertension can be expected when intracranial hypertension is corrected either medically or following surgery. Usually, low BP prior to evacuation of a mass lesion suggests a systemic disorder (e.g., blood loss) requiring urgent attention (also see Chap. 8). In general, no attempt should be made to lower BP with anesthestic agents or vasodilators; if autoregulation (AR) is defective, cerebral blood flow (CBF) will passively decrease and cerebral ischemia may result. In contrast, if AR is intact, vasodilation will result, leading to increased ICP and attenuated CPP.[16]

In most patients with mass lesions requiring surgical evacuation, good venous access will have been established in the Emergency Dept. Two large-bore IVs are a minimum. In addition an arterial catheter should be inserted for direct BP monitoring. Other monitors, including ECG, esophageal stethoscope, and Foley catheter, are also important (see Chap. 8). Recent experimental evidence suggests that small differences in brain temperature are critical in determining outcome after cerebral ischemia.[17] Consequently, core body temperature should be monitored. Similarly, a retrograde jugular catheter, to assess jugular venous oxygen saturation, can help identify patients with compensated cerebral hypoperfusion who are at risk for infarction, and, therefore, Pa_{CO_2} can be set for optimal CBF. Furthermore, calculation of AVD_{O_2} can be of prognostic value; i.e., failure of AVD_{O_2} to improve >1 vol percent after decompression of a traumatic mass lesion is associated with secondary cerebral infarction and poor outcome.[18]

Once airway and venous access are secure, the patient should be carefully positioned on the OR table (Fig. 6-2). Up to 30 percent of patients coming to surgery may have concomitant cervical spine injuries.[19] The neck, therefore, should be maintained in a neutral position by avoiding excessive flexion or rotation. Maintenance of the neutral position minimizes the risk of spinal

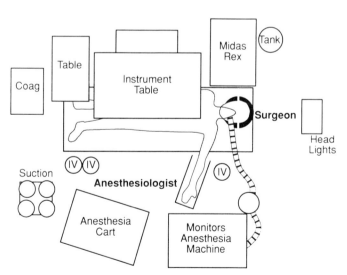

Figure 6-2 Operating room set up for acute head trauma illustrated from above. The neck should be maintained in the neutral position; this improves venous return from the head and minimizes the risk of spinal cord damage.

cord damage and also improves venous drainage from the head. Because significant cerebral swelling can result from impeding venous return, it is preferable to affix the endotracheal tube (ETT) to the face with sticky tape and not use the tie. Intraoperatively, in addition to determination of levels of blood gases, tests for normal levels of electrolytes, glucose and coagulation should be performed. Hyperglycemia is common after severe head injury and significantly worsens the effect of ischemia.[20] Similarly, disseminated intravascular coagulation (DIC) and the presence of any clotting abnormality may complicate severe head injury and make surgical hemostasis difficult or increase the risk of a delayed lesion.[21, 22] Obviously, blood products should be available to replace blood loss and, if any coagulation parameters are abnormal, active treatment should be begun, even if surgical hemostasis appears normal.

Finally, we routinely give all patients with traumatic mass lesions 500 ml of mannitol (20 percent Osmitrol), or approximately 1.5 gm/kg. Even though smaller doses may decrease ICP, this can be safely attempted only if an ICP monitor is in place. There is a limited role for other diuretics in acute head injury. Although mannitol can transiently increase ICP and cerebral blood volume and can even lead to further bleeding, its overall protective effects far outweigh its side effects until surgical decompression can be achieved.

Craniotomy Technique

Many operative approaches have been described for traumatic lesions, but we believe that a large frontal-parietal temporal free flap or "trauma craniotomy" optimizes surgical therapy for a number of reasons. First, rotational forces are a common mechanism of injury.[23] Such injuries result in frontal-temporal contusions and disruption of bridging veins to the sagittal, petrosal, or transverse sinuses. Therefore, surgical exposure should ideally allow access to the epi- and subdural spaces, entire temporal and inferior frontal lobes as well as bridging veins in the midline or middle fossa. Second, a large craniotomy minimizes the risk of brain strangulation and infarction if herniation were to occur during surgery.

The operative technique is depicted in Fig. 6-3. In the rapidly deteriorating patient an immediate temporal decompression is performed by incising the

---

Figure 6-3 Diagrams illustrating the operative technique for an acute subdural hematoma. (*A*) Outline of the skin incision; this flap allows access to the areas likely to be injured following rotational acceleration/deceleration injuries. (*B*) In the rapidly deteriorating patient, a subtemporal decompression may be necessary before completing the craniotomy. (*C*) The dural opening should provide access to basal, anterior, and midline structures. (*D*) The hematoma is removed with careful irrigation and suction. (*E*) Following dural closure, back-up sutures are inserted to prevent hematoma reaccumulation.

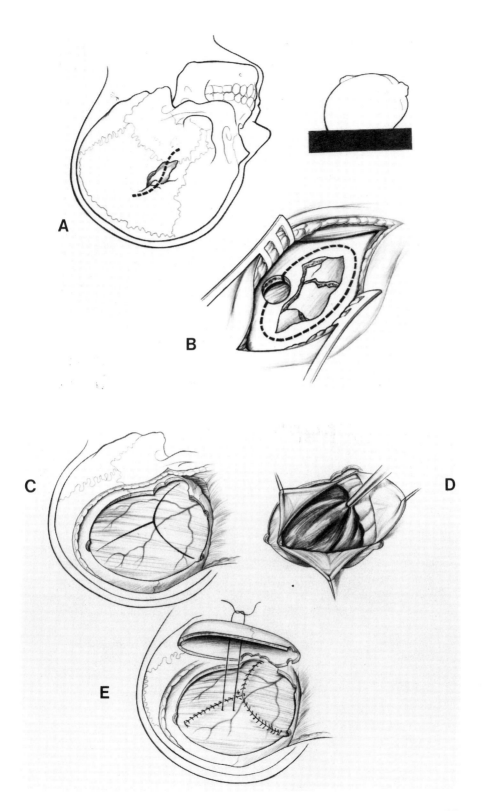

skin and temporalis muscle down to the bone just anterior to the ear and above the zygoma. A burr hole, and, if necessary, a small craniectomy is created to partially decompress the temporal lobe, following which the craniotomy can be carefully completed. A large C-shaped incision is made, starting just anterior to the tragus and above the zygoma, coursing posterior superior to the pinna, across the parietal region, to the midline where it is carried forward to the hairline and crossed over to the opposite side in a curvilinear fashion. A subtemporal craniectomy augments the exposure. We routinely preserve the pericranium, in case it is needed to augment the dura.

The dural opening is curved anteriorly in a gentle C in the temporal region from underneath the initial burr hole. The hematoma should be removed, using gentle irrigation, which may prevent further bleeding. No attempt should be made to chase elusive pieces of clot. Once hemostasis is ensured, dural closure is imperative, if necessary with dural augmentation using pericranial or temporalis fascia graft. Dural closure prevents oozing into the subdural space and CSF leaking and, in the event of wound infection, can isolate the brain from contamination. Peripheral and central tack-up sutures are used to obliterate the epidural space and prevent the development of a delayed hematoma. The bone flap is then secured in place with wire or micro-internal fixation plates. A subgaleal drain is left in place and a two-layer scalp closure performed. Most patients should have an intracranial pressure monitor inserted.[7,8]

Prior to the use of CT scanning, exploratory burr holes were routinely performed, but now are only occasionally necessary. Without localizing signs (e.g., ipsilateral dilated pupil), bilateral temporal, frontal, and parietal burr holes are necessary. The first burr hole should be placed in the temporal region ipsilateral to the dilated pupil, or, if both pupils are dilated, on the side of external trauma or skull fracture. In the head-injured patient needing emergency laparotomy who is too hemodynamically unstable for a CT scan to be obtained, burr-hole exploration has been advised. These patients often demonstrate bilaterally fixed and dilated pupils and despite burr hole placement, reported mortality exceeds 95 percent.[24] The diagnostic yield from burr holes in these patients is also very low. Therefore, an alternate approach to bilateral burr holes is the placment of an ICP monitor and a CT scan after laparotomy.

If there is an isolated head injury with evidence of brain stem compression, burr hole exploration has been suggested as a means to improve outcome by avoiding the critical delay in CT.[24–26] Under these circumstances, particularly in an elderly person who has fallen, extraaxial hematomas, especially SDH, are common.[24,27] Intraoperative ultrasound (IOUS) may be utilized to identify ICH. If a lesion is identified, a craniotomy should be performed. The patients most likely to benefit from immediate burr hole exploration are those with evidence of brainstem compression who respond to mannitol. However, analysis of the technique described above, in both adults and children, is far from encouraging.[24,26] Only 10 to 20 percent of patients are able to make a functional recovery. The presence of hypotension is again an adverse factor; mortality exceeds 95 percent. Although burr hole exploration alone may benefit a select subset of head-injured patients, in almost all circumstances we believe that preoperative CT scanning is essential.

Extradural Hematoma

Extradural hematomas (EDH) are potentially lethal but, in the absence of other pathology, should rarely cause death. The single most common cause of preventable mortality and morbidity is a delay in diagnosis and surgical decompression.[27]

Extradural hematomas account for 0.2 to 6 percent of all head injuries, up to 12 percent of severe head injuries and are more commonly found in males. These hematomas are usually encountered in the second and third decade of life, whereas few are found at the extremes of age because of the increased adherence of the dura to the inner table of the skull.[28–31] Most EDH are unilateral and are located in the temporal region secondary to laceration of the middle meningeal artery that follows skull fracture or deformation. At impact, the dura is stripped from the inner table allowing blood to collect in the extradural space. Once the hematoma is >6 to 8 mm thick it will continue to strip dura.[32] Linear or depressed skull fractures are commonly found with EDH. Hemorrhage from venous sources, such as diploic or meningeal veins or a sinus, accounts for one-third of EDH. A blow to the vertex or in the anterior-posterior direction can result in bilateral EDH as a result of sagittal sinus bleeding. Although rare, these lesions are often not suspected clinically and are associated with a higher mortality than unilateral pathology.[33]

Epidural hematomas were thought to reach their maximum size immediately,[32] but since the advent of CT scanning, it is clear that as many as 20 percent develop in a delayed fashion, usually within 12 h of trauma.[10,31] Evolving EDH are often of venous origin and can be associated with coagulopathy or can follow the release of tamponade after hyperventilation, osmotic diuresis, surgical decompression, or even CSF otorrhea. In addition, delayed EDH may develop after the successful resuscitation from shock. Therefore, a repeat CT scan should be obtained 12 h after admission in all patients with a skull fracture and decreased GCS score, even if the initial scan was normal. The fact that EDH can develop after hyperventilation or osmotic diuresis emphasizes the need for an ICP monitor in the management of suspected intracranial hypertension if no mass lesion is apparent. Associated intradural pathology, usually a contusion or SDH, can be seen in as many as one-third of patients and is recognized as a poor prognostic indicator.[28,30,34,35] Usually these patients are older, have a lower admission GCS score and a greater incidence of extracranial injuries.

The clinical presentation depends on the size, location, and rate of formation of the EDH. Neurologic sequelae result from both the initial impact and brain stem compression. There is no single clinical finding that is specific for EDH. Furthermore, the classic presentation of a lucid interval followed by a decline in consciousness is present in only a third of patients.[28,31] Altered consciousness is the most important clinical finding. Features of brain stem compression (hemiparesis and anisocoria) may be present, particularly with low temporal EDH.

The diagnostic procedure of choice is CT scan. Once identified, almost all EDH require surgery although conservative management has been advocated in neurologically normal patients with small CT lesions. In the only prospective study addressing this issue, Knuckey and coworkers,[36] found that 32 percent of patients with small (<40 ml) EDH eventually came to require operation. The likelihood of surgery was doubled if a small EDH was discovered in the temporal region within 6 h of injury. Lucency in the hematoma, indicating ongoing bleeding, and shift of midline structures are additional ominous signs and mitigate against conservative management.[37] Large EDH (>80 ml) usually lead to coma secondary to increased ICP; ICP monitoring can thus be useful in predicting which patients with small EDH may require surgery. However, the effects of a temporal clot on cerebral dynamics may be undetected with standard monitoring until clinical deterioration has occurred. Conservative management is thus appropriate only for isolated, small, high-convexity EDH without shift, which are discovered more than 24 h after injury.

The type of craniotomy performed is determined by the presence of other structural lesions as seen on CT and by the patient's neurologic status. If the patient's neurologic status is good and there are no associated changes on CT, the flap may be placed directly over the EDH. In all other circumstances, we prefer a large free flap. In the herniating patient, partial removal of the clot through the initial burr hole is mandatory before completing the full craniotomy. Usually, there is no need to open the dura. The exception occurs when significant intradural pathology has been identified on CT or inappropriate swelling occurs following EDH evacuation. Intracranial hypertension and swelling may result from development of a contralateral extraaxial hematoma or development of a second lesion. Meticulous hemostasis, including the bone edges, is necessary prior to closure.

In the pre-CT era, mortality following EDH was 15 to 40 percent; since the widespread use of CT, <5 percent of patients die.[28,31,38] Numerous factors affect outcome, including age, size, and rate of development of the hematoma; the presence of associated intradural pathology; neurologic condition; and time to surgery.[27-31, 38] Younger patients tend to do better, whereas older patients are more likely to have associated intradural pathology and thus have a poorer outcome. In the comatose patient, poor outcome correlates well with greater hematoma size.[31] A particularly ominous CT sign is the presence of mixed density within the hematoma. It is believed that this signifies ongoing bleeding, and, therefore, the hematoma is likely to increase further. Neurologic status at admission is an important determinant of outcome. Coma is associated with 15 percent mortality, whereas noncomatose individuals rarely, if ever, die. The presence of hemiparesis or unilateral pupillary dilation does not correlate with outcome; in contrast, the presence of posturing and bilateral dilated pupils is strongly associated with mortality. Finally, early surgical treatment improves outcome. For example, Mendelow and coworkers found that those who died had surgery an average of 15 h after injury whereas survivors were usually operated on within 2 h.

Subdural Hematoma

Acute subdural hematoma (SDH) represents the most common traumatic lesion in severe head injury that requires surgery. In contrast to EDH, which is usually not associated with severe structural injury, SDH is a marker of severe brain injury. The mechanisms behind this are not known in detail, but clinical and experimental evidence suggests that delayed ischemia may be partly responsible. Brain injury after SDH is not solely due to impact because biomechanical studies indicate that the pattern of deceleration leading to SDH is different from that causing diffuse axonal injury.[39] Similarly, mass effect is not the sole determinant of neurologic dysfunction; even with prompt surgical evacuation only one-third of patients with SDH recover to functional independence.[40,41] Moreover, in those who subsequently die, ischemic damage is observed at neuropathologic evaluation, even in patients with a lucid interval,[42] suggesting that a delayed phenomenon is partly responsible for the severe brain injury. Experimental observations are consistent with this theory. For example, in a rat model of SDH developed by Bullock and colleagues, qualitative neuropathologic examination demonstrated a zone of ischemia closely related to the SDH even in the face of normal CPP.[43] Furthermore, autoradiographic assessment of the same area indicated that CBF is subthreshold for ischemia.[44] Local pressure gradients or the release of toxic substances from blood breakdown are postulated to lead to the ischemia. This belief is in accordance with Mendelow and coworkers'[45] finding that autologous blood leads to greater ischemic damage than do other substances in an animal model of ICH.

Excitatory amino acids may be responsible for the phenomenon above. Ligand-gated channels, primarily those associated with excitatory amino acids, are activated leading to ionic destabilization.[46] In experimental head injury, excitatory amino acids are markedly increased. For example, Bullock and coworkers[47] measured levels of aspartate and glutamate with in vivo microdialysis after SDH in the rat. Beneath the lesion both levels were elevated to 750 percent of their normal value. Although there was no threshold relationship between excitatory amino acid release and CBF, the extent of the ischemic zone correlated well with the level of both glutamate and aspartate. In addition, ischemic damage can be lessened in the experimental setting by blocking the effect of excitatory amino acids with specific antagonists.[44,48] These experimental studies reinforce the clinical observation that the foundation of surgical treatment of SDH is the avoidance of secondary insults, such as hypoxia or hypotension.

Subdural hematomas are found in 5 to 8 percent of patients admitted to hospital with head injury, in 22 percent of patients with severe head injury, and they represent 60 percent of intracranial lesions needing surgery.[39,49] Males, particularly in the 5th and 6th decade are affected, especially after a fall or assault rather than a motor vehicle accident.[39,41,49] Bleeding in the subdural space develops from one of several mechanisms: arterial laceration, torn Sylvian or cortical veins, or torn bridging veins either to the sagittal sinus in the midline or to the petrosal and transverse sinuses in the middle fossa. However, at surgery it is often difficult to identify the specific source of bleeding. Almost all SDH are found over the convexities, and half are associated with parenchymal contusion or hemorrhage.[49] Bilateral and interhemispheric SDH are rare. The latter may result after relatively minor trauma in anticoagulated patients and has been reported in infants that are vigorously shaken.[50]

The clinical course of SDH is determined by the severity of the brain injury and the rate of development of the hematoma. Half of the patients are comatose from outset and 90 percent of comatose patients coming to surgery after head injury harbor an SDH. In the conscious individual, severe headache and restlessness often indicate the presence of SDH.

Once an SDH is identified, craniotomy is needed unless the patient is flaccid and without any brainstem function. Management should be individualized according to age, neurologic status, and the presence of other injuries, but delaying surgical evacuation can adversely affect outcome.[40] Burr hole drainage is inadequate; most clots are solid, and the source of bleeding cannot be controlled. However, in the patient who is *in extremis* with a severe coagulopathy, burr hole drainage may provide temporary relief. In these circumstances the hematoma is often of varying densities as seen on CT. The primary goal of craniotomy is to decompress the brain. A secondary objective is to remove the clot to minimize the deleterious effects of blood-breakdown products.[45] Contusions or ICH are frequently associated with SDH and may require debridement simultaneous with SDH removal.

A large craniotomy, as previously described, is the recommended approach. In the deteriorating patient, partial evacuation of the clot is prudent before completing the craniotomy. A free bone flap, taking advantage of fracture lines if present, is quicker and may be less likely to bleed in the postoperative period than an osteoplastic flap. The dura is often tense and bulging despite hyperventilation and administration of mannitol. A wide dural opening is necessary; this prevents strangulation of a bulging brain and allows access to bleeding both at the base and along the midline without excess retraction. The hematoma is first removed with gentle irrigation and suction. Bleeding points are controlled with bipolar coagulation or tamponade using gelfoam,

Surgicel, or Avitene. Small pieces of clot should not be pursued where exposure is inadequate. Once the SDH is removed, the brain is systematically inspected for contusion and hemorrhagic necrosis.

Significant brain swelling may occur after hematoma evacuation and, if established, mortality can exceed 85 percent.[51] Experimental work suggests that this swelling may be secondary to increased ischemia rather than hyperemia.[52] Under these circumstances barbiturates (if BP is normal) may help alleviate swelling; otherwise, a lobectomy may be required. In addition, dural augmentation may be performed and the bone flap not replaced. The benefits of such an approach are controversial.[53] Closure of the craniotomy is performed as previously described. An ICP monitor is usually placed as half the patients develop increased ICP. A CT scan should be obtained immediately after surgery. Up to 60 percent of patients may develop other lesions, including contralateral extraaxial hematoma or ICH, some of which require immediate surgical evacuation. The presence of hypoxia and coagulopathy increases the risk of developing these delayed lesions.[54]

Mortality after SDH is higher than with other intracranial mass lesions and is reported to be 40 to 90 percent in most series.[39–41,55] Just as with EDH, it appears that the single most preventable cause of death and disability may be a delay in surgical decompression[40]; however, there are numerous other factors that can affect outcome.[55] First, patients more than 60 years of age[56] and motorcyclists, particularly those not wearing a helmet,[55] have poor outcomes. Second, preoperative neurologic status is an accurate predictor of outcome. The highest mortality is seen in those with a GCS score of 3 to 5, whereas nearly all patients with a GCS score >12 may make a functional recovery. Decerebrate rigidity and pupillary abnormalities, especially fixed and dilated pupils, are ominous findings. Third, intracranial hypertension following surgery has a profound effect on outcome. If ICP is normal, mortality is <30 percent and up to 80 percent of survivors can make a functional recovery. However, if uncontrollable intracranial hypertension results, particularly if ICP >45 mmHg, death is inevitable.[7,8,40,41,55] Finally, hypotension and hypoxemia, are well documented to adversely affect survival.[12,13] It is unclear whether the presence of other intracranial lesions[40,41] affects outcome.

Intracerebral Hematoma

Although small hemorrhagic parenchymal lesions are the commonest focal finding on CT after head injury, space-occupying contusions or intracerebral hematomas (ICH) are uncommon, being identified in about 10 percent of patients with severe head injury.[5] Generally, intracerebral hematomas are well circumscribed, homogeneous collections of blood >2 cm in diameter, whereas large contusions are a heterogeneous mixture of hemorrhage, edema, and normal brain. Although it is useful to think of large contusions and discrete ICH as separate entities, they represent a spectrum of the same disorder.

Both affect the brain by similar mechanisms leading to direct destruction of neural tissue, local mass effect, and intracranial hypertension. In addition, blood breakdown appears to be toxic and can lead to profound ischemic changes independent of CPP.[45] Despite the ease with which these lesions can be identified using CT, their management remains controversial.

Large contusions are seen most commonly in young males following a motor vehicle accident.[57,58] Other lesions, particularly SDH, are commonly associated with ICH or contusion. The parenchymal lesions are inevitably found in the frontal or temporal lobes and develop when the head in motion strikes a stationary object such as occurs in an MVA or fall. Under these circumstances, the brain continues to move and is traumatized by the irregular surface of the anterior fossa or sphenoid wing. Blood vessels can also be torn by the movement with resulting hemorrhage. More discrete hematomas may develop under a depressed skull fracture or after penetrating injuries of the skull, such as stab or gunshot wounds. However, ICH may also develop in a delayed fashion, usually within 48 h of injury. The exact pathogenesis of delayed ICH is unclear but could be secondary to defective autoregulation. Decreased cerebral vascular resistance and increased pressure in the capillaries may lead to leakage of blood through damaged vessel walls. Risk factors for delayed traumatic intracranial hemorrhage (DTICH) include hypoxia and coagulopathy.[21,54] In addition, DTICH may result after releasing tamponade, such as when evacuating other mass lesions. DTICHs are more commonly found in older patients or alcoholics in whom cerebral atrophy is prominent.[59]

The clinical presentation of ICH is dependent on both size and location of the hemorrhage and the effect of the primary injury. Thirty to 50 percent of the patients are unconscious at hospital admission. Features of intracranial hypertension and herniation can result in which case ICH is indistinguishable from extra-axial hematoma (EAH). Temporal and cerebellar hematoma are most likely to cause early brain stem compression. In contrast, other patients may be fully conscious but have profound focal neurologic deficits because of the hematoma location. Neurologic dysfunction may also progress secondary to hematoma enlargement or the development of edema. Failure to improve or improvement followed by sudden deterioration suggests the development of a DTICH.

CT scanning is the diagnostic procedure of choice. Although MRI, particularly T_2-weighted images, may detect areas of contusion more readily and help predict the development of delayed hematoma, its use is limited in the acute stage as both hemorrhagic and nonhemorrhagic lesions appear isointense with brain. CT-detected lesions may vary from inhomogeneous, poorly defined areas of mixed high and low density surrounded by edema (contusions), to homogeneous, circumscribed areas of high density (hematomas) that can reach considerable size. In the patient who does not go immediately to surgery, a single CT scan is insufficient to fully evaluate intraparenchymal lesions as they may evolve with time.[11] Even the smallest contusion can mature into a life-threatening hematoma. A follow-up CT scan is indicated in all patients who show evidence of a parenchymal lesion, irrespective of the clinical condition. The peak incidence of delayed hemorrhage occurs in the first 24 to 48 h after injury. Therefore, subsequent CTs should be obtained during this time.[11,54] Any increase in ICP, deterioration in neurologic status, or failure to improve should prompt earlier CT evaluation.

It is unclear which patients with traumatic ICH require surgical treatment.[9,11,57,58] In fact most patients with ICH do not require surgical intervention. Care must be individualized, and the factors favoring hematoma evacuation must be carefully weighed against the risks and potential benefits of surgery.

The fully conscious and neurologically intact patient is rarely a surgical candidate. In contrast to extraaxial hematoma, coma is not always an indication for surgical evacuation of an ICH. Experimental models suggest that early removal is optimal as ischemic damage can be reduced and outcome improved.[60] Therefore, neurologic deterioration is probably the strongest indicator for surgical evacuation of ICH. Hematomas greater than 3 cm in diameter or 30 ml in volume should be removed, if accessible, as they are most likely to lead to deterioration, particularly if associated with edema. Lesion size alone does not signify increased ICP, especially in the older patient with an atrophic brain. Increased ICP is most reliably indicated by shift, obliterated perimesencephalic cisterns, or in the case of a cerebellar hematoma resulting in upward herniation, obliterated quadrigeminal cisterns.[5] When these features are present, surgical treatment should be strongly considered. Temporal or cerebellar hematomas are more likely to cause rapid compression because of their proximity to the brainstem, and therefore, often require early evacuation. Hematomas in eloquent areas, such as speech or motor cortex, are relative contraindications to surgery unless they are life threatening. Lesions in the basal ganglia are often part of diffuse axonal injury (DAI) and usually indicate a poor prognosis.[61] They are usually small and, because of their location, do not often warrant evacuation. However, stereotactic techniques can be used to achieve decompression if significant mass effect is observed on CT. Large bifrontal contusions or hematomas often pose a problem. Removal of one lesion in the face of an already injured contralateral frontal lobe can leave the patient with profound abulia. However, intracranial hypertension can develop in a delayed fashion and complicate the course of these patients. While medical managment can be successful, some patients may benefit from a large bifrontal decompressive craniotomy.[62] Associated injuries such as extraaxial hematomas, depressed skull fractures, or penetrating wounds may warrant surgery in their own right. It is logical to remove an ICH simultaneously, as the abnormality is usually a single entity. Angiography may first be necessary to exclude vascular injuries after stab or shrapnel wounds.

When doubt exists about the indications for surgery, an ICP monitor can be valuable in deciding management. For example, Galbraith and Teasdale[9] found that all patients requiring surgical evacuation of an ICH had ICPs >30 mmHg within 6 h after monitoring was initiated. In contrast, only 10 percent of patients whose initial ICP <10 mmHg eventually needed surgery. A late rise in ICP, 5 to 7 days after injury, can occur in up to 20 percent of patients because of delayed swelling. Patients with ICH should therefore be monitored for a minimum of 5 days and evacuation considered if ICP progressively increases. Before making a final decision to operate under these circumstances, follow-up CT scan is indicated. Burr-hole exploration and drainage alone has not been found to be helpful.

At surgery it is best to perform a large frontal-temporal craniotomy as described in a preceding section. Almost all traumatic ICH are accessible through this approach, and with a few modifications, lesions situated more posteriorly can be removed. The principles of evacuation are similar for both contusions and hematomas; i.e., they should be gently irrigated and aspirated until a circumferential margin of normal tissue is encountered. A specimen should be sent for histologic analysis as occasionally an arteriovenous malformation (AVM) or tumor can bleed, precipitating an MVA or fall. Care must be taken not to damage or remove viable brain, particularly in eloquent regions. Thus, the surgical approach should be limited to the confines of the lesion itself. Absolute hemostasis is essential. Occasionally massive cerebral swelling can occur at the time of dural opening or after removal of the clot. Intraoperative ultrasound is useful to exclude the development of another mass lesion in this circumstance. (Management of this problem is discussed in more detail below.) Postoperatively, all patients should have an ICP monitor placed, especially those in coma, because many will develop intracranial hypertension. An immediate postoperative CT scan is useful as a baseline to exclude reaccumulation of the clot, the development of new lesions, and to determine the extent of cerebral swelling. Insertion of a ventriculostomy can be helpful when the ICH extends into the ventricles. In contrast, ventricular drainage does not appear to be of benefit in primary traumatic intraventricular hemorrhage. In part, this may be due to the association of traumatic intraventricular hemorrhage and diffuse axonal injury.[63]

Outcome is affected by both the severity of the primary injury and presence of the hematoma; between 25 to 50 percent of patients with traumatic ICH die. Outcome is also poor in cases of DTICH where mortality can approach 75 percent. The strongest prognostic indicator is the patient's initial neurologic condition. Comatose patients often do poorly whereas those who are conscious at admission can usually be expected to make a good recovery. Outcome is also adversely affected by the presence of large deep hematomas, particularly those associated with intracranial hypertension and other hemorrhagic or nonhemorrhagic lesions. Increased age, systemic disease, and the presence of extracranial injuries similarly impact recovery.

Despite the ease with which traumatic ICH can be identified, these hematomas continue to adversely impact the outcome after head injury. Prompt identification and evacuation may lessen this effect, but presently criteria identifying those patients who will benefit from surgery are unclear.

Posterior Fossa Hematoma

Traumatic posterior fossa hematomas are uncommon but important to recognize as sudden rapid deterioration from brain stem compression can occur. No specific clinical picture is associated with these lesions, therefore their identification and localization immediately after trauma can be difficult. The presence of occipital abrasions, nuchal rigidity, respiratory irregularity, hypertension, and an occipital fracture, particularly if it extends through the foramen magnum, should alert the clinician to the possible presence of a posterior fossa lesion. Very few patients have cerebellar findings in the acute phase.

Posterior fossa EDH account for <10 percent of EDH but are the commonest traumatic posterior fossa lesion. Arterial sources of bleeding are rare; the hematoma usually originates from venous bleeding from the diploic space, emissary veins, transverse or sigmoid sinus and is frequently associated with a fracture extending from the inion to the foramen magnum.[29,64] The same fracture may be seen with an SDH that results from torn bridging veins. Less than 3 percent of SDH are found in the posterior fossa.[41,49] Intracerebral hematomas are also rare but potentially dangerous because of their proximity to the brainstem.

CT scan with fine cuts of the posterior fossa is the diagnostic procedure of choice. EDH may cross the level of the tentorium; in contrast, SDH do not. The latter can be associated with cerebellar contusions. Obliteration and displacement of the fourth ventricle indicate severe compromise of intracranial compliance, and obliteration of the quadrigeminal cisterns signifies upward ventral herniation. Obstructive enlargement of the lateral and third ventricles can often be seen.

Hematomas in the posterior fossa are poorly tolerated because of the small size of the posterior compartment. Any lesion >30 ml in volume or 3 cm in diameter should be evacuated irrespective of the clinical condition as they invariably lead to significant brainstem compression. Smaller lesions in which the fourth ventricle or quadrigeminal cisterns or both are obliterated should be considered for surgery. Hematomas resulting in coma or the presence of clinical findings suggesting brainstem compression require urgent evacuation.

Surgery is best performed in the prone or modified park-bench position through a large suboccipital craniectomy. The posterior ring of the foramen magnum and arch of C1 should be removed to provide adequate decompression and to attenuate the effects of postoperative swelling. Dural augmentation can be useful also. Ventriculostomy is often required and, if inserted first, care should be taken not to overdrain CSF and precipitate upward herniation.

Mortality in patients with posterior fossa hematomas is usually high, even for EDH in which 30 to 40 percent of patients die. Coma and the presence of a supratentorial lesion are predictive of a poor prognosis. However, patients with posterior fossa lesions diagnosed and treated before the development of brainstem compression can be expected to make an excellent recovery.[64]

Cerebral Swelling

Cerebral swelling can occur at any time, but it is most often encountered while a traumatic mass lesion is being removed or shortly after evacuation. The exact mechanism is unclear; such intraoperative or postoperative edema may be secondary to impaired autoregulation and increased cerebral blood volume. Alternatively, experimental work by Kuroda and coworkers[52] suggests that ischemia could contribute to this problem. Cerebral swelling may also be secondary to the development of another lesion, such as a contralateral hematoma. This should be suspected after evacuating a large hematoma when there is a contralateral temporal fracture or a fracture that crosses a sinus. Both coagulopathy and hypoxia increase the risk of developing secondary ICH. Intraoperative ultrasound can be helpful in determining whether cerebral swelling is due to a surgical lesion. Irrespective of the cause, cerebral swelling must be dealt with expeditiously to prevent further brain injury. Large craniotomies are preferable as the risk of brain strangulation and infarction is less. The anesthesiologist should immediately check head position to ensure that venous return is not impeded. Excessive rotation or tight tapes about the neck may obstruct venous drainage, thereby increasing ICP. Similarly the endotracheal tube and ventilator should be immediately assessed for obstruction, disconnection, or malfunction. Risk factors, such as hypoxia, hypercarbia, hypotension, hypovolemia, hyponatremia, and coagulopathy must be excluded and preferably prevented from happening. Initial treatment of intraoperative swelling requires head elevation 15 to 20° and hyperventilation, preferably by increasing the tidal volume instead of rate to maximize venous return. The level of CO_2 can be optimized by calculating retrograde jugular venous oxygen saturation as an estimate of relative CBF. A 500 ml, 20 percent mannitol bolus is essential, followed by thiopental, if necessary. The thiopental should be given only in the case of normal BP and normovolemia. As AR is frequently impaired, induced hypotension has been suggested as a last resort to control swelling but is mentioned only to be condemned. In most instances, the treatment outlined here will be sufficient. Occasionally, lobectomy or a large decompressive craniotomy is necessary. The use of the latter is controversial in the acute phase, but it appears to be of some benefit in patients who develop delayed cerebral swelling in the postoperative period.[53] Mortality from established cerebral swelling is high.[51]

CRANIECTOMY FOR LESIONS OF THE SKULL AND MENINGES

Injuries of the skull and meninges may occur in isolation, concurrently with, or as contributions to injuries of the brain. This section will deal with depressed skull fractures, craniofacial injuries, and penetrating or missile wounds. Controversies exist as to the correct treatment, particularly as many of these problems are dealt with in conjunction with other specialties, such as plastic surgery or otolaryngology. The restoration of normal anatomy and prevention of infection are the primary goals of surgery. However, in many instances a mass lesion and neurologic compromise are present, and prevention of CNS deterioration must take precedent.

Depressed Skull Fracture

A skull fracture is depressed if the outer table of the fracture segment lies below the inner table of the surrounding intact skull. The position of the bone fragments identified radiologically obviously indicates only the final position of the fragments. During the moment of impact the bone fragments may have been driven into the brain and then subsequently repelled to a more benign-appearing position. As a result, the dura can be lacerated with even benign-appearing fractures.

Previously, it was thought that all fragments should be elevated to improve neurologic function and prevent posttraumatic epilepsy, but several large series have demonstrated that removal of the bone neither significantly alleviates neurologic compromise, nor minimizes the risk of epilepsy.[65,66] The bone fragment, instead of acting as a mass lesion, causes damage by lacerating and bruising the underlying brain during impact. The indications for surgery are, thus, the prevention of infection and restoration of normal anatomy. The latter, when there is significant cosmetic deformity, such as on the forehead, can sometimes be of primary importance.

As with fractures elsewhere, depressed skull fractures are classified primarily as open or closed. Open or compound fractures are more common. A scalp laceration may lie directly over the fracture or, because of the scalp's mobility, lie distant from it. Fractures involving an air sinus are also regarded as open. If dural integrity is breached, foreign bodies and contaminated material are introduced into the intracranial cavity. Bacterial infection leading to a brain abscess, and less commonly, meningitis, may then develop in the ensuing weeks. Bone fragments often lacerate the brain, and significant ICH can be found in 5 to 10 percent of depressed skull fractures. Closed depressed skull fractures result in noticeable cosmetic deformity when the fragment is depressed 3 to 4 mm below the inner table. Injuries to the forehead and orbital rim, where about half of depressed skull fractures are seen, are particularly disfiguring. Radiologic investigations, including skull x-rays and CT, are necessary to evaluate the extent of deformity because scalp swelling precludes accurate clinical evaluation.

The primary goal of surgery in open skull fractures is to remove all foreign and contaminated material, debride the wound, and repair dural integrity. Restoration of cosmetic appearance, although important, is a secondary goal. Until recently, surgeons debrided and removed the bone fragments and performed cranioplasty several months later. However, recent studies suggest that immediate replacement of the bone fragments does not carry an increased risk of infection and can produce an acceptable cosmetic result. For optimal success, the wound should be adequately debrided, dural integrity restored, and surgery performed within 24 h of injury.[66,67] The use of mini- and micro-internal fixation plates (Fig. 6-4 *A,B,C*), autologous bone grafts, and IV antibiotics may facilitate the operative technique and outcome.

Craniectomy Technique

The operative technique is depicted in Fig. 6-5. The scalp incision must be large enough to allow access to the periphery of the fracture, allow room to harvest pericranial graft as needed, or enlarge the craniectomy if an intracranial procedure is required. Head pin fixation should not be used because it limits scalp mobility and prevents the use of rotation flaps if a large skin defect is present. If an intracranial mass lesion complicates the depressed skull fracture, a trauma craniotomy is preferable, and the fracture should be dealt with secondarily.

A linear or curvilinear incision over the fracture or a scalp flap can be used for closed fractures. As the operative indication is cosmetic, the incision must be placed behind the hairline. Compound wounds are dirty, contaminated, and foreign material may often be driven into the brain. Therefore, simple debridement of the wound in the Emergency Dept is inadequate treatment. Intravenous antibiotics, to cover both gram-positive and -negative organisms are essential. Devitalized tissue requires debridement. All contaminated material must be removed, and intensive irrigation must be performed before attending to the fracture. Coverage of the fracture site with full thickness skin is desirable; extensive scalp mobilization, galea-splitting incisions, or even rotation flaps may, therefore, become necessary. Provision should be made to cover any exposed bone with pericranium to allow skin grafting, if required. It is beyond the scope of this chapter to discuss the plastic surgical techniques needed for such grafting.

Surgical exposure should reveal normal skull around the fracture and should attempt to preserve pericranium. The fracture is often comminuted and fragments are impacted, resulting in dural laceration. Instead of levering the fragments, which can lead to further damage, a burr hole should be placed at the fracture margin and normal dura identified. Each fragment should be carefully loosened and then extracted. Any fragment close to a major sinus should be assumed to have lacerated it. Before removing such fragments, adequate exposure must be obtained to control bleeding. In addition, a contingency for rapid and massive transfusion must be available. Although removal of all foreign or contaminated material and devitalized tissue is fundamental, bone removal must be continued until circumferential normal dura is identified. In-driven bone fragments often tear the dura and are associated with cortical lacerations and contusions. Even if the dura is intact, an underlying cortical contusion or laceration can be found nearly half the

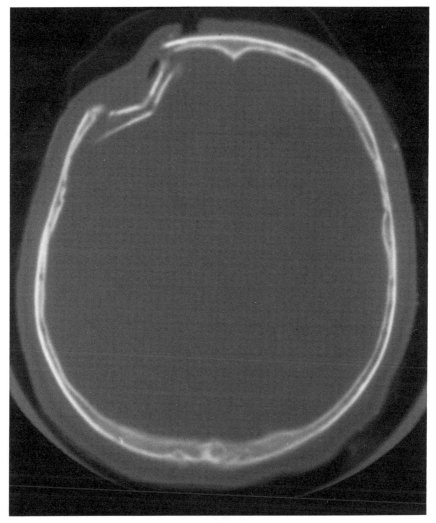

A

Figure 6-4 Head CT scan demonstrating a right frontal depressed skull fracture (*A*) and subsequent repair (*B*) using plate and screw fixation. Extensive craniofacial injuries can be repaired using this technique (*C*). Note the intracranial pressure monitor and reinforced endotracheal tube.

time. The decision to open intact dura should be based on the preoperative CT or the presence of inappropriate swelling. Careful cortical debridement and hemostasis is performed prior to dural closure, which is achieved either primarily, or with a pericranial or fascia lata patch. Dural closure decreases the incidence of CSF leak and is the single most important factor in preventing intracranial infection after compound injuries.

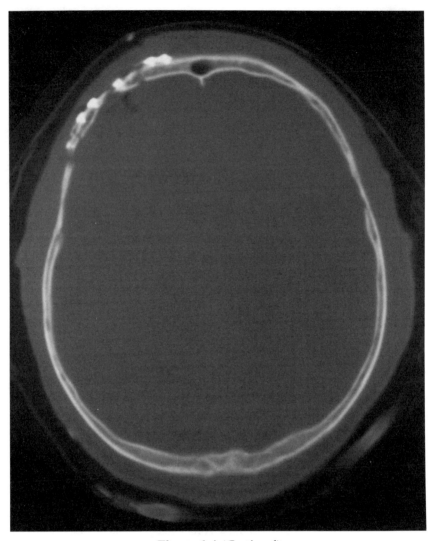

B

Figure 6-4 (*Continued*)

Bone fragments can be replaced if the wound is < 24 h old.[67] Although cosmetic repair is best achieved at the primary operation, there does not appear to be a role for early cranioplasty. An ICP monitor should be placed if intracranial debridement was performed or an intracranial lesion was identified on preoperative CT scan. Postoperative skull x-rays and CT are a useful baseline for further care.

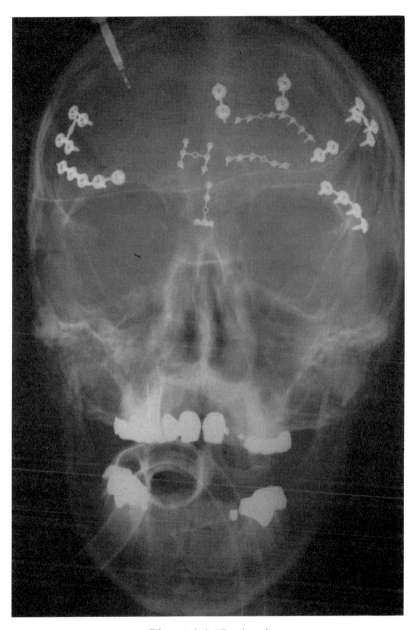

C

Figure 6-4 (*Continued*)

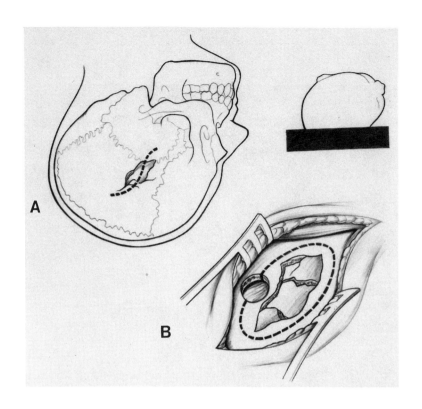

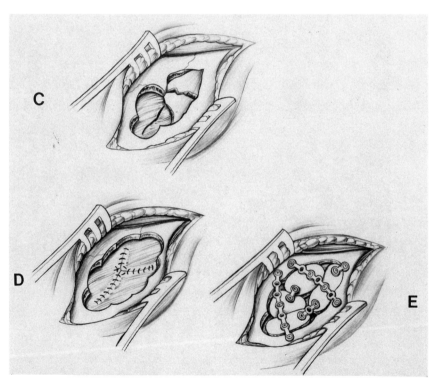

Stab Wounds

Stab wounds to the head are uncommon. Even with an innocuous scalp wound, all knife or penetrating injuries should be regarded as compound, and dural laceration should be assumed. Wounds are commonly found in the left frontal or temporal region because most assailants are right handed. Falls or accidental penetration may occur through cryptic entry sites, such as the orbit and nose, by breaking the thin floor of the anterior cranial fossa. Most injuries are localized in nature; therefore, disturbances in consciousness are uncommon unless a large ICH results. Usually patients exhibit no neurologic findings, or focal findings only.

Even if there is no neurologic compromise, a full radiologic investigation is required in all patients with a stab wound to the head (Fig. 6-6). CT scan is the investigation of choice because it can delineate the extent of intracranial injury and the tract of the penetrating object. Density settings may have to be altered to identify relatively radiolucent objects, such as wood. The presence of pneumocephalus indicates loss of dural integrity. In addition to CT, all patients should have skull x-rays, because a slot fracture (Fig. 6-6) may otherwise be missed with disastrous consequences. Angiography is indicated if a large ICH is found or the knife tract transgresses the region of major vessels.

The principles outlined in the previous section for depressed skull fractures apply to the management of stab wounds. However, no attempt should be made to remove any protruding object until radiologic investigation is complete and sufficient operative exposure has been performed. This may require innovative planning in the OR. Occasionally a traumatic aneurysm requires early operative repair.

Gunshot Wounds

In contrast to stab wounds, gunshot wounds (GSW) to the head are a major social problem and are among the 10 leading causes of death in the United States. Many victims do not reach neurosurgical care and of those who do, approximately half die.[68-70] Since World War II more people have been

---

Figure 6-5 Diagrams illustrating the surgical technique for a compound depressed skull fracture. (A) Devitalized scalp is removed as part of the skin incision, which should be designed to ensure full thickness scalp closure over the fracture. (B) A burrhole is created to identify normal dura, and the full extent of dural or parenchymal injury or both is exposed either through a craniotomy (dotted line) or (C) after careful removal of the bone fragments. (D) Following debridement of the injured brain, the dura is closed, if necessary, with a pericranial patch. Dural integrity is critical to the long-term success of this procedure. (E) Bone fragments are replaced using plate and screw fixation.

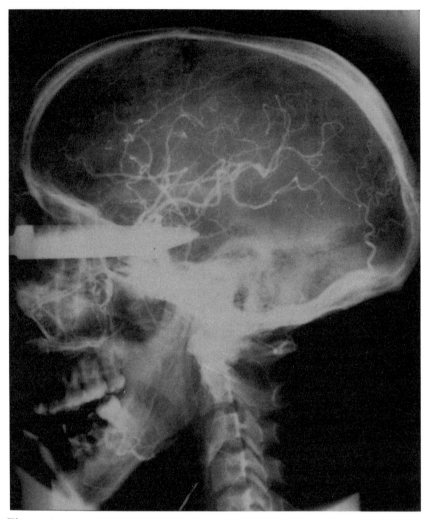

Figure 6-6 Penetrating trauma, such as a knife wound, requires full radiologic evaluation. If the knife blade is retained, angiography is necessary before surgical removal is attempted.

killed by missile injury in civilian life than in the Korean and Vietnam wars combined. Every year it is estimated that 0.2 percent of the Los Angeles population is shot, emphasizing the enormity of the social problem.[71] Furthermore, 50 percent of suicides and homicides are firearm related.[72]

Unlike other penetrating injuries, missile wounds involve injury to both the brain and skull/meninges. The severity of the resultant injury is determined principally by the velocity of the bullet. At 500 ft/s (low velocity) primary damage is limited to local injury along the tract. Once the velocity exceeds 1000 ft/s (high velocity) damage is caused by two further mechanisms: shock waves spreading in front of the bullet and cavitation. Both lead to compression and stretching of neural tissue remote from the missile tract and result in a secondary loss of autoregulation in addition to intracranial hypertension and hematoma formation. Neurologic damage can be compounded when multiple bone fragments are driven into the brain at the entry site. There is great variation in the characteristics of the entry and exit wounds because of (1) the type of weapon used; (2) the size, shape, and trajectory of the bullet; and (3) the way it makes contact with the skull. In tangential wounds, extensive bony comminution and underlying brain injury can result even though the bullet does not enter the skull, because significant energy is imparted by the impact. Of particular importance is the immense soft tissue injury that can occur from this type of wound. Although small entry wounds are found in high-velocity injuries, a tremendous force is delivered to the brain, and death is invariable. In contrast, low-velocity injuries, which are most commonly encountered in civilian practice, tend to cause a single tract and local injury.[73] However, extensive, severe injury can result if the bullet tumbles or ricochets within the skull.

Rapid, early resuscitation, and definitive treatment have been instrumental in improving outcome after GSW. The risk of edema, ICH formation, and the subsequent development of infection are all decreased by early surgery. Rapid treatment, however, may result in preservation of patients incapable of making a functional recovery. Therefore, triage is important prior to committing a patient to surgery. After full resuscitation, a neurologic evaluation and CT scan will provide the best means of assessment. GSW appear to be an all-or-none phenomena.[71] Mortality is inevitable in patients with a postresuscitation GCS score of 3 to 5. An exception to this is the individual with a discrete unilateral ICH. Therefore, no management decision should be made without a CT scan. Patients with less severe injuries (GCS score >5) can make striking recoveries and, therefore, should receive urgent operative attention.

The basic principles of emergency care apply to missile injuries. It is important to look elsewhere because GSW are often multiple. The wound should be inspected, bleeding should be controlled, and sterile dressings placed prior to obtaining a CT scan. CT defines the presence and extent of extraaxial or intracerebral hematoma, the missile tract, and the presence and depth of bony or metal fragments (Fig. 6-7). Angiography may be necessary to exclude the rare traumatic aneurysm that can develop within 2 h of injury and is most often seen following shrapnel or low-velocity injuries involving the middle cerebral artery (MCA) distribution.[74] High-velocity injuries tend to tear the entire vessel rather than injure the vessel wall.

Because of the great hazard of infection, intravenous antibiotics, to cover both gram-positive and -negative organisms should be administered as soon

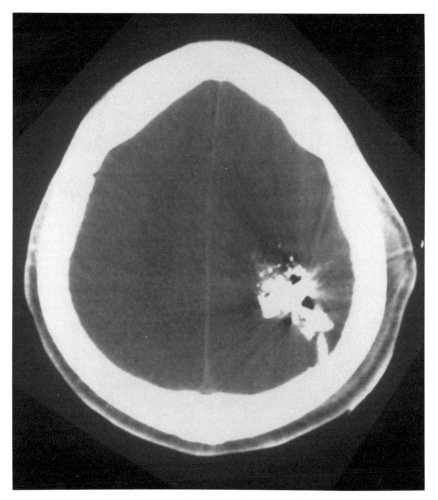

Figure 6-7 Head CT scan depicting intraparenchymal bone and metallic fragments following a gun shot wound to the head. Surgical debridement and restoration of the normal anatomy are required; however, removal of deep-seated fragments is not always indicated.

as possible and preferably before surgery. Although the use of antibiotics is generally accepted, it must be remembered that early and thorough debridement with complete dural closure are central to preventing infection. Consistent with this statement is the observation by Carey and coworkers[75] that 90 percent of bullet tracts and 75 percent of the bone fragments are sterile, when cultured within a few hours of injury. The missile tract is then sealed by brain swelling. Therefore, instead of being caused by primary contamination of the intracranial tract, subsequent infection results from secondary bacterial contamination from the scalp. Support for this belief is provided by Taha and coworkers[76] who observed that 75 percent of organisms causing intracranial infections after GSW were identical to organisms identified in the scalp wound. Seizures complicate 30 percent of GSW and, therefore, antiepileptic drugs should be started. In addition, mannitol should be given to all patients with significant cerebral swelling or a mass lesion.

Surgery of GSW to the head has several goals: (1) debridement and removal of necrotic tissue in addition to bone and metal fragments, (2) closure of the dura to prevent infection, and (3) evacuation of extraaxial or intracerebral hematomas. Hematomas can complicate about 50 percent of GSW; therefore, contingency planning is important when operating on missile wounds to the head. The principles described previously for craniotomy and craniectomy apply. Provision should be made for scalp mobilization, rotation flaps, and harvesting of pericranial grafts. Even the smallest-appearing scalp wound can have extensive necrosis beyond its edges from blast effect. Curvilinear incisions that incorporate an elliptical excision of the entry site are preferable because of the scalp's limited mobility. Alternatively, a flap can be used, particularly if there is a mass lesion.

As with depressed skull fractures, a burr hole should be placed in normal skull adjacent to the fracture, and comminuted fragments should be carefully removed to expose the dura. Alternatively, a craniotomy around the fracture can be made; this is particularly useful if a large hematoma requires evacuation. The dura is opened in a stellate fashion, starting from the entry site. A combination of pulped, tense, bulging brain, clot, bone fragments, and metallic fragments is usually encountered. After careful inspection and surface debridement, debris and clot can be removed from the depths of the tract with a small sucker and irrigation by staying within the damaged areas. Fragments of bone and metal should be saved, counted and sent for forensic analysis. The walls of an adequately debrided tract stay open and pulsate. If the tract closes, further pulped brain or an ICH distal to the tract require removal. Coagulopathy is common after missile injury to the brain and should be aggressively corrected to prevent the development of a delayed hemorrhage.

There is extensive debate on how much brain requires debridement and the amount of vigor with which bone and metal fragments need to be removed. Removal of all necrotic brain tissue can limit extensive edema formation. However, this may not be necessary in all low-velocity injuries and must be balanced against initiation of further bleeding. Simple irrigation may be sufficient to remove debris. The routine use of antibiotics has decreased the incidence of postoperative meningitis, but brain abscess still complicates about 5 to 10 percent of GSW and is clearly related to the presence of devitalized tissue, particularly bone. Military experience indicates that infection is tenfold more likely around a retained bone fragment. Thus for combat-related injuries, removal of all accessible bone at primary surgery and immediate reoperation if retained fragments are identified postoperatively, are advised; however, such an aggressive approach may not be required for civilian GSW. Certainly, all accessible fragments should be removed. Based on combat experience, Carey and coworkers[75] suggested that clusters of small fragments were more likely to lead to infection than were large fragments. By contrast, Taha and coworkers,[76] found that fragments <1 cm in size were unlikely to cause an infection. In their study 600 cases of missile wounds to the head were analyzed; only 30 of these developed intracranial infection. Dural integrity was the strongest predictor of delayed infection; the risk of infection was 1.8 percent in the absence of retained bone fragments, 20.6 percent if bone was present, and 84 percent if a CSF leak and wound dehiscence developed. Unlike bone, metallic fragments are not believed to contribute to infection and, therefore, do not need aggressive removal unless readily accessible.

Once debridement and hemostasis are complete, dural closure is necessary. This is a fundamental step in preventing CSF leak and decreasing the risk of infection.[76] Pericranial or fascia lata patch graft may be necessary, particularly for extensive wounds. We prefer to avoid dural substitutes. Cranioplasty, if needed, should only be considered in a delayed fashion at least 3 to 6 months after injury. The scalp is closed in two layers. An ICP monitor should be inserted in all patients and postoperative CT obtained.

Mortality after GSW remains high (50 to 60 percent), despite advances in medical care.[71,72] There are multiple variables which can be correlated with outcome. For example, mortality is higher in older individuals, after suicide attempts, and almost inevitable if GCS score is <5 after resuscitation. Multilobed, bihemispheric injuries that cross the midline (transventricular) are similarly fatal. Patients with anterior bifrontal injury, however, are likely to survive and should not be excluded from treatment. Intracranial infection develops in about 5 percent of survivors. Factors that predict infection include (1) extensive wounds, (2) involvement of the sinuses, (3) inadequate debridement, (4) dural closure, and (5) the development of a CSF leak.[76]

CRANIOFACIAL INJURIES

The management of craniofacial injuries has evolved substantially over the last decade, in part because of better diagnosis and improvement in surgical technique. Many of these injuries are best treated in a combined approach involving plastic surgeons, otolaryngologists, and neurosurgeons. There is a high frequency of injury to the frontal sinus and associated intracranial cerebral injury pathology.

Frontal Sinus Fracture

The anterior cranial vault is extremely strong and withstands forces 2 to 3 times greater than other facial bones without breaking. High-speed MVAs are the commonest cause of frontal sinus fractures, and when present, intracranial pathology is usually found.

Anterior wall fractures are the domain of the otolaryngologist, but once the integrity of the posterior wall is disturbed, the condition requires neurosurgical attention. Although the presence of intracranial pathology (hematoma or contusion) takes precedence, the goals of surgery are to prevent a CSF leak and infection, correct cosmetic deformity, and prevent longterm complications, such as mucocele formation or osteomyelitis.

Removal of sinus mucosa and closure of dural tears are central to the long-term success of the operation. Unlike mucosa elsewhere, mucosa in the frontal sinus does not regenerate after injury but tends to form cysts that later develop into mucoceles or mucopyoceles. There is relatively little information about long-term outcome with nonsurgical treatment. In contrast to displaced fractures, linear, nondisplaced fractures may be adequately treated with IV antibiotics and follow-up CT scans. Displacement of bone fragments, pneumocephalus, or parenchymal contusion indicates dural laceration and requires operative intervention (Fig. 6-8).

Surgical treatment of posterior wall fracture is usually performed by means of a bicoronal incision. Careful positioning and administration of mannitol are helpful to allow brain relaxation and thereby improve exposure. Brain retraction should be avoided as the traumatized brain is particularly susceptible to a second insult. The dura should be carefully inspected, initially extradurally; if damaged, intradural debridement of contused brain and removal of contaminated material are necessary. Primary dural closure should follow, if necessary, with a patch. Remaining bone fragments at the fracture site should be then removed. If the injury is extensive, the posterior wall should be cranialyzed; this also provides room for secondary cerebral swelling. To prevent regrowth, all mucosa should be removed, the inner aspect of the sinus burred with a high-speed drill and the frontal nasal duct plugged with muscle.

At closure, a vascularized pedicle of pericranium is placed subfrontally to provide an additional barrier between the sinus and dura. The orbital rim and anterior frontal bone are then restored using microplates and autologous bone graft if necessary. An ICP monitor should be inserted because cerebral swelling causing frontal dysfunction can be clinically silent.

Facial Injuries

Complex craniofacial injuries have traditionally been managed in three stages: (1) early craniotomy to treat intracranial pathology and repair the dura,

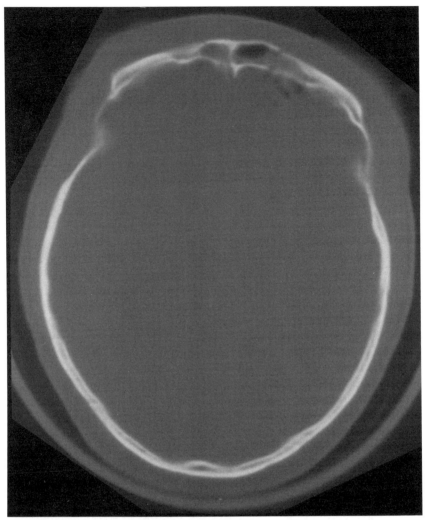

A

Figure 6-8 Head CT scan illustrating a nondisplaced fracture of both the anterior and posterior walls of the frontal sinus (*A*). The underlying pneumocephalus and parenchymal contusions (*B*) suggest a dural tear that requires surgical repair.

(2) orbitofacial repair 7 to 10 days later, and (3) delayed cranioplasty 6 months following injury. To improve long-term results, however, early single-stage repair within 24 h of injury is now often advocated. This increases demands on the anesthesiologist because approximately half the patients with facial fractures have associated intracranial pathology.[77] The combination of

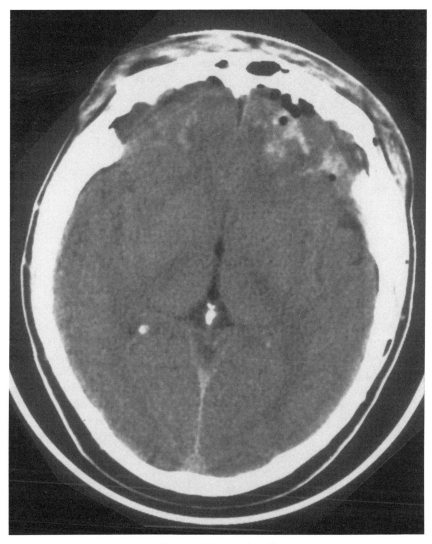

B

Figure 6-8 (*Continued*)

facial and intracranial pathology is most commonly seen following an MVA, particularly in patients with Le Fort type III, orbitoethmoid, or upper-face fractures.[78] Although distinct advantages may be offered by early surgery, namely, better bony alignment, lower incidence of CSF leak and infection, less scar tissue, and better long-term cosmesis, the prevention of neurologic compromise or brain injury takes precedence. Contraindications to an early, single-stage repair include GCS score <8, ICP >15, and a large ICH with shift.[78] When indicated, close cooperation among neurosurgeons, plastic surgeons, otolaryngologists, and ophthalmologists is needed. Intracranial pathology and dural repair should be dealt with first and an ICP monitor placed before attempting craniofacial repair, the details of which are beyond the scope of this chapter. If intracranial hypertension results, it is prudent to postpone surgery. However, in carefully selected patients, excellent results can be achieved.[77,79]

VASCULAR INJURIES

Traumatic Intracranial Aneurysms

Traumatic intracranial aneurysms are rare but can have devastating consequences. They are most commonly found after penetrating injuries, fractures involving the skull base, or injuries involving shrapnel or low velocity missiles, particularly if they cross the distribution of the middle cerebral artery.[74] When a traumatic intracranial aneurysm is suspected, angiography is necessary. To prevent disastrous enlargement or rupture, it is important to treat these lesions as soon as they are discovered; in some cases, this may be within 2 h of injuries. Unlike berry aneurysms, traumatic aneurysms are often found along the peripheral course of vessels rather than basal bifurcations. In addition, they are false aneurysms and have no neck, thereby making clip obliteration difficult. Trapping and excision is preferable if it can be safely performed.

Dural Sinus Injuries

Injury to the dural sinus poses a great technical challenge to surgeons and anesthesiologists alike. Prediction of sinus injury, control of hemorrhage, and reestablishment of venous drainage are critical to successful management. Sinus injury should be suspected when a depressed fracture lies over a major vascular sinus (Fig. 6-9). Bony elevation should not be attempted if mass effect is not seen on CT or only minimal cosmetic deformity is present. The presence of cerebral swelling on CT may indicate sinus occlusion/laceration and the need for surgical treatment. Although a "delta" sign on contrast-enhanced CT often predicts an occluded sinus, angiography is essential to fully delineate the pathology. When the transverse sinus is injured, sufficient views should be obtained to determine which transverse sinus is dominant. MR angiography (MRA) may have a role to play in the future in evaluating sinus injury.

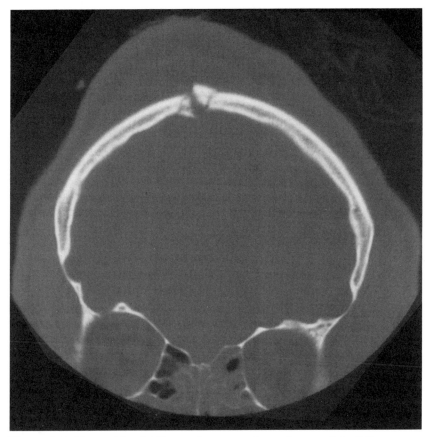

Figure 6-9 Coronal head CT scan demonstrating a depressed skull fracture adjacent to the superior sagittal sinus. Surgical treatment should only be undertaken when the entire operating team is able to deal with massive hemorrhage.

When sinus injury is suspected, surgical treatment should only be undertaken when the operative team is prepared to deal with massive hemorrhage. Careful positioning is needed so that head tilt can prevent or minimize hemorrhage. Taking precautions against venous air embolism and ensuring reliable venous access are essential. The neck should be inspected to prevent any obstruction to venous return. The fragment of bone that is thought to have injured the sinus should be removed after a suitable exposure to control hemorrhage has been created. Sinus repair can be achieved by simple ligation or reconstruction. In the anterior third of the superior sagittal sinus or the nondominant transverse sinus, ligation can be accomplished because adequate collaterals usually exist to provide venous drainage. Injury to other areas requires reconstruction. This can be achieved with direct suture, oversewing with muscle, patch graft, or interposed vein graft. The major complication of sinus injury is loss of venous drainage, which results in venous infarction and cerebral swelling. Consequently, postoperative ICP monitoring is strongly suggested.

OTHER OPERATIONS

During the acute phase after head injury, patients may require further cranial procedures, such as removal of DTICH or decompression for cerebral swelling. In addition, they frequently require surgery for other extracranial injuries. In these circumstances, neurologic function should take precedence, and clear communication should occur between anesthesiologists, neurosurgeons, and operating surgeons. A follow-up CT scan can help determine surgical risk, and the use of ICP monitoring may provide vital information to improve intraoperative care.

In the subacute or chronic phase, other operations such as tracheostomy, jejunostomy, ventriculoperitoneal (VP) shunt, cranioplasty, or burr holes for chronic SDH may be necessary. Although beyond the scope of this book, the same principles of care apply.

CONCLUSIONS

Head injury is a significant cause of death and disability; surgery plays a critical role in reversing this. It is incumbent upon both the neurosurgeon and anesthesiologist to fully evaluate the patient, prevent secondary complications, and treat the brain with care to achieve optimal results. A systematic approach with meticulous attention to detail is central to the successful treatment of patients with head injury.

REFERENCES

1. Jenkins LW, Moszynski K, Lewelt W, et al: Increased vulnerability of the mildly traumatized rat brain to cerebral ischemia: The use of controlled secondary ischemia as a research tool to identify common or different mechanisms contributing to mechanical and ischemic brain injury. *Brain Res* 477:211, 1988.

2. Miller JD, Murray LS, Teasdale GM: Development of a traumatic intracranial hematoma after a "minor" head injury. *Neurosurg* 27:669, 1990.

3. Gutman MB, Moulton RJ, Sullivan I, et al: Risk factors predicting operable intracranial hematomas in head injury. *J Neurosurg* 77:9, 1992.

4. Teasdale GM, Jennett B: Assessment of coma and impaired consciousness. A practical scale. *Lancet* 2:81, 1974.

5. Eisenberg HM, Gary Jr HE, Aldrich EF, et al: Initial CT scan findings in 753 patients with severe head injury: A report from the NIH Traumatic coma data bank. *J Neurosurg* 73:688, 1990.

6. Ropper AH: Lateral displacement of the brain and level of consciousness in patients with an acute hemispheral mass. *N Engl J Med* 314:953, 1986.

7. Miller JD, Becker DP, Ward JD, et al: Significance of intracranial hypertension in severe head injury. *J Neurosurg* 47:503, 1977.

8. Miller JD, Sullivan HG: Severe intracranial hypertension. In Trubuhovich RV (ed): *Management of Acute Intracranial Disasters (International Anesthesiology Clinics)*. Boston, Little, Brown 1979; 19–75.

9. Galbraith SL, Teasdale GM: Predicting the need for operation in a patient with an occult traumatic intracranial hematoma. *J Neurosurg* 55:75, 1981.

10. Poon WS, Rehman SU, Poon CYF, et al: Traumatic extradural hematoma of delayed onset is not a rarity. *Neurosurg* 30:681, 1992.

11. Soloniuk D, Pitts LH, Lovely M, et al: Traumatic intracerebral hematomas: Timing of appearance and indications for operative removal. *J Trauma* 26:787, 1986.

12. Miller JD, Sweet RC, Narayan R, et al: Early insults to the injured brain. *JAMA* 20:439, 1978.

13. Newfield P, Pitts LH, Kaktis J, et al: Influence of shock on survival after head injury. *Neurosurg* 6:596, 1980.

14. Froman C: Alteration of respiratory function in patients with severe head injuries. *Br J Anaesth* 40:354, 1968.

15. Williams G, Roberts PA, Smith S, et al: The effect of apnea on brain compliance and intracranial pressure. *Neurosurg* 29:242, 1991.

16. Bouma GJ, Muizelaar JP, Bandoh K, et al: Blood pressure and intracranial pressure-volume dynamics in severe head injury: Relationship with cerebral blood flow. *J Neurosurg* 77:15, 1992.

17. Busto R, Dietrich WD, Globus M-T: The importance of brain temperature in cerebral ischemic injury. *Stroke* 20:1113, 1989.

18. LeRoux P, Cooper J, Slee T, et al: The role of cerebral arteriovenous difference of oxygen in predicting ischemia and outcome after craniotomy for head injury. *Proceedings of the Congress of Neurological Surgeons*, 1991.

19. Kalsbeck WD, McLaurin RI, Harris BSH, et al: The national head and spinal cord injury survey: Major findings. *J Neurosurg* 53:S19, 1980.

20. Lam AM, Winn HR, Cullen BF, et al: Hyperglycemia and neurological outcome in patients with head injury. *J Neurosurg* 75:545, 1991.

21. Kaufman H, Hui K, Mattson J, et al: Clinical pathologic correlations of disseminated intravascular coagulation in patients with head injury. *Neurosurg* 15:34, 1984.

22. Stein SC, Young GS, Talucci RC, et al: Delayed brain injury after head trauma: Significance of coagulopathy. *Neurosurg* 30:160, 1992.

23. Holbourn AHS: Mechanisms of brain injuries. *Lancet* 2:438, 1943.

24. Andrews BT, Pitts LH, Lovely MP, et al: Is computed tomographic scanning necessary in patients with tentorial herniation? Results of immediate surgical exploration without computed tomography in 100 patients. *Neurosurg* 19:408, 1986.

25. Andrews BT, Bederson JB, Pitts LH: Use of intraoperative ultrasonography to improve the diagnostic accuracy of exploratory burr holes in patients with traumatic tentorial herniation. *Neurosurg* 24:345, 1989.

26. Johnson DL, Duma C, Sivit C: The role of immediate operative intervention in severely head-injured children with a Glasgow Coma Scale score of 3. *Neurosurg* 30:320, 1992.

27. Hoff JT, Spetzler R, Winestock D: Head injury and early signs of tentorial herniation—a management dilemma. *West J Med* 128:112, 1978.

27. Mendelow AD, Karmi MZ, Paul KS, et al: Extradural haematoma: Effect of delayed treatment. *Br Med J* 1:1240, 1979.

28. Bricolo AP, Pasut LM: Extradural hematoma: Toward zero mortality. A prospective study. *Neurosurg* 63:30, 1985.

29. Jamieson KG, Yelland JDN: Extradural hematoma. *J Neurosurg* 29:13, 1968.

30. Phonprasert C, Suwanwela C, Hongsaprabhas C, et al: Extradural hematoma: Analysis of 138 cases. *J Trauma* 20:679, 1980.

31. Rivas JJ, Lobato RD, Sarabia, et al: Extradural hematoma: Analysis of factors influencing the courses of 161 patients. *Neurosurg* 23:44, 1988.

32. Ford LE, McLaurin RL: Mechanism of extradural hematomas. *J Neurosurg* 20:760, 1963.

33. Dharker SR, Bhargava N: Bilateral epidural haematoma. *Acta Neurochir (Wien)* 110:29, 1991.

34. Jamjoom A: The influence of concomitant intradural pathology on the presentation and outcome of patients with acute traumatic extradural haematoma. *Acta Neurochir (Wien)* 115:86, 1992.

35. Ericson K, Kahansson S: Computed tomography of epidural hematomas. Association with intracranial lesions and clinical correlation. *Acta Radiol* 22:513, 1981.

36. Knuckey NW, Gelbard, Epstein MH: The management of "asymptomatic" epidural hematomas. *J Neurosurg* 70:392, 1989.

37. Hamilton M, Wallace C: Nonoperative management of acute epidural hematoma diagnosed by CT: The neuroradiologist's role. *Am J Neuroradiol* 13:853, 1992.

38. Cordobes F, Lobato RD, Rivas JJ, et al: Observations on 82 patients with extradural hematoma. *J Neurosurg* 54:179, 1981.

39. Gennarelli TA, Thibault LE: Biomechanics of acute subdural hematoma. *J Trauma* 22:680, 1982.

40. Seelig JM, Becker DP, Miller JD, et al: Traumatic acute subdural hematoma: Major mortality reduction in comatose patients treated within four hours. *N Engl J Med* 304:1511, 1981.

41. Stone JL, Rifai MHS, Sugar O, et al: Subdural hematomas. Acute subdural hematoma: Progress in definition, clinical pathology and therapy. *Surg Neurol* 19:216, 1983.

42. Adams JH, Graham DI, Gennarelli TA: Head injury in man and experimental animals: Neuropathology. *Acta Neurochir Suppl* 32:15, 1983.

43. Miller JD, Bullock R, Graham DI, et al: Ischemic brain damage in a model of acute subdural hematoma. *Neurosurg* 27:433, 1990.

44. Inglis FM, Bullock R, Chen MH, et al: Ischaemic brain damage associated with tissue hypermetabolism in acute haematoma: Reduction by a glutamate antagonist. In Reulen HJ, Baethmann A, Fenstermacher J, et al (eds): *Brain Oedema. Proceedings of the VIII Congress of Brain Oedema.* Wein: Springer-Verlag, p. 277, 1990.

45. Mendelow AD, Bullock R, Nath FP, et al: Experimental intracerebral haemorrhage: Intracranial pressure changes and cerebral blood flow. In Miller JD, Teasdale GM, Rowan JO, et al (eds): Intracranial Pressure. *Proceedings of the Sixth International Symposium on Intracranial Pressure.* Berlin, Springer-Verlag, p. 515, 1986.

46. Hovda DA, Becker DP, Katayama Y: Secondary injury and acidosis. *J Neurotrauma* 9:547, 1992.

47. Bullock R, Butcher SP, Chen MH, et al: Correlation of the extracellular glutamate concentration with extent of blood flow reduction after subdural hematoma in the rat. *J Neurosurg* 74:794, 1991.

48. Chen M, Bullock R, Graham D, et al: Ischemic neuronal damage after acute subdural hematoma in the rat: Effects of pretreatment with glutamate antagonist. *J Neurosurg* 74:944, 1991.

49. Jamieson KG, Yelland JDN: Surgically treated traumatic subdural hematomas. *J Neurosurg* 37:137. 1972.

50. Vaz R, Duarte F, Oliveira J, et al: Traumatic interhemispheric subdural haematomas. *Acta Neurochir (Wien)* 111:128, 1991.

51. Lobato RD, Sarabia R, Cordobes F, et al: Post traumatic cerebral hemispheric swelling: Analysis of 55 cases studied with computerized tomography. *J Neurosurg* 68:417, 1988.

52. Kuroda Y, Bullock R: Local cerebral blood flow mapping before and after removal of acute subdural hematoma in the rat. *Neurosurg* 30:687, 1992.

53. Elliott JP, LeRoux P, Howard M, et al: Outcome following decompressive craniectomy for acute intraoperative brain swelling associated with head trauma. *Surg Forum* 1992

54. LeRoux P, Haglund M, Hope A, et al: Delayed traumatic intracranial hemorrhage: An analysis of risk factors. *J Neurosurg* 74:348, 1991.

55. Wilberger JE, Harris M, Diamond DL: Acute subdural hematoma. *J Trauma* 30:733, 1990.

56. Howard MA, Gross AS, Dacey RG, et al: Acute subdural hematoma: An age dependent clinical entity. *J Neurosurg* 70:858, 1989.

57. Jamieson K, Yelland J: Traumatic intracerebral hematoma. Report of 63 surgically treated cases. *J Neurosurg* 37:528, 1972.

58. Papo I, Caruselli G, Luongo A, et al: Traumatic cerebral mass lesions: Correlation between clinical intracranial pressure and computed tomographic data. *Neurosurg* 7:337, 1980.

59. Bullock R, Hannemann C, Murray L, et al: Recurrent hematomas following craniotomy for traumatic intracranial mass. *J. Neurosurg.* 72:9, 1990.

60. Nehls DG, Mendelow AD, Graham DI, et al: Experimental intracerebral hemorrhage: Early removal of a spontaneous mass lesion improves late outcome. *Neurosurg* 27:674, 1990.

61. MacPherson P, Teasdale E, Khaker S, et al: The significance of traumatic hematoma in the region of the basal ganglia. *J Neurol Neurosurg Psychiatry* 49:29, 1986.

62. Kjellberg RN, Prieto A Jr: Bifrontal decompressive craniotomy for massive cerebral edema. *J Neurosurg* 34:488, 1971.

63. LeRoux P, Haglund M, Newell D, et al: Intraventricular hemorrhage in blunt head trauma: An analysis of 43 cases. *Neurosurg* 31:678, 1992.

64. Garza-Mercado R: Extradural hematoma of the posterior cranial fossa. Report of seven cases with survival. *J Neurosurg* 59:664, 1983.

65. Jennett B, Miller JD, Brackman R: Epilepsy after non-missile depressed skull fracture. *J Neurosurg* 41:208, 1974.

66. Van den Heever HG, Van der Merwe JJ: Management of depressed skull fractures: Selective conservative management of nonmissile injuries. *J Neurosurg* 71:186, 1989.

67. Jennett B, Miller JD: Infection after depressed fracture of the skull. Implications for management of non-missile injuries. *J Neurosurg* 36:333, 1972.

68. Kaufman HH, Makela ME, Lee KF, et al: Gunshot wounds to the head: A perspective. *Neurosurg* 18:689, 1986.

69. Benzel EC, Day WT, Kesterson L, et al: Civilian craniocerebral gunshot wounds. *Neurosurg* 29:67, 1991.

70. Grahm TW, Williams FC Jr, Harrington T, et al: Civilian gunshot wounds to the head: A prospective study. *Neurosurg* 27:696, 1990.

71. Ordog GJ (ed): *Management of Gunshot Wounds*. New York, Elsevier, 1988, p. 14.

72. Kellermann AL, Rivara FP, Somes G, et al: Suicide in the home in relation to gun ownership. *N Engl J Med* 327:467, 1992.

73. Raimondi AI, Samuelson GH: Craniocerebral gunshot wounds in civilian practice. *J Neurosurg* 17:483, 1970.

74. Haddad FS, Haddad GF, Taha J: Traumatic intracranial aneurysms caused by missiles: Their presentation and management. *Neurosurg* 28:1, 1991.

75. Carey M, Young H, Mathis J, et al: A bacteriological study of craniocerebral missile wounds from Vietnam. *J Neurosurg* 34:145, 1971.

76. Taha JM, Haddad FS, Brown JA: Intracranial infection after missile injuries to the brain: Report of 30 cases from the Lebanese conflict. *Neurosurg* 29:864, 1991.

77. Brandt KE, Burruss GL, Hickerson WL, et al: The management of mid-face fractures with intracranial injury. *J Trauma* 31:15, 1991.

78. Derdeyn C, Persing JA, Broaddus WK, et al: Craniofacial trauma: An assessment of risk related to the timing of surgery. *Plast Reconstr Surg* 86:238, 1990.

79. Benzil DL, Robotti E, Dagi TF, et al: Early single-stage repair of complex craniofacial trauma. *Neurosurg* 30:166, 1992.

CHAPTER 7

Influence of Anesthetic Agents and Techniques on Intracranial Hemodynamics and Cerebral Metabolism

Alan A. Artru

THE UNINJURED BRAIN: METABOLISM AND REGULATION OF THE CEREBRAL VASCULATURE AND RECOMMENDATIONS FOR PATIENT CARE

The Cerebral Vessels

The cerebral vascular and perivascular structures constitute a complex system that regulates the delivery of oxygen and substrate to the brain. This delivery is modulated by a constantly adjusting cerebral vascular resistance (CVR) that regulates both the cerebral blood flow (CBF) to the whole brain (global control) and the local distribution of CBF (regional control). The cerebral vascular and perivascular structures are composed of three distinct anatomic and functional "layers" (Fig. 7-1). The endothelial cells of the cerebral vessels and the underlying internal elastic membrane comprise the intima. The intima constitutes the innermost of the three layers of the cerebral vasculature. These endothelial cells are unlike those of the systemic circulation because they are connected by tight junctions. Tight junctions between the cells prevent large and/or polar molecules in blood from diffusing across the endothelial cells into the middle layer that contains the vascular smooth muscle. Diffusion of substances is further limited by desmosomes at the tight junctions, enzymes in the endothelial cells that degrade drugs and chemicals before they can diffuse across the cells, and by a paucity of pinocytotic vesicles.

The middle of the three layers of the cerebral vasculature is the media containing smooth muscle cells, fibroblasts, and elastic fibers. The term "basement membrane" has been used to refer to the internal elastic membrane, the media, and an external elastic membrane. In the large arteries the media contains substantial amounts of elastic fibers along with approximately six layers of smooth muscle cells. As the arteries branch and become smaller, the proportion of elastic fibers decreases so that the media is composed chiefly of smooth muscle cells. The number of layers of smooth muscle cells decreases to one or two in small arterioles. Receptors on these smooth muscle cells permit an influx of calcium through potential-operated channels when receptor activation leads to membrane depolarization. The classic effector acting on potential-operated channels is potassium. Membrane depolarization results in calcium influx, which in turn, releases some sequestered intracellular calcium. Calcium influx alone is insufficient for contraction of the actin-myosin complex within smooth muscle cells. Activation of receptor-operated channels permits an influx of calcium and other ions. Neurotransmitter interaction with receptors does not lead to membrane depolarization. The classic effector acting on receptor-operated channels is norepinephrine. The influx of calcium and other ions releases greater amounts of sequestered intracellular calcium. Whether caused by potential-operated or receptor-operated mechanisms, the result of calcium activation is development of muscle tension and increased CVR (Fig. 7-2).

In the extraparenchymal and large arteries, the adventitia, which contains

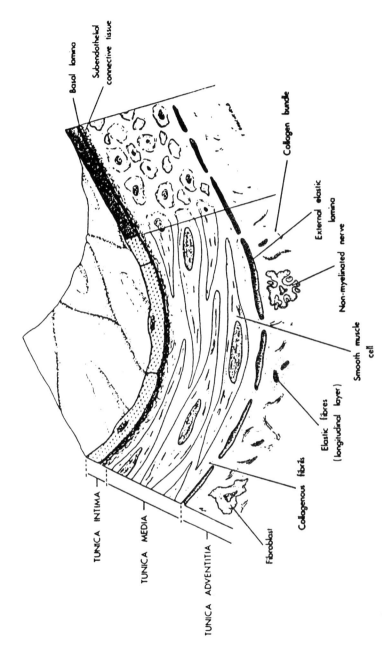

Figure 7-1 The three anatomical and functional "layers" of cerebral vessels: the intima, media, and adventitia. In small arterioles and capillaries, the adventitia is replaced by astrocyte foot processes. [*From Edvinson L, MacKenzie ET, McCulloch J: The Blood Vessel Wall. In Edvinson L, MacKenzie ET, McCulloch J (eds): Cerebral Blood Flow and Metabolism, New York, Raven Press, 1993, with permission.*]

Basal lamina

Subendothelial connective tissue

Collagen bundle

External elastic lamina

Non-myelinated nerve

Smooth muscle cell

Elastic fibres (longitudinal layer)

Collagenous fibris

Fibroblast

TUNICA INTIMA

TUNICA MEDIA

TUNICA ADVENTITIA

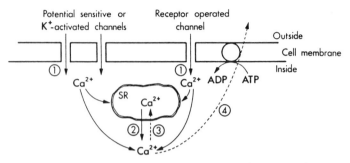

Figure 7-2 The two types of calcium channels on vascular smooth muscle cell membranes. Potential-operated channels permit influx of calcium in response to cell membrane depolarization. Receptor-operated channels permit influx of calcium and other ions without cell membrane depolarization. [*From Edvinson L, MacKenzie ET, McCulloch J: The Blood Vessel Wall. In Edvinson L, MacKenzie ET, McCulloch J, (eds): Cerebral Blood Flow and Metabolism, New York, Raven Press, 1993, with permission.*]

collagen and elastic fibers with an underlying external elastic membrane, comprises the outer layer of the cerebral vasculature. In the intraparenchymal small arteries and capillaries, there is no adventitia and the astrocyte foot processes comprise the outer layer. These form a "casing" around the basement membrane layer and minimize diffusion of large and/or polar molecules from the brain extracellular space into the middle layer that contains the vascular smooth muscle. Either gaps in this astrocyte casing or specialized sites on the astrocyte foot processes allow neurotransmitters and chemical/metabolic substances in the brain to reach receptor sites on the cerebral vascular smooth muscle.

Myogenic Influences

Cerebral vascular smooth muscle constricts in response to increase of transmural pressure, i.e., the difference between arterial blood pressure and intracranial pressure (ICP).[1-4] It is believed that increased transmural pressure causes vascular contraction because the stretch of the smooth muscle cell membrane increases the frequency of spontaneous membrane depolarizations and/or because the stretch of the actin-myosin complex increases its contractility. When transmural pressure is decreased, the stimulus for constriction weakens, and cerebral vascular smooth muscle relaxes. Rhythmic spontaneous activity of smooth muscle cells provides the basal tone of the cerebral vessels.[5-7] Rhythmic contraction increases when transmural pressure increases.

CBF is directly related to cerebral perfusion pressure (CPP) and inversely related to CVR. CPP is defined as the difference between mean arterial blood pressure and the pressure in the small cerebral veins just before they enter the dural sinuses. Cerebral venous pressure is about 2 to 5 mmHg more than ICP up to pressures of 100 mmHg.[8,9] Proximal dural sinus pressure is close to cerebral venous pressure, but dural sinus pressure decreases as the sinuses course toward the internal jugular vein. Simultaneous measurement of cerebral venous pressure and internal jugular vein pressure shows that jugular vein pressure remains a few mmHg greater than atmospheric pressure and much less than cerebral venous pressure when cerebral venous pressure increases in response to elevation of ICP.[10] Because CVR is high when intravascular pressure is high, and CVR is low when intravascular pressure is low, CBF remains constant over the wide range of blood pressures at which myogenic regulation operates. This constancy of CBF is termed autoregulation of CBF (Fig. 7-3).

The cerebral vascular responses to intravascular pressure change consist of two components. The first is a rate-dependent, rapid reaction that is sensitive to pressure pulsations. These rapid responses begin within 0.4 to 1.0 s after a sharp step increase in pressure. The second component is a rate-independent, slower reaction to change of mean pressure. It is generally believed that these slower responses begin within several seconds and are complete within 90 to 120 s.[11,12] However, recent studies of CBF velocity as measured by transcranial Doppler have reported restoration of CBF velocity and recovery from subsequent overshoot of flow velocity by 15 s following vascular compression or abrupt step decrease of arterial blood pressure.[13,14] Others believe the slower responses are the ones responsible for autoregulation of CBF.[15] The vessels

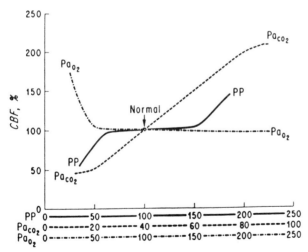

Figure 7-3 CBF as a function of cerebral perfusion pressure (CPP), Pa_{CO_2} and Pa_{O_2}. [*From Michenfelder JD: Cerebral Blood Flow and Metabolism. In Cucchiara RF, Michenfelder JD (eds): Clinical Neuroanesthesia, New York, Churchill Livingstone, 1990, with permission.*]

controlled primarily by myogenic regulation are believed to be located chiefly at the arteriolar level within the pia or just within the cortex.[16]

Recommendations for Patient Care

Autoregulation of CBF normally occurs over CPPs ranging from 50 to 70 mmHg to 130 to 150 mmHg.[17-20] When CPP exceeds 130 to 150 mmHg, the cerebral vascular smooth muscle constrictor responses fall. As a result, the cerebral vasculature is passively dilated by high intravascular pressure. At some critical level of dilation, cerebral vascular endothelial cells become so "stretched" that the tight junctions between cells are lost, and the endothelial cells separate, thereby increasing the risk for vasogenic cerebral edema and intracerebral hemorrhage.[21] Vasodilating influences, such as hypoxia and high levels of Pa_{CO_2} or inhalational anesthetics, impair autoregulation and increase the risk for edema and hemorrhage.[19,22-24] Hyperventilation and intravenous drugs of the sedative-hypnotic and benzodiazepines classes augment the autoregulatory vasoconstrictor response to high CPP and may decrease the risks of edema and hemorrhage.

As CPP decreases, cerebral vascular smooth muscle relaxes. The rate of dilation of cerebral arterioles of >200 μm increases at 80 to 90 mmHg, then increases logarithmically at pressures near 70 mmHg becoming 6 to 20 times more rapid than at 80 to 90 mmHg.[21] Cerebral arterioles of <70 μm dilate at <60 mmHg.[21] When CPP decreases to 50 to 70 mmHg, relaxation of cerebral vascular smooth muscle approaches but does not reach its maximum.[25] At lower CPPs the force "driving" blood through the vessels is not adequate to maintain normal CBF.[26-28] At some critical CPP value, the decreases in CBF cannot be compensated for by the increased cerebral extraction of oxygen and substrate, and cellular metabolism and function deteriorate (Table 7-1). A decrease of CPP to less than 50 to 70 mmHg with vasodilators is reported to cause less neurologic damage than when CPP is decreased to similar values with combination of vasodilators, hemorrhage, and head tilt.[29] A decrease of CPP to less than 50 to 70 mmHg with isoflurane or desflurane is reported to cause lsss disturbance of cerebral metabolites than when CPP is decreased with nonanesthetic vasodilator drugs, presumably because isoflurane and desflurane decrease cerebral metabolic needs.[30,31]

Rheologic Influences

While intravascular pressure provides the "driving force" for blood to flow through cerebral vessels, the amount of flow for any given CPP is a function of the ease of flow and deformation of blood as it passes through those vessels. CBF is inversely proportional to the viscosity of blood. Viscosity is a measure of friction and correlates shear stress to shear rate,[32] which, for practical purposes, is synonymous with velocity gradient.[33] When the velocity

Table 7-1 Cerebral blood flow thresholds for alteration of cerebral metabolism and function

Ischemic threshold for:	Cerebral blood flow ml/100 g per min	Effect
Brain tissue oxygen inadequacy	30	Reduced brain PCr and increased lactate
Onset of cortical failure	20	Decreased EEG, brain pH and evoked cortical response
Ischemic penumbra	15–20	No neuronal function but maintain cell integrity
Complete electrical silence	15	No EEG or evoked potential response; risk for permanent neurologic damage if long duration
Metabolic failure	10	Massive increase of brain K, decreased cellular ATP, irreversible damage even if short duration

gradient is high, axial flow (blood flow in the center of the vessel) is high relative to peripheral flow (blood flow at the edge of the vessel). Thus, the conditions favoring high CBF are low viscosity and high shear rate or velocity gradient.

The previous section considered the effects of CPP and cerebral vascular constriction or dilation on CBF. The change in vessel size determined CVR. The relationship between CBF, CPP, and CVR is expressed by the following: flow equals perfusion pressure divided by resistance (analogous to Ohm's law). As regards hemorheology, the equation relating to CBF is expressed by the following: flow is proportional to perfusion pressure divided by viscosity (a simplification of the Hagen-Poiseuille equation). Blood viscosity is determined by several factors including hematocrit, erythrocyte aggregation, erythrocyte flexibility, platelet aggregation, and plasma viscosity.[34,35] In addition, cerebral vessels dilate when viscosity increases and constrict when viscosity decreases.[10]

Recommendations for Patient Care

Hematocrit is the single most important factor influencing blood viscosity. The steepest portion of the blood viscosity-hematocrit curve occurs within the hematocrit range of 30 to 50 percent.[36] Reduction of hematocrit within this range by hemodilution with crystalloid, dextran, autologous plasma, etc.[37] significantly decreases viscosity and increases CBF. Whereas some authors report no associated improvement of oxygen transport or tissue oxygenation,[37] others report that hemodilution increased oxygen delivery and decreased the volume of poorly perfused (CBF <20 ml/100g per min) brain tissue during focal cerebral ischemia.[38,39] At a level of hematocrit of about 30 percent, reduction of hematocrit causes little decrease of viscosity or increase of CBF.

Aggregation of erythrocytes is a reversible process influenced by shear rate and erythrocyte surface characteristics. Disaggregation is promoted by normalization of blood osmolarity and pH.[36,40,41] In contrast to erythrocyte aggregation, platelet aggregation usually is irreversible. Platelet aggregation can be prevented by treatments that interfere with the ability to aggregate (dextran[42–44]) and by treatments that inhibit platelet-activating factor (BN50739, Apafant[45]). Erythrocyte flexibility decreases with hypoxia and acidosis, but is restored to normal with correction of Pa_{O_2} and pH.[10] The importance of manipulating plasma viscosity as a means of producing clinically important changes in blood viscosity remains theoretical at present.

Endothelial Influences

The tight junctions between cerebral vascular endothelial cells restrict large and/or polar molecules in blood from gaining access to receptor sites on cerebral vascular smooth muscle cells in the media. Thus, vasoactive substances with free access to systemic vascular smooth muscle by their passage across the fenestrated systemic endothelium might be expected to exert minimal vascular effects on the cerebral circulation. The observation that certain vasoactive substances with potent effects systemically exert potent effects also on the cerebral circulation suggests that in the brain they act by a route or routes other than by passage across the cerebral vascular endothelium.

One mechanism that may contribute to the cerebral vascular responses to substances in blood is the release of endothelium-derived factors in response to the action of vasoactive substances on the luminal border of the endothelial cells.[46] Cerebral endothelial cells release a variety of factors that produce relaxation of cerebral vascular smooth muscle. These factors include prostacyclin, a lipid-like relaxing factor, hydroxyl radicals, and nitric oxide.[47] Cerebral endothelial cells also release factors that produce constriction of cerebral vascular smooth muscle. These include endothelin and other, uncharacterized constricting factors.[48,49]

Endothelial-derived relaxing factors appear to relax cerebral vascular smooth muscle by stimulating guanyl cyclase to form cGMP. Endothelial-derived relaxing factors may reach smooth muscle cells by diffusion across the internal elastic lamina and media or via endothelial cell projections that extend to the smooth muscle cell membrane. Endothelial-derived factors cause dilation or contraction of the portion of the cerebral vessels where vasoactive substances in blood interact with the endothelium. In addition, the response to activation of one site on the luminal side of the endothelial cell is propagated longitudinally along the vessel so that dilation or contraction occurs over a greater length of the vessel than the site of initial interaction. Endothelial factors appear to mediate not only responses to substances in blood (such as so-called direct acting smooth muscle dilators, such as sodium nitroprusside), but also some (but not all) of the neurotransmitters and chemical-metabolic substances released on the "brain side" of the media. These latter substances presumably interact with receptors on the contraluminal side of the endothelial cells. The major endothelial-derived relaxing factor is now thought to be nitric oxide.

Recommendations for Patient Care

Endothelial-derived factors are reported to participate in the cerebral vascular responses to a number of familiar substances, including histamine, serotonin, acetylcholine (systemic or topically applied), adenosine, substance P, neurokinin A, vasopressin, and bradykinin.[46] In cerebral vessels with intact endothelium, histamine and serotonin cause vascular contraction. The endothelium-derived constricting factor(s) responsible for these responses is uncharacterized. When the endothelium is removed, histamine acts directly on receptor sites of cerebral vascular smooth muscle and causes vasodilation, similar to its action in the systemic circulation. Acetylcholine in blood or when applied topically to exposed cerebral arteries causes relaxation of cerebral vessels reportedly via endothelium-derived nitric oxide.[50,51] In contrast, the dilating action of acetylcholine released from parasympathetic nerve terminals at the media-adventitia border is endothelium independent. In cerebral vessels with intact endothelium, adenosine causes more vessel dilation than in cerebral vessels with the endothelium removed.[52,53] Prophylactic treatment with histamine receptor blockers in patients with a history consistent with histamine-mediated drug responses and avoidance of cholinomimetic drugs may be useful to prevent unwanted vascular effects from endothelial-derived factors.

Metabolic and Chemical Influences

In the brain tissue extracellular space are chemicals and metabolites derived from neurons (40 percent of brain mass) and glial cells.[10] Also in this space are small and/or polar molecules that are able to pass from the blood across the cerebral vascular endothelium. From this space also, chemicals and metabolites derived from neurons, glial cells, or blood cross the astrocyte foot process that separates brain tissue from the media of the cerebral vasculature in order to interact with receptor sites on cerebral vascular smooth muscle. These chemicals and metabolites play a principal role in maintaining the close relationship of regional CBF to brain metabolism (so-called flow-metabolism coupling) as well as maintaining the CBF response to Pa_{CO_2}, hypoxia and, presumably, anesthetics.

The brain normally extracts 33 to 50 percent of the available oxygen and 10 percent of the available glucose supplied by the cerebral circulation.[54] About 75 percent of the metabolic oxygen use occurs in neurons, and the remaining 25 percent occurs in glial cells. In normal resting brain, 5 to 10 percent of glucose use occurs anaerobically resulting in cerebral lactate formation.[55] Lactate is just one of a number of cerebral vasodilators and vasoconstrictors that are believed to participate in the chemical-metabolic regulation of the cerebral vasculature (Table 7-2).

Some act rapidly with transient effect whereas others produce prolonged effects. The effects of some chemical-metabolic regulators, such as potassium ion in brain extracellular fluid, cause dilation at certain concentrations and constriction at others.[56] The substances that link CBF with metabolism are believed to be adenosine, hydrogen ion and/or potassium ion. Histamine, dopamine, and GABA are released from nerve terminals located in brain tissue and not at the media-adventitia border of cerebral vessels. Thus, they are considered to be neuropharmacologic rather than vasoactive neurotransmitters. The concentration of histamine in brain is low relative to the neurotransmitters. While about 50 percent of histamine is in nerves and 50 percent of histamine is in mast cells, the latter is the major source of functionally

Table 7-2 Chemical-metabolic regulators*

Dilation	Contraction
H (acid CSF)	K (>10 mmol/liter)
Adenosine	PGE_2, $PGF_{2\alpha}$
K ($<$mol/liter 10 mm)[†]	TXA_2, TXB_2
Lactate	LKC_4, LKD_4
PGI_2 (prostacyclin)	Low osmolarity of ECF
Histamine H_1 (c), H_2 (d), H_3 (r)	Increase of Ca in ECF
Bradykinin B_1 (c), B_2 (d)	Alkaline CSF
High osmolarity of ECF	Dopamine (n), D_1, D_2 (m)
Decrease of Ca in ECF	

* Membrane depolarization allows calcium influx through potential-operated channels; blocked by calcium channel blockers (such as nimodipine, nifedipine, diltiazem, verapamil) and by NMDA receptor antagonists (such as dizocilpine maleate, formerly known as MK-801). Arachidonic acid is formed by action of phospholipase on membrane phospholipids. Leukotrienes (LK) are formed by action of lipoxygenase on arachidonic acid. Prostaglandins (PG) and thromboxanes (TX) are formed by action of cyclooxygenase on arachidonic acid. (c) = constriction, (d) = dilation, (r) = regulatory, (n) = neuropharmacologic, (m) = metabolic.

† Extracellular potassium concentrations approaching 0 mmol/liter cause contraction. Normal CSF potassium concentration is 3 mmol/liter.[179–181]

active histamine in the brain. High concentrations of histamine can constrict cerebral vessels by acting at H_1 receptors to inhibit formation of cAMP. Low concentrations of histamine can dilate cerebral vessels by acting at H_2-receptors to stimulate formation of cAMP. H_3-receptors regulate histamine synthesis. Dopamine affects CBF secondarily by altering the cerebral metabolic rate for glucose and oxygen via D_1- and D_2-receptors. GABA may act via postsynaptic $GABA_A$-receptors to cause vasodilation and via presynaptic $GABA_B$ receptors to inhibit sympathetic nerve activity. Bradykinin may act via B_1-receptors to cause vasoconstriction and via B_2-receptors to cause vasodilation.

Inhalational anesthetics increase CBF and decrease the cerebral metabolic rate for oxygen ($CMRO_2$). Among the inhalational anesthetics in clinical use for many years, isoflurane is a less potent cerebral vasodilator and more potent depressor of $CMRO_2$ than halothane or enflurane.[57] The cerebral metabolic and vascular effects of the newer inhalational anesthetics, desflurane and sevoflurane, appear to be similar to those of isoflurane. Nitrous oxide is most commonly reported to increase both CBF and $CMRO_2$.[57] Barbiturates, such as thiopental, decrease CBF and $CMRO_2$ by 50 to 60 percent.[58,59] Etomidate induces similar decreases in CBF and $CMRO_2$.[60] Propofol also decreases CBF and $CMRO_2$ although the magnitude of those changes (20 to 55 percent) is somewhat less than those reported with barbiturates and etomidate.[61] Hypothermia to 27°C causes a reduction of CBF and $CMRO_2$ that is similar to that reported with thiopental and etomidate.[57]

Recommendations for Patient Care

The cerebral vascular response to Pa_{CO_2} is mediated by chemical-metabolic regulation. CO_2 in blood rapidly equilibrates with CO_2 in brain tissue extracellular fluid where, in combination with water, it dissociates to hydrogen and bicarbonate ions. Increase of Pa_{CO_2} increases the hydrogen ion in brain tissue extracellular fluid, which acts on cerebral vascular smooth muscle sites to cause vasodilation. Conversely, when Pa_{CO_2} decreases, the reduction of hydrogen ion leaves unopposed the action of chemical-metabolic constrictors, and cerebral vascular smooth muscle contracts (Fig. 6-3). CBF is reported to change approximately 2 to 6 percent for each 1 mmHg alteration change of Pa_{CO_2} over the range of 20 to 60 mmHg.[10] Classic studies on pial vessels indicate that CBF begins to change within 20 to 120 s of altering Pa_{CO_2} and reaches a new steady level within 12 min.[62] More recent flow velocity studies suggest this process may be complete in the order of seconds. In contrast, brain extracellular fluid hydrogen ion concentration changes little with metabolic acidosis or alkalosis.[63] Regulation of Pa_{CO_2} can be employed to influence regional CBF (as during carotid endarterectomy) or cerebral blood volume (as in patients with increased ICP). An increase of Pa_{CO_2} in addition to intravenous administration of acetazolamide or papaverine can be used to determine underlying vascular insufficiency, revealed as subnormal augmentation of flow, in cases of suspected ischemic penumbra.[64] With prolonged change of Pa_{CO_2}, regulation of brain extracellular fluid ionic composition restores pH so that CBF normalizes within 24 to 36 h.[65] In patients with chronic bronchitis or emphysema, it is not recommended to abruptly reduce Pa_{CO_2} to normal because of the potential that CBF may fall to ischemic levels.[10]

The cerebral vascular response to hypoxia is also mediated by chemical metabolic regulation. A decrease of Pa_{O_2} to less than 50 to 60 mmHg causes an increase of brain tissue adenosine that acts on cerebral vascular smooth muscle to cause cerebral vasodilation.

Chemical-metabolic regulation couples CBF to cerebral metabolism. Increase of brain tissue cell activity results in increased output of vasodilating metabolites. Conversely, when brain tissue cell activity decreases, the reduced output of vasodilating metabolites leaves unopposed the action of chemical-metabolic constrictors, and cerebral vascular smooth muscle contracts. Usually, intravenous anesthetics preserve flow-metabolism coupling while inhalational anesthetics disturb it.

Hypothermia, isoflurane, and potent sedative/hypnotic drugs, such as thiopental, have all been reported to improve the brain's tolerance for conditions of reduced oxygen and substrate delivery.[66]

Neurogenic Influences

Axons that release neurotransmitters acting on the cerebral circulation are located in the adventitia or adventitia-media border.[67] These neurotransmitters are considered to be vasoactive although some serve a neuropharmacologic role as well. When the cell bodies of these axons are located systemically, these neurogenic influences are termed "extrinsic." When the cell bodies are located within the brain itself, these neurogenic influences are termed "intrinsic." The principal classes of vasoactive nerves are sympathetic, parasympathetic, and sensory (Table 7-3). Although sympathetic nerves generally cause cerebral vessels to constrict, their action may vary with vessel size, type, location, and the circumstances under which sympathetic stimulation occurs. In humans, receptors for norepinephrine have been characterized as being chiefly of the alpha 1-adrenoceptor type.[68] Cell bodies of intrinsic cholinergic vasodilator nerves are located in the fastigial nucleus, substantia inominata and/or sphenopalatine ganglia.[69] Sensory nerves are often also referred to as peptidergic nerves. Some extrinsic norepinephrine-releasing neurons may interact with beta 1-adrenoceptors to cause cerebral vasodilation.[70] Some classes of nerves innervate both arteries and veins, others innervate arteries and/or capillaries.[67] Some neurotransmitters are more effective when applied on the contraluminal side of the blood-brain barrier (such as vasoactive intestinal peptide,[71,72] and others lose effectiveness when the endothelium is stripped (such as substance P).[73,74]

Table 7-3 Neurogenic regulators*

Sympathetic	Parasympathetic	Sensory (Peptidergic)
NE (v) constrictor, $\alpha1,2,\beta1,2$ mainly extr. (sup. cer. g., some stellate g.) intr. from locus ceruleus	ACh (v,n) dilator extr. (sphenopalatine g., otic g.) intr. (fastigial n.)	Sub P/Neurokinin A (tachykinins) dilator, NK1,2,3, extr. (trigem. g.) CGRP dilator, CGRP1,2 extr. (trigem. g.)
Neuropep Y (v) constrictor, V1,2 50% extr. (sup. cer. g.) 50% intr. (fastigial n.)	VIP/PHI (v,n) dilator extr. (sphenopalatine g., otic g.) PACAP 27,38 dilator	
5HT (v,n) constrict or dilate, 5HT 1,2,3,β 50% extr. (sup. cer. g.) 50% intr. (raphae n.)	Prevent excessive constriction	
Prevent excessive dilation		

* Neurotransmitters, like norepinephrine, activate receptor-operated channels to release sequestered intracellular calcium; they may also cause a lesser influx of extracellular calcium via potential-operated channels. Gastrin-releasing peptide, somatostatin, neurotensin, dynorphin B, galanin, vasopressin, and cholecytokinin are neurotransmitters in cerebral blood vessels; however, their effects are incompletely understood. Gamma aminobutyric acid (GABA) and dopamine may also possess cerebral vasoactive properties. v = vasoactive, n = neuropharmacologic, extr. = extrinsic, intr. = intrinsic.[26,182–189]

Recommendations for Patient Care

Many investigators believe that neurogenic regulation plays an important role in most of the characteristic responses of the cerebral circulation. One example is the neurons originating from the trigeminal ganglia. These form the so-called trigemino-cerebrovascular system containing substance P, neurokinin A, and calcitonin gene-related peptide. These potent dilators are released to "protect" the brain from vasoconstriction following subarachnoid hemorrhage.[75,76] Cholinomimetics, unlike other neurotransmitters, are reported to produce an increase of CBF in a variety of species following parenteral administration that is blocked by intravenous atropine.[77-81] Possible explanations include failure of the blood-brain barrier to exclude cholinomimetrics, action via endothelial-derived factors, and stimulation of muscle spindle afferents.

One well-recognized function of neurogenic regulation of cerebral vessels is that it "protects" the cerebral circulation from abrupt increases in CPP. Sudden, large increases in arterial blood pressure result in increased activity of adrenergic nerves ascending through the superior cervical ganglia and along the internal carotid arteries. This extrinsic adrenergic activity contracts cerebral arterioles preventing excessive surges of blood through the cerebral microvasculature.[82,83] When such surges are not prevented, they dilate the cerebral vessels, increasing the risk for cerebral edema and hemorrhage. Infiltration of local anesthetic for cervical plexus or other nerve block, which may be used alone or in combination with general anesthesia during surgery on the carotid artery, cervical vertebral disc, etc. may block adrenergic nerve activity ascending through the superior cervical ganglia and impair its "protective" effect.

THE INJURED BRAIN: METABOLISM AND REGULATION OF THE VASCULATURE AND RECOMMENDATIONS FOR PATIENT CARE

Myogenic Influences

Head injury results in some or all of the following sequelae: cerebral ischemia, brain tissue edema, vascular occlusion, brain tissue contusion or infarction, subarachnoid hemorrhage, cerebral vasospasm, and brain tissue hypoxia. The magnitude of these sequelae generally is proportional to the severity of head trauma. These sequelae reduce oxygen and substrate delivery to the brain and disturb the ability of cerebral vascular smooth muscle to contract when intravascular pressure increases. As a result, autoregulation of CBF is impaired. The degree of impairment is a function of the magnitude of the reduction of oxygen and substrate delivery and the limit on CBF imposed by the insult.[10] In conditions that limit CBF, such as ischemia, vascular occlusion, and subarachnoid hemorrhage, autoregulation is partially preserved (though at lower CBFs) when the insult is mild (flow 20 to 40 percent of basal flow). The partial preservation of autoregulation occurs via intracortical collaterals.[16] Intravascular pressure in pial arterioles, normally about 80 percent of systemic pressure, decreases to 20 percent of systemic pressure with vascular occlusion.[84,85] The observation that vascular occlusion doesn't affect intravascular pressure in collaterals suggests that the decrease of pial arteriole pressure to 20 percent of systemic pressure is due to the pressure gradient between the arteriole and its collateral circulation. When flow-limiting conditions, such as ischemia, vascular occlusion, and subarachnoid hemorrhage are severe and reduce CBF to <20 percent of basal flow, autoregulation is completely lost.[86]

In conditions that do not reduce CBF to ischemic levels, such as mild to moderate head trauma, cerebral edema, affected regions peripheral to contusion or infarction, and diabetes (even when no other signs of autonomic neuropathy are present), autoregulation is partially preserved, and flows are low, normal, or elevated depending on the degree of insult.[87] In conditions that increase CBF, such as hypoxia, hypercapnia, and seizures, autoregulation is partially preserved and flows are increased.

Inhalational anesthetics, vasodilators, and opiate antagonists also may impair autoregulation of CBF.[88] CBF usually becomes more pressure dependent as the concentration of inhalational anesthetic increases (Fig. 7-4). In contrast,

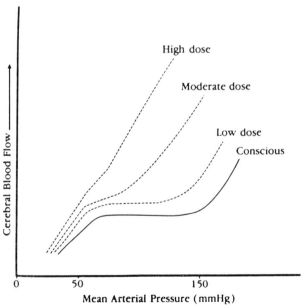

Figure 7-4 CBF as a function of cerebral perfusion pressure. Intravenous anesthetics depress the autoregulatory curve. Inhalational anesthetics cause a concentration-related straightening of the autoregulatory curve. [*From Donegan J: Effect of Anesthesia on Cerebral Physiology and Metabolism. In Newfield P, Cottrell JE (eds): Neuroanesthesia: Handbook of Clinical and Physiologic Essentials, Boston, Little, Brown, 1991, with permission.*]

intravenous anesthetics, except perhaps ketamine, usually don't impair autoregulation of CBF at clinically relevant doses.

With long-standing hypertension, a rightward shift of the autoregulatory curve occurs[89] (Fig. 7-5). With antihypertensive therapy, the autoregulatory curve may shift back to normal within several days.[90] However, the return to a normal autoregulatory curve is not observed in all patients, and in elderly hypertensive patients, particularly, reduction of CPP to less than 80 to 90 mmHg may decrease CBF. The excessive sympathetic nervous system activity that may result following head injury may also cause a rightward shift of the autoregulatory curve so that the threshold for brain tissue oxygen inadequacy occurs at a CPP of 60 mmHg rather than at 40 mmHg.[11,91,92] Conversely, bilateral sympathectomy may cause a leftward shift of the autoregulatory curve, decreasing both the lower and upper limits of autoregulation.[93] Hypotension may cause constriction of pial arterioles due to stimulation of extrinsic sympathetic innervation but dilation of intracortical vessels due to chemical-metabolic regulation.[94]

The term "false autoregulation" is applied to conditions of severe brain damage where there is no increase of CBF when CPP is increased, but instead, a decrease of CBF occurs when CPP is decreased.[95–100] Such conditions usually are characterized by a decreased or absent vasodilatory response to Pa_{CO_2}.[97–102] Suggested explanations for false autoregulation are that increase of mean arterial blood pressure is matched by equal increases of ICP or that endothelial damage and sludging of cellular elements prevent any increase of CBF.

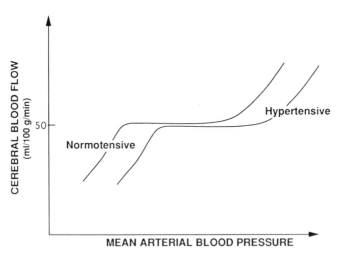

Figure 7-5 CBF as a function of cerebral perfusion pressure. In hypertensive patients the autoregulatory curve is shifted to the right of that in normotensive patients.

Recommendations for Patient Care

During conditions of reduced oxygen and substrate delivery that may occur following head injury, if CPP is maintained at a low value, the insult will be worsened because that low pressure provides inadequate CBF. On the other hand, if CPP is maintained at a value that would be at the high end of the autoregulatory range for normal vessels, there is an increased risk for vasogenic cerebral edema or intracerebral hemorrhage in vessels where autoregulation has been lost. Because of the low likelihood of salvaging brain tissue in the area of severe insult, it is often recommended that CPP be maintained at a value most likely to provide adequate CBF to the areas of mild and modest insult without overdistending the vasculature of the severely ischemic areas. This effect may be achieved by maintaining CPP at the breakpoint of the CBF/CPP slope for the area of modest insult, usually about 90 mmHg.[86] Noninvasive measures of CBF, such as Doppler, and electrical techniques, such as central conductance time, may be of assistance in guiding blood pressure management.[103]

When brain injury causes hypertension, computed tomography (CT) may aid blood pressure management. The finding of cerebral edema with normal blood pressure is a contraindication to intentional elevation of blood pressure.[86] The same finding with increased blood pressure suggests that blood pressure should be decreased to 150 to 180 mmHg systolic using treatments that do not dilate cerebral vessels. Computed tomography may also aid in the management of patients with neurologic deficits and normal blood pressure following subarachnoid hemorrhage with vasospasm. If CT scanning following blood pressure elevation with dopamine, or its equivalent, and volume expansion with low-molecular-weight dextran, or its equivalent, reveals no swelling or mild swelling without midline shift, therapy should be continued for 2 to 14 days with titration of blood pressure against the neurologic deficit.[86,104] If CT scanning reveals swelling and a midline shift, intentional elevation of blood pressure and volume expansion should be discontinued.

During conditions of reduced oxygen and substrate delivery that may occur following head injury, it is often recommended that concentrations of inhalational anesthetics be limited to those at which CBF is not significantly increased in order to prevent overdistention of cerebral vessels and also to prevent regional "steal" of CBF. Providing that patients are hyperventilated and intravenous anesthetics are used, a significant increase of CBF usually does not occur if the concentration of halothane and enflurane are limited to 0.5 minimum alveolar concentration (MAC) and the concentration of isoflurane is limited to 1.0 MAC. However, even with such precautions, inhalational anesthetics have been reported to increase ICP in conditions of brain injury or intracranial space-occupying lesion[105,106] although there have been no outcome studies on the influence of anesthetic agents on patients with head trauma.

Rheologic Influences

Under normal conditions in healthy brain, CPP and the radius of cerebral arteries, which determines cerebral vascular resistance, are the major factors that determine CBF. In areas of focal cerebral ischemia, cerebral vessels are near maximally dilated, autoregulation of CBF is impaired, and blood viscosity becomes an important determinant of CBF.[107-110]

The shear rate of cerebral blood decreases in areas of ischemia.[36,111] Low shear rate enhances erythrocyte aggregation, which in turn, increases the viscosity of blood causing regional CBF to decrease and ischemia to worsen. In patients with cerebral vascular disease, hematocrit correlates positively with blood viscosity,[112] and viscosity is significantly increased in those who develop neurological deficits secondary to ischemia.[34,113-116] Hematocrit or serum fibrinogen correlate negatively with CBF in stroke patients[113] and hematocrit greater than 50 percent correlates positively with infarct size in patients with occlusive cerebrovascular disease.[117] Aging decreases erythrocyte flexibility, which in turn, increases the viscosity of blood.[34] Platelet aggregation, another cause for increased blood viscosity, is greater in patients with stroke than in age-matched volunteers.[118] However, with chronic hyperviscosity states, such as in patients with chronic bronchitis or emphysema, CBF returns to normal.[119]

Recommendations for Patient Care

Administration of autologous plasma or low-molecular-weight dextran decreases viscosity and improves regional CBF in ischemia.[42-44,120] As a result, the mean power frequency increased and the slowing decreased as seen on the electroencephalogram, the neurological status improved, and the volume of hemispheric infarction decreased.[36,121-124] Reduction of hematocrit to 33 percent is considered to provide the optimum decrease of viscosity without reducing oxygen delivery.[125-127] Raising hematocrit more than 33 percent not only produces a modest increase of the oxygen-carrying capacity of blood (due to increased hemoglobin) but also produces an enormous increase of viscosity, which decreases CBF and, hence, net oxygen transport capacity. Decreasing hematocrit to less than 33 percent produces a negligible improvement of CBF but decreases oxygen-carrying capacity (due to decreased hemoglobin) and, therefore, decreases net oxygen transport capacity (Fig. 7-6). Infarct size increased and regional CBF decreased when packed erythrocyte transfusions were used to elevate hematocrit in ischemia.[128]

Hypervolemic hemodilution improves regional CBF and cortical oxygen transport in ischemic but not in nonischemic brain.[42,123,129] Hydroxyethyl starch decreases erythrocyte aggregation but only at a blood concentration of greater than 4 percent.[130] Pentoxifylline, an inhibitor of fibrinogen synthesis, decreases blood viscosity and promotes platelet disaggregation in patients with cerebral vascular disease.[131]

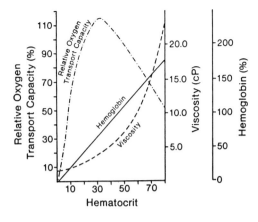

Figure 7-6 Relative oxygen transport capacity, viscosity and hemoglobin as a function of hematocrit. (*From Kee DB Jr, Wood JH: Influence of Blood Rheology on Cerebral Circulation. In Wood JH (ed): Cerebral Blood Flow, New York, McGraw-Hill, 1987, with permission.*)

Endothelial Influences

When head injury causes subarachnoid hemorrhage, the extravasated blood stimulates release of endothelin and other endothelium-derived constricting factors from cerebral endothelial cells. These endothelial-derived factors initiate constriction of cerebral vessels within a number of hours after subarachnoid hemorrhage.[55,132] This constrictor response is termed "cerebral vasospasm." Endothelin-induced constriction occurs chiefly in large cerebral arteries (conducting vessels). The smaller arteries (resistance vessels) dilate, presumably due to the local action of chemical-metabolic vasodilators. As a result, CBF decreases but cerebral blood volume increases (in one study by about 60 percent). Vasospasm may persist for up to several weeks.[133]

Endothelin and other endothelium-derived constricting factors also are released in response to other conditions of decreased cerebral oxygen and substrate delivery.[134] Constriction initiated by these factors may continue for hours or days after cerebral oxygen and substrate delivery is restored. This constrictor response may play a role in the failure of reflow through cerebral vessels after a period of reversible insult.

The so-called direct-acting smooth muscle dilators may be used to control systemic blood pressure or may be used in an attempt to improve regional CBF when either cerebral vasospasm is present or when it is believed there has been a failure of reflow after cerebral ischemia. The cerebral vascular dilating action of these drugs appears to be mediated, in part, by release of endothelium-derived relaxing factors. The vascular relaxation associated with these factors continues while the drug is administered. When administration of the drug is discontinued, cerebral vascular tone returns to normal as the drug effect dissipates.

Recommendations for Clinical Practice

When cerebral vasospasm is present, autoregulation of CBF is impaired and CBF is decreased. The slope of the relationship between CBF and CPP is flattened, and the threshold for cerebral ischemia occurs at a CPP that is greater than normal (Fig. 7-7). As long as CPP is maintained at normal or greater than normal values, CBF generally is adequate. Even small decreases of CPP may decrease CBF enough to disturb cerebral metabolism. Often, when CPP is permitted to decrease and CBF decreases proportionately, restoration of CPP is not accompanied by restoration of CBF.

Attempts have been made to increase CPP to supranormal values when it was suspected that there was a failure of reflow after reversible cerebral ischemia. Increased CPP may not restore CBF and increases the risk for vasogenic cerebral edema and intracerebral hemorrhage. Success has been reported at treating failure of reflow with drugs that antagonize endothelium-derived constricting factors.

One treatment that has repeatedly been shown to reverse endothelin-induced vasoconstriction is prostacyclin. Another treatment that has been used to treat vasospasm is calcium channel-blocking drugs. Nimodipine has been reported to improve neurological outcome from cerebral vasospasm without improving CBF. Presumably the beneficial effect of nimodipine is attributable to its interruption of the calcium-dependent cascade of neuronal damage and not to reversal of cerebral vasoconstriction. So-called direct-acting smooth muscle dilators such as sodium nitroprusside and hydralazine

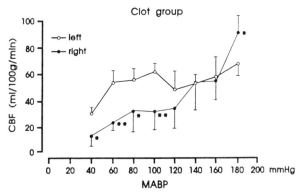

Figure 7-7 CBF as a function of mean arterial blood pressure after subarachnoid hemorrhage with unilateral clots. Open circles depict data from cerebral hemispheres where no blood clot was present after subarachnoid hemorrhage, and solid circles depict data from cerebral hemispheres where blood clot was present following subarachnoid hemorrhage. [*Reproduced from: Edvinson L, MacKenzie ET, McCulloch J: The Blood Vessel Wall. In Edvinson L, MacKenzie ET, McCulloch J (eds): Cerebral Blood Flow and Metabolism, New York, Raven Press, 1993, with permission.*]

have also been used in an attempt to treat vasospasm. With release of endothelium-derived relaxing factors by these smooth muscle dilators, CBF at CPPs less than the lower limit of autoregulation remains proportionate to CPP and, at any given perfusion pressure in that range, may be increased as compared with flows when no hypotensive drug is administered. CBF at CPPs more than the lower limit of autoregulation also become proportionate to CPP although the slope of the CBF/CPP relationship is less steep than at CPPs less than the lower limit of autoregulation. Inhalational anesthetics also cause relaxation of cerebrovascular smooth muscle. It is not certain whether the dilating effects of inhalational anesthetics are mediated by endothelium-derived factors, or are direct effects of the anesthetics on smooth muscle, or are mediated by other regulators of the cerebral vasculature. As a result of their dilating action, the inhalational anesthetics impair autoregulation of CBF much in the same way as do the smooth muscle dilator drugs. Use of smooth muscle dilators (such as sodium nitroprusside, nitroglycerin, etc.) or inhalational anesthetics to control blood pressure at CPPs greater than the lower limit of autoregulation increases the risk for cerebral steal, increased ICP, vasogenic edema, and hemorrhage. Better alternatives may be ganglionic blockers, such as trimethaphan or adrenergic blockers, such as labetalol. On the other hand, smooth muscle dilators and inhalational anesthetics may improve cerebral oxygen and substrate delivery at CPPs less than the lower limit of autoregulation.

Metabolic and Chemical Influences

Conditions that reduce oxygen and substrate delivery to brain tissue cause release of chemical-metabolic vasodilators. The resultant imbalance between dilating and constricting factors influences the cerebrovascular response to chemical-metabolic conditions. The degree of impairment is a function of the magnitude of oxygen impairment and glucose excess or inadequacy. Moderate oxygen and glucose insufficiency causes the hypoxic/ischemic release of dilators, such as adenosine and hydrogen ion. With moderate oxygen insufficiency and excess glucose, lactate formation may be so great as to reach neurotoxic levels. Increase of ischemic lactate formation is greater when glucose is given and ischemia is incomplete than when subjects are starved and ischemia is complete.[29]

In severe ischemia, dilation of cerebral vessels adjacent to the ischemic area causes a "bleed out" regionally, defined as "intracerebral steal."[109,135] After ischemia sufficient to cause neurological damage, the acute increase of CBF upon restoration of flow is termed "initial hyperemia." Subsequent decreased CBF lasting for several days after reversible cerebral ischemia is termed "post-ischemic hypoperfusion" and is characterized by a lesser depression of the cerebral metabolic rate for glucose than of the cerebral metabolic rate for oxygen or of regional CBF, thereby indicating anaerobic glycolysis. A following secondary increase of CBF is termed "delayed hyperemia.[136] Impairment of autoregulation of CBF may persist for as long as 3 years after brain injury.[137]

The cerebral vascular response to chemical-metabolic conditions is affected also by anesthetics and other vasoactive drugs that may exert their effects as a result of direct effects on the cerebral vasculature and as a result of regulatory responses to decreased arterial blood pressure. Chemical-metabolic responses may be altered by inhalational anesthetics secondary to anesthetic-induced impairment of flow-metabolism coupling, dose-dependent cerebral vasodilation, and reduction of arterial blood pressure. In global ischemia followed by recirculation, inhalational anesthetics cause heterogeneous CBF with regional areas of hypo- and hyperperfusion.[29] Chemical-metabolic responses may be altered by intravenous anesthetics secondary to cerebral vasoconstriction and hypotension. Responses may be altered by direct-acting hypotensive drugs secondary to cerebral vasodilation and hypotension and by adrenergic- and ganglionic-blocking hypotensive drugs secondary to hypotension.

Recommendations for Patient Care

The CBF response to Pa_{CO_2}, mediated by chemical-metabolic regulation, often is partially or wholly preserved when other cerebrovascular responses, mediated by other regulatory systems, such as autoregulation, are lost.[29,132–143] CBF responses to Pa_{CO_2} may be partially impaired by head trauma with or without vascular occlusion, hypotension, or subarachnoid hemorrhage, as well as by atherosclerosis and intracranial surgery with or without manipulation of cerebral vessels.[97,99,137,142,144–146] Preserved reactivity to Pa_{CO_2} with loss of autoregulation is termed "dissociated vasoparalysis."[132] Loss of both reactivity to Pa_{CO_2} and autoregulation is termed "total vasoparalysis."[132] Some CO_2 reactivity usually persists following head trauma. Hyperventilation usually remains an effective treatment to cause cerebral vasoconstriction and, hence, reduction of cerebral blood volume and ICP. Hypercapnia due to inadequate ventilation may produce the opposite effects. Hyperventilation also may restore autoregulation of CBF by correcting brain extracellular fluid acidosis.[147] When head trauma is complicated by subarachnoid hemorrhage, some CO_2 reactivity may persist even though CBF is decreased. Hyperventilation should be used with caution because hypocapnia-induced vasoconstriction superimposed on an already-decreased CBF may cause ischemia. Hypercapnia is reported to be minimally effective in increasing regional CBF in areas where cerebral vessels are constricted as a result of hemorrhage and may worsen ischemia by producing intracerebral steal.[148]

During ischemia, high blood glucose values, i.e., levels approaching 200 mEq/liter or greater, may result in formation of lactate in brain tissue that is neurotoxic (>15 to 20 mmol/liter). Blood glucose values in this range may occur when intravenous fluids contain dextrose or may occur in response to steroid administration in the absence of exogenous glucose. Insulin therapy and monitoring of blood glucose values may be helpful in such situations.

It should be remembered that, upon institution of insulin therapy, brain tissue glucose levels do not decrease as quickly as blood levels.

CBF increases when Pao_2 decreases to less than 50 mmHg, and CBF doubles at Pa_{O_2} of 30 mmHg. The CBF response to hypoxia is lost with severe hypoglycemia.[149] Reactivity to Pa_{O_2} also is impaired by the same insults that impair reactivity to Pa_{CO_2}.[144,150]

During inhalational anesthesia, hyperventilation usually remains an effective treatment to cause cerebral vasoconstriction and, hence, reduction of cerebral blood volume and ICP (Fig. 7-8). Whereas this fact appears true for all currently used inhalational anesthetics, differences may exist between anesthetics with regard to the magnitude of vasoconstriction caused by hypocapnia. With intravenous anesthetics, there is no conclusive evidence that hyperventilation combined with anesthetic-induced cerebral vasoconstriction causes a potentially hazardous decrease of CBF.

When mean arterial blood pressure is decreased to 50 mmHg using high concentrations of isoflurane, the cerebral metabolic rate for oxygen decreases significantly.[151] Hyperventilation to Pa_{CO_2} of 20 mmHg increases CVR and decreases CBF as compared with values at hypotension and normocapnia.[152] However, the magnitude of the constrictor response is not as great as during normotension and with lower concentrations of isoflurane. When mean arterial blood pressure is decreased to 50 mmHg using trimethaphan, sodium nitroprusside, or nitroglycerin, the cerebral metabolic rate for oxygen does not decrease significantly.[153,154] Hyperventilation to Pa_{CO_2} of 20 mmHg causes no significant change of cerebral vascular resistance or CBF.[155,156] These results suggest that, in these circumstances, chemical-metabolic regulation (which acts to preserve CBF adequate for metabolic needs) influences the cerebral vasculature more than direct drug effects (mediated here, in part, by endothelial-derived factors) or blood pressure effects (mediated here, in part, by myogenic regulation).

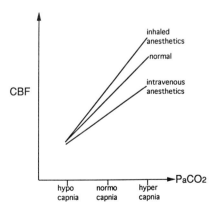

Figure 7-8 CBF as a function of Pa_{CO_2}. Inhalational anesthetics elevate the CO_2 response curve whereas intravenous anesthetics depress it.

Neurogenic Influences

Head injury frequently triggers an acute increase of systemic blood pressure. Extrinsic adrenergic innervation to the cerebral circulation is stimulated in response to acute systemic hypertension. Increased plasma neuropeptide Y and norepinephrine may be involved in increased systemic blood pressure.[157] Activation of extrinsic sympathetic nerves prevents excessive systemic blood pressure from being applied to the cerebral microvasculature and decreases blood brain barrier breakdown and local infarct volume.

Intrinsic adrenergic and dopaminergic innervation is stimulated also in response to ischemia. Activation of intrinsic vasoconstrictor nerves decreases regional flow in the ischemic area. Adrenergic nerves also take up serotonin after subarachnoid hemorrhage.[158] Stimulation of adrenergic nerves releases serotonin, worsening cerebral vasoconstriction. Intrinsic cholinergic innervation is also stimulated in response to ischemia. Activation of intrinsic vasodilator nerves improves regional flow in ischemic areas.

There are many more amino acid-releasing nerves with terminals in brain tissue and having neuropharmacologic action than there are sympathetic, parasympathetic, or sensory (peptidergic) nerves with nerve terminals on cerebral vessels and having vasoactive action. Amino acid neurotransmitters may be inhibitory or excitatory and play a critical role in cellular events leading to neuronal injury. Inhibitory amino acid neurotransmitters include gamma-aminobutyric acid (GABA), glycine, taurine, and beta alanine. Excitatory amino acid neurotransmitters include glutamic, aspartic, and homocysteic acid. Intrinsic GABA-ergic and taurinergic neurons (inhibitory neurotransmitter neurons) are stimulated by ischemia and reduce neuronal survival.[159,160] Intrinsic glutaminergic innervation is stimulated in response to hypoxia, hypoglycemia, and ischemia. The excitatory neurotransmitters act at three receptor subtypes: the N-methyl-D-aspartate (NMDA)-, kainate (KAIN)-, and quisqualate (QUIS)-preferring subtypes (Table 7-4). NMDA-receptor antagonists may be competitive such as CGP 39551, APV, APH, CGS 19755, and CPP (formerly known as SDZ EAA 494), or noncompetitive, such as dizocilpine (formerly MK-801), PCP, dextrorphan, dextromethorphan, ketamine (SKF 10,047), and MDL 27,266. QUIS subtypes may be of the α-amino-3-hydroxy-5-methyl-4-isoxasole proprionic acid (AMPA) and metabotropic types. Metabotropic receptors regulate phosphatidyl inositol turnover

Table 7-4 Excitatory amino acid receptors

NMDA (memb. chan.)
blockers-comp. or noncomp.
KAIN (memb. chan.)
QUIS
AMPA (memb. chan.)
metabotropic (phosphatidyl inositol turnover)

whereas NMDA, KAIN, and AMPA receptors regulate membrane channels. QUIS-AMPA competitive antagonists include GDEE and NBQX or DNQX (formerly FG 9202).[161]

Recommendations for Patient Care

Blockade of the superior cervical ganglia may occur during infiltration of local anesthetics to produce cervical plexus block. The resulting impairment of extrinsic adrenergic innervation may increase the risk for cerebral edema and hemorrhage on the ipsilateral cerebral hemisphere. Interruption of cholinergic innervation to the circle of Willis (as may occur with block of the sphenopalatine ganglia or when anticholinergic drugs reach the central nervous system) increases infarct size following carotid occlusion. Interruption of peptidergic nerves (as may occur with block of the trigeminal ganglia) abolishes reperfusion hyperemia postischemia.

Catecholamines in blood normally are prevented entry into brain tissue by the tight junctions and enzymes contained in the cerebral vessels. Increased permeability of the "blood-brain barrier" following head trauma may allow circulating epinephrine and norepinephrine passage into brain tissue, increasing CBF and cerebral metabolic rate for oxygen.[162] Monoamine oxidase inhibitors decrease dopamine metabolism and prevent ischemia-induced neuronal necrosis.[163] Idazoxan, an α-adrenergic receptor antagonist reduces the size of ischemic infarct after ligation of the middle cerebral artery.[164]

Blockers of the $GABA_A$ chloride channel and, also, non-GABA chloride channel blockers reduce neuronal death.[165,166] Dizocilpine decreases histopathologic damage and deterioration of evoked potentials in some but not all models of ischemia (though perhaps not when ischemia is severe), decreases spreading depression caused by cortical electrical stimulation, and increases regional CBF after ischemia.[167-170] Dextrorphan decreases neuronal damage after focal ischemia and also after hypoxia/hypoglycemia.[171] Dextromethorphan improves regional CBF after ischemia.[172] SKF 10,047 reduces hippocampal damage and improves motor function after ischemia.[173] MDL 27,266 reduces hippocampal damage after moderate ischemia. CGS-19755 improves regional CBF and decreases infarct volume after ischemia.[174,175] CPP decreases the volume of neuronal damage after ischemia and also after subarachnoid hemorrhage.[176,177] DNQX decreases neuronal damage after severe transient ischemia.[178] Clinical applications of these drugs, however, remain to be explored.

REFERENCES

1. Bayliss WM: On the local reactions of the arterial wall to changes of internal pressure. *J Physiol (Lond)* 28:220, 1902.

2. Ekstrom-Jodal B: On the relation between blood pressure and blood flow in

the canine brain with particular regard to the mechanism responsible to cerebral blood flow autoregulation. *Acta Physiol Scand Suppl* 350:1, 1970.

3. Farrar JK, Roach MR: The effects of increased intracranial pressure on flow through major cerebral arteries in vitro. *Stroke* 4:795, 1973.

4. Folkow B: Intravascular pressure as a factor regulating the tone of the small vessels. *Acta Physiol Scand* 17:289, 1949.

5. Nicoll PA, Webb RL: Vascular patterns and active vasomotion as determiners of flow through minute vessels. *Angiography* 6:291, 1955.

6. Wiedeman MP: Effect of venous flow on frequency of venous vasomotion in the bat wing. *Circ Res* 5:641, 1957.

7. Wiedeman MP: Contractile activity of arterioles in the bat wing during intraluminal pressure changes. *Circ Res* 19:559, 1966.

8. Johnston IH, Rowan JO: Raised intracranial pressure and cerebral blood flow: III. Venous outflow tract pressures and vascular resistances in experimental intracranial hypertension. *J Neurol Neurosurg Psychiatry* 37:392, 1974.

9. Yada K, Nakagawa Y, Tsuru M: Circulatory disturbance of the venous system during experimental intracranial hypertension. *J Neurosurg* 39:723, 1973.

10. Miller JD, Bell BA: Cerebral blood flow variations with perfusion pressure and metabolism. In Wood JH (ed): *Cerebral Blood Flow*. New York, McGraw-Hill, 1987: 119–130.

11. Miller JD, Stanek A, Langfitt TW: Concepts of cerebral perfusion pressure and vascular compression during intracranial hypertension. *Prog Brain Res* 35:411–432, 1972.

12. Symon L, Held K, Dorsch NWC: A study of regional autoregulation in the cerebral circulation to increased perfusion pressure in normocapnia and hypercapnia. *Stroke* 4:139, 1973.

13. Aaslid R, Lindegaard K-F, Sorteberg W, et al: Cerebral autoregulation dynamics in humans. *Stroke* 20:45, 1989.

14. Aaslid R, Newell DW, Stoos R, et al: Assessment of cerebral autoregulation dynamics from simultaneous arterial and venous transcranial Doppler recordings in humans. *Stroke* 22:1148, 1991.

15. Held K, Gottstein U, Niedermayer W: CBF in non-pulsatile perfusion. *Cerebral Blood Flow*. New York, Springer-Verlag, 1969.

16. Date H, Hossman K-A, Shima T: Effect of middle cerebral artery compression on pial artery pressure, blood flow, and electrophysiological function of cerebral cortex of cat. *J Cereb Blood Flow Metab* 4:593, 1984.

17. Harper AM: Autoregulation of cerebral blood flow: Influence of the arterial blood pressure on the blood flow through the cerebral cortex. *J Neurol Neurosurg Psychiatry* 29:398, 1966.

18. Lassen NA: Cerebral blood flow and oxygen consumption in man. *Physiol Rev* 39:183, 1959.

19. Rapela CE, Green HD: Autoregulation of canine cerebral blood flow. *Circ Res* 15(suppl. 1):205, 1964.

20. Schneider M: Critical blood pressure in the cerebral circulation. In Schade JP, McMenemy WH (eds): *Selective Vulnerability of the Brain in Hypoxaemia*. Oxford, Blackwell Scientific, 1963: 7–20.

21. Kontos HA, Wei EP, Navari RM, et al: Responses of cerebral arteries and arterioles to acute hypotension and hypertension. *Am J Physiol* 234:H371, 1978.

22. Harper AM: Physiology of cerebral blood flow. *Br J Anaesth* 37:225, 1965.

23. Hirsch H, Körner K: Über die Druck-Durchblutung—Relation der Gehirngefasse. *Pflugers Arch Ges Physiol* 280:316, 1964.

24. Lassen NA: Autoregulation of cerebral blood flow. *Circ Res* 15(suppl 1):201, 1964.

25. Mackenzie ET, Farrar JK, Fitch W, et al: Effects of hemorrhagic hypotension on the cerebral circulation. I. Cerebral blood flow and pial arteriolar caliber. *Stroke* 10:711, 1979.

26. Fog M: Cerebral circulation: The reaction of the pial arterial to a fall in blood pressure. *Arch Neurol Psychiatry* 37:351, 1937.

27. Fog M: Cerebral circulation. II. Reaction of pial arteries to increase in blood pressure. *Arch Neurol Psychiatry* 41:260, 1939.

28. Forbes HS, Cobb SS: Vasomotor control of cerebral vessels. *Brain* 61:221, 1938.

29. Gamache FW Jr: Comparison of global and focal cerebral ischemia. In Wood JH (ed): *Cerebral Blood Flow*. New York, McGraw-Hill, 1987: 518–530.

30. Newberg LA, Milde JH, Michenfelder JD: Systemic and cerebral effects of isoflurane-induced hypotension in dogs. *Anesthesiology* 60:541, 1984.

31. Milde LN, Milde JH: The cerebral and systemic hemodynamic and metabolic effects of desflurane-induced hypotension in dogs. *Anesthesiology* 74:513, 1991.

32. Dintenfass L: Inversion of the Fåhraeus-Lindqvist phenomenon in blood flow through capillaries of diminishing radius. *Nature* 215:1099, 1967.

33. Kee DB Jr, Wood JH: Influence of blood rheology on cerebral circulation. In Wood, JH (ed): *Cerebral Blood Flow*. New York, McGraw-Hill, 1987: 173–185.

34. Sakuta S: Blood filtrability in cerebrovascular disorders, with special reference to erythrocyte deformability and ATP content. *Stroke* 12:824, 1981.

35. Tohgi H, Uchiyama S, Ogawa M, et al: The role of blood constituents in the pathogenesis of cerebral infarction. *Acta Neurol Scand* 72 (Suppl):616, 1979.

36. Kee DB Jr, Wood JH: Rheology of the cerebral circulation. *Neurosurgery* 15:125, 1984.

37. Hino A, Ueda S, Mizukawa N, et al: Effect of hemodilution on cerebral hemodynamics and oxygen metabolism. *Stroke* 23:423, 1992.

38. Kee DB Jr, Wood JH: Experimental isovolemic haemodilution-induced augmentation of carotid body flow and oxygen transport through graded carotid stenoses. *Neurol Res* 13:205, 1991.

39. Cole DJ, Schell RM, Przybelski RJ, et al: Focal cerebral ischemia in rats: Effects of hemodilution with α-α cross-linked hemoglobin on CBF. *J Cereb Blood Flow Metab* 12:971, 1992.

40. Chien S, Vsami S, Taylor HM, et al: Effects of hematocrit and plasma proteins on human blood rheology at low shear rates. *J Appl Physiol* 21:81, 1966.

41. Schmid-Schonbein H: Factors promoting and preventing the fluidity of blood. In Effrons RM, Schmid-Schonbein H, Ditzel J (eds): *Microcirculation*. New York, Academic Press, 1981: 249–266.

42. Wood JH, Simeone FA, Fink EA, et al: Hypervolemic hemodilution in experimental focal cerebral ischemia: Elevations of cardic output, regional cortical blood flow, and ICP after intravascular volume expansion with low molecular weight dextran. *J Neurosurg* 59:500, 1983.

43. Wood JH, Simeone FA, Fink EA, et al: Correlative aspects of hypervolemic hemodilution with low-molecular-weight dextran after experimental cerebral arterial occlusion. *Neurology* 34:24, 1984.

44. Wood JH, Simeone FA, Snyder LL, et al: Hemodilutional and non-hemodilutional hypervolemia in treatment of focal cerebral ischemia. *J Cereb Blood Flow Metab* 1(suppl 1):S178, 1981.

45. Bielenberg GW, Wagener G, Beck T: Infarct reduction by the platelet activating factor antagonists Apafant in rats. *Stroke* 23:98, 1992.

46. Kanamaru K, Waga S, Fujimoto K, et al: Endothelium-dependent relaxation of human basilar arteries. *Stroke* 20:1208, 1989.

47. González C, Estrada C: Nitric oxide mediates the neurogenic vasodilation of bovine cerebral arteries. *J Cereb Blood Flow Metab* 11:366, 1991.

48. Kobayashi H, Hayashi M, Kobayashi S, et al: Effect of endothelin on the canine basilar artery. *Neurosurgery* 27:357, 1990.

49. Yoshimoto S, Ishizaki Y, Sasaki T, et al: Effect of carbon dioxide and oxygen on endothelin production by cultured porcine cerebral endothelial cells. *Stroke* 22:378, 1991.

50. Parsons AA, Schilling L, Wahl M: Analysis of acetylcholine-induced relaxation of rabbit isolated middle cerebral artery: effects of inhibitors of nitric oxide synthesis, Na, K-ATPase, and ATP-sensitive K channels. *J Cereb Blood Flow Metab* 11:700, 1991.

51. Koźniewska E, Oseka M, Styś T: Effects of endothelium-derived nitric oxide on cerebral circulation during normoxia and hypoxia in the rat. *J Cereb Blood Flow Metab* 12:311, 1992.

52. Faraci FM, Mayhan WG, Heistad DD: Responses of rat basilar artery to acetylcholine and platelet products in vivo. *Stroke* 22:56, 1991.

53. Kovách AGB, Szabó C, Faragó M, et al: Effect of hemorrhagic hypotension on cerebrovascular reactivity and ultrastructure in the cat. *Stroke* 22:1541, 1991.

54. Siesjö BK: *Brain Energy Metabolism.* New York, John Wiley, 1978.

55. Powers WJ, Grubb RL Jr: Hemodynamic and metabolic relationships in cerebral ischemia and subarachnoid hemorrhage. In Wood JH ed: *Cerebral Blood Flow.* New York, McGraw-Hill, 1987: 387–401.

56. Pickard JD, Simeone FA, Spurway NC, et al: Mechanism of the pH effect on tone of bovine middle cerebral arterial strips in vitro. In Harper AM, Jennett WB, Miller JD, et al (eds): *Blood Flow and Metabolism in the Brain.* Edinburgh, Churchill Livingstone, 1975: 9.17–9.18.

57. Michenfelder JD: Cerebral blood flow and metabolism. In Cucchiara RF, Michenfelder JD (eds): *Clinical Neuroanesthesia.* New York, Churchill Livingstone, 1990: 1–40.

58. Michenfelder JD: The in vivo effects of massive concentrations of anesthetics on canine cerebral metabolism. In Fink BR (ed): *Molecular Mechanisms of Anesthesia.* New York, Raven Press, 1975: 537–543.

59. Pierce EC Jr, Lambertsen CJ, Deutsch S, et al: Cerebral circulation and metabolism during thiopental anesthesia and hyperventilation in man. *J Clin Invest* 41:1664, 1962.

60. Milde LN, Milde JH, Michenfelder JD: Cerebral functional, metabolic, and hemodynamic effects of etomidate in dogs. *Anesthesiology* 63:371, 1985.

61. Artru AA, Shapira Y, Bowdle TA: Electroencephalogram, cerebral metabolic, and vascular responses to propofol anesthesia in dogs. *J Neurosurg Anesth* 4:99, 1992.

62. Raper AJ, Kontos HA, Patterson JL: Response of pial precapillary vessels to changes in arterial carbon dioxide tension. *Circ Res* 28:518, 1971.

63. Harper AM, Bell RA: The effect of metabolic acidosis and alkalosis on the blood flow through the cerebral cortex. *J Neurol Neurosurg Psychiatry* 26:341, 1963.

64. Lassen NA, Astrup J: Ischemic penumbra. In Wood JH (ed): *Cerebral Blood Flow.* New York, McGraw-Hill, 1987: 458–466.

65. Bode ET: Neurointensive care. In Cucchiara RF, Michenfelder JD (eds): *Clinical Neuroanesthesia.* New York, Churchill Livingstone, 1990: 437–472.

66. Milde LN: Cerebral protection, In Cucchiara RF, Michenfelder JD (eds): *Clinical Neuroanesthesia.* New York, Churchill Livingstone, 1990: 171–222.

67. Edvinsson L, Mackenzie ET, McCulloch J, et al: Perivascular innervation and receptor mechanisms in cerebrovascular bed, In Wood JH (ed): *Cerebral Blood Flow.* New York, McGraw-Hill, 1987: 145–172.

68. Edvinsson L: Sympathetic control of cerebral circulation. *Trends Neurosci* 5:425, 1982.

69. Hardebo JE, Arbab M, Suzuki N, et al: Pathways of parasympathetic and sensory cerebrovascular nerves in monkeys. *Stroke* 22:331, 1991.

70. Edvinsson L, Owman C: Pharmacological characterization of adrenergic a- and b-receptors mediating the vasomotor responses of cerebral arteries in vitro. *Circ Res* 35:835, 1974.

71. McCulloch J, Edvinsson L: Cerebral circulatory and metabolic effects of vasoactive intestinal polypeptide. *Am J Physiol* 238:H449, 1980.

72. Wilson DA, O'Neill JT, Said SI, et al: Vasoactive intestinal polypeptide and the canine cerebral circulation. *Circ Res* 48:138, 1981.

73. Dahlöf C, Dahlöf P, Tatemoto K, et al: Neuropeptide Y (NPY) reduces field stimulation evoked release of noradrenaline and enhances force of contraction in the rat portal vein. *Naunyn Schmiedebergs Arch Pharmacol* 328:327, 1985.

74. Edvinsson L, Fredholm BB, Hamel E, et al: Perivascular peptides relax cerebral arteries concomitant with stimulation of cyclic adenosine monophosphate accumulation or release of an endothelium-derived relaxing factor in the cat. *Neurosci Lett* 58:213, 1985.

75. McCulloch J, Uddman R, Kingman TA: Calcitonin gene-related peptide: Functional role in cerebrovascular regulation. *Proc Natl Acad Sci U S A* 83:5731, 1986.

76. Moskowitz MA: The neurobiology of vascular head pain. *Ann Neurol* 16:157, 1984.

77. Heistad DD, Marcus ML, Said SL, et al: Effects of acetylcholine and vasoactive intestinal peptide on cerebral blood flow. *Am J Physiol* 239:H73, 1980.

78. Lowe RF, Gilboe DD: Canine cerebrovascular response to nitroglycerin, acetylcholine, 5-hydroxytryptamine and angiotensin. *Am J Physiol* 225:1333, 1973.

79. Matsuda M, Stirling MJ, Deshmukh VD, et al: Effect of acetylcholine on cerebral circulation. *J Neurosurg* 45:423, 1976.

80. Reynier-Rebuffel AM, Lacombe P, Aubineau P, et al: Multiregional cerebral blood flow changes induced by a cholinomimetic drug. *Eur J Pharmacol* 60:237, 1979.

81. Scremin OU, Rovere AA, Raynald AC, et al: Cholinergic control of blood flow in the cerebral cortex of the rat. *Stroke* 4:232, 1973.

82. Bill A, Lunder J: Sympathetic control of cerebral blood flow in acute arterial hypertension. *Acta Physiol Scand* 96:114, 1976.

83. Edvinsson L, Owman C, Siesjö BK: Physiological role of cerebrovascular sympathetic nerves in the autoregulation of cerebral blood flow. *Brain Res* 117:519, 1976.

84. Jansen J, Kanzow E: Pressure drop and vascular resistance in cerebral circulation. In Klug W, Brock M, Klinger M, et al (eds): *Advances in Neurosurgery, Vol. II.* New York, Springer-Verlag, 1975: pp. 314–315.

85. Symon L: A comparative study of middle cerebral pressure in dogs and macaques. *J Physiol* 191:449, 1967.

86. Symon L: Pathologic regulation in cerebral ischemia. In Wood JH (ed): *Cerebral Blood Flow*. New York, McGraw-Hill, 1987: 413–424.

87. Dandona P, James IM, Newbury PA, et al: Cerebral blood flow in diabetes mellitus: Evidence of abnormal cerebrovascular reactivity. *Br Med J* 2:325, 1978.

88. Turner DM, Kassell NF, Sasaki T, et al: High dose naloxone produces cerebral vasodilation. *Neurosurgery* 15:192, 1984.

89. Strandgaard S, Jones JV, MacKenzie ET, et al: Upper limit of cerebral blood flow autoregulation in experimental renovascular hypertension in the baboon. *Circ Res* 37:164, 1975.

90. Strandgaard S: Autoregulation of cerebral blood flow in hypertensive patients: The modifying influence of prolonged antihypertensive treatment on the tolerance to acute, drug-induced hypotension. *Circulation* 53:720, 1976.

91. Heistad DD, Marcus ML, Sandberg S, et al: Effect of sympathetic nerve stimulation on cerebral blood flow and on large cerebral arteries of dogs. *Circ Res* 41:342, 1977.

92. Miller JD, Stanek AE, Langfitt TW: Cerebral blood flow regulation during experimental brain compression. *J Neurosurg* 39:186, 1973.

93. Thomas D, Bannister RG: Preservation of autoregulation of cerebral blood flow in autonomic failure. *J Neurol Sci* 44:205, 1980.

94. Symon L: Regional vascular reactivity in the middle cerebral arterial distribution: An experimental study in baboons. *J Neurosurg* 33:532, 1970.

95. Enevoldsen EM, Jensen FT: Autoregulation and CO_2 responses of cerebral blood flow in patients with acute severe head injury. *J Neurosurg* 48:689, 1978.

96. Enevoldsen EM, Cold G, Jensen FT, et al: Dynamic changes in regional CBF, intraventricular pressure, CSF pH and lactate levels during the acute phase of head injury. *J Neurosurg* 44:191, 1976.

97. Miller JD, Garibi J, North JB, et al: Effects of increased arterial pressure on blood flow in the damaged brain. *J Neurol Neurosurg Psychiatry* 38:657, 1975.

98. Miller JD, Reilly PL, Farrar JK, et al: Cerebrovascular reactivity related to focal brain edema in the primate. In Pappius HM, Feindel W (eds): *Dynamics of Brain Edema*. Berlin, Springer-Verlag, 1976: 68–76.

99. Overgaard J, Tweed WA: Cerebral circulation after head injury. I. Cerebral blood flow and its regulation after closed head injury with emphasis on clinical correlations. *J Neurosurg* 41:531, 1974.

100. Reilly PL, Farrar JK, Miller JD: Vascular reactivity in the primate brain after acute cryogenic injury. *J Neurol Neurosurg Psychiatry* 40:1092, 1977.

101. Frei HJ, Wallenfang T, Poll W, et al: Regional cerebral blood flow and regional metabolism in cold induced edema. *Acta Neurochir (Wien)* 29:15, 1973.

102. Marmarou A, Poll W, Shapiro K, et al: The influence of brain tissue pressure upon local cerebral blood flow in vasogenic edema. In Beks JWF, Bosch DA (eds): *Intracranial Pressure, Vol. III*. Berlin, Springer-Verlag, 1976: 10–13.

103. Symon L, Hargadine J, Zawirski M, et al: Central conduction time as an index of ischaemia in subarachnoid haemorrhage. *J Neurol Sci* 44:95, 1979.

104. Kassell NF, Peerless SJ, Durward QJ, et al: Treatment of ischemic deficits from vasospasm with intravascular volume expansion and induced arterial hypertension. *Neurosurgery* 11:337, 1982.

105. Newfield P, McKay RD: Head trauma; anesthesia. In Newfield P, Cottrell JE (eds): *Neuroanesthesia: Handbook of Clinical and Physiologic Essentials*. Boston, Little, Brown, 1991: 311–337.

106. Lanier WL, Weglinski MR: Intracranial pressure. In Cucchiara RF, Michenfelder JD (eds): *Clinical Neuroanesthesia*. New York, Churchill Livingstone, 1990: 77–115.

107. McHenry LD, West JW, Cooper ES, et al: Cerebral autoregulation in man. *Stroke* 5:695, 1974.

108. Meyer JS, Shimazu K, Fukuuchi Y, et al: Impaired neurogenic cerebrovascular control and dysautoregulation after stroke. *Stroke* 4:169, 1973.

109. Symon L, Branston NM, Strong AJ: Autoregulation in acute focal ischemia. An experimental study. *Stroke* 7:547, 1976.

110. Yatsu FM: Acute medical therapy of strokes. *Stroke* 13:524, 1982.

111. Wood JH, Kee DB: Clinical rheology of stroke and hemodilution. In Barnett HJM, Mohr JP, Stein BM, et al (eds): *Stroke: Pathophysiology, Diagnosis and Management*. New York, Churchill Livingstone, 1986: 97–108.

112. Prats AR, Wood JH, Kron RE, et al: Relative influences of hematocrit and plasma fibrinogen as determinants of fresh blood viscosity during hemodilution therapy in stroke patients. *Neurology,* 1988, in press.

113. Grotta J, ASckerman R, Correia J, et al: Whole blood viscosity parameters in cerebral blood flow. *Stroke* 13:296, 1982.

114. Kee DB Jr, Wood JH: Blood viscosity and cerebral blood flow, In Plum F, Pulsinelli WA (eds): *Cerebrovascular Diseases: Fourteenth Princeton-Williamsburg Conference*. New York, Raven Press, 1985: 107–177.

115. Ott EO, Ladurner G, Lechner H: Relationship between disturbed rheological properties and cerebral hemodynamics in recent cerebral infarction. *Prog Biochem Pharmacol* 13:349, 1977.

116. Thomas DJ, Duboulay GH, Marshall J, et al: Effect of haematocrit on cerebral blood flow in man. *Lancet* 2:941, 1977.

117. Harrison MJ, Pollock S, Kendall BE, et al: Effect of haematocrit on carotid stenosis and cerebral infarction. *Lancet* 2:114, 1981.

118. Couch JR, Hassanein RS: Platelet aggregation, stroke and transient ischemic attack in middle-aged and elderly patients. *Neurology* 26:888, 1976.

119. Wade JPH: Transport of oxygen to the brain in patients with elevated haematocrit values before and after venesection. *Brain* 106:513, 1983.

120. Wood JH, Simeone FA, Kron RE, et al: Relationship of cortical blood flow and cardiovascular responses to alterations in fresh blood viscosity as determined by capillary step-response viscometry. *J Cereb Blood Flow Metab* 1(suppl 1):S233, 1981.

121. Strand T, Splund K, Eriksson S, et al: A randomized controlled trial of hemodilution therapy in acute ischemic stroke. *Stroke* 15:980, 1984.

122. Wood JH, Polyzoidis KS, Epstein CM, et al: Quantitative EEG alterations after isovolemic hemodilutional augmentation of cerebral perfusion in stroke patients. *Neurology* 34:764, 1984.

123. Wood JH, Simeone FA, Kron RE, et al: Experimental hypervolemic hemodilution: Physiological correlations of cortical blood flow, cardiac output, and intracranial pressure with fresh blood viscosity and plasma volume. *Neurosurgery* 14:709, 1984.

124. Goslinga H, Eijzenbach V, Heuvelmans JHA, et al: Custom-tailored hemodilution with albumin and crystalloids in acute ischemic stroke. *Stroke* 23:181, 1992.

125. Du Boulay GH, Symon L: The anaesthetist's effect upon the cerebral arteries. *Proc R Soc Med* 64:77, 1971.

126. Gottstein U: Therapie der Zerebralen Zirkulationsstörungen. *Dtsch Med Wochenschr* 93:1815, 1968.

127. Gottstein U, Held K: Effekt der Hämodilution nach intravenser infusion von neidermolekularen Dextranen auf die Hunzirkulation des menschen. *Dtsch Med Wochenschr* 94:522, 1969.

128. Sundt TM, Waltz AC, Sayre GP: Experimental cerebral infarction: Modification by treatment with hemodilution, hemoconcentrating and dehydrating agents. *J Neurosurg* 26:46, 1967.

129. Wood JH, Simeone FA, Kron RE, et al: Rheological aspects of experimental hypervolemic hemodilution with low-molecular-weight dextran. Relations of cortical blood flow, cardiac output and intracranial pressure to fresh blood viscosity and plasma volume. *Neurosurgery* 11:739, 1982.

130. Corry WD, Jackson LJ, Seaman GVF: The effect of hydroxyethyl starch on the rheological properties of human erythrocyte suspension. *Biorheology* 18:517, 1981.

131. Ott E, Lechner H: Changes of flow properties of the blood in cerebrovascular disease and medical treatment with pentoxifylline. *J Cereb Blood Flow Metab* (*Suppl*) 3:S530, 1977.

132. Volby B: Alterations in vasomotor reactivity in subarachnoid hemorrhage. In Wood JH (ed): *Cerebral Blood Flow*. New York, McGraw-Hill, 1987: 402–412.

133. Heilbrun MP, Olesen J, Lassen NA: Regional cerebral blood flow studies in subarachnoid hemorrhage. *J Neurosurg* 37:36, 1972.

134. Kadel KA, Heistad DD, Faraci FM: Effects of endothelin on blood vessels of the brain and choroid plexus. *Brain Res* 518:78, 1990.

135. Sengupta D, Harper M, Jennett B: Effect of carotid ligation on cerebral blood flow in baboons: 1. Response to altered arterial pCO_2. *J Neurol Neurosurg Psychiatry* 36:736, 1973.

136. Pulsinelli WA, Levy DE, Duffy TE: Regional cerebral blood flow and glucose metabolism following transient forebrain ischemia. *Ann Neurol* 11:499, 1982.

137. Symon L, Crockard HA, Dorsch NWC, et al: Local cerebral blood flow and vascular reactivity in a chronic stable stroke in baboons. *Stroke* 6:482, 1975.

138. Hashi K, Meyer JS, Shinmaru S, et al: Changes in cerebral vasomotor reactivity to CO_2 and autoregulation following experimental subarachnoid hemorrhage. *J Neurosci* 17:15, 1972.

139. Heilbrun MP, Olesen J, Lassen NA: Regional cerebral blood flow studies in subarachnoid hemorrhage. *J Neurosurg* 37:36, 1972.

140. Boisvert DPJ, Pickard JD, Graham DI, et al: Delayed effects of subarachnoid haemorrhage on cerebral metabolism and the cerebrovascular response to hypercapnia in the primate. *J Neurol Neurosurg Psychiatry* 42:892, 1979.

141. Mendelow AD, McCalden TA, Hattingh J, et al: Cerebrovascular reactivity and metabolism after subarachnoid hemorrhage in baboons. *Stroke* 12:58, 1981.

142. Jacubowski J, Bell BA, Symon L, et al: A primate model of subarachnoid hemorrhage: Change in regional cerebral blood flow, autoregulation, carbon dioxide reactivity, and central conduction time. *Stroke* 12:601, 1982.

143. Kamiya K, Kuyama H, Symon L: An experimental study of the acute stage of subarachnoid hemorrhage. *J Neurosurg* 59:917, 1983.

144. Lewelt W, Jenkins LW, Miller JD: Effects of experimental fluid percussion injury of the brain on cerebrovascular reactivity to hypoxia and hypercapnia. *J Neurosurg* 56:332, 1982.

145. Saunders ML, Miller JD, Stablein D, et al: The effects of graded experimental trauma on cerebral blood flow and responsiveness to CO_2. *J Neurosurg* 51:18, 1979.

146. Bell BA, Foubister GC, Neto NGF, et al: Effect of experimental common carotid arteriotomy on cerebral blood flow in rats. *Neurosurgery* 16:322, 1985.

147. Paulson OB, Olesen J, Christensen MS: Restoration of autoregulation of cerebral blood flow by hypocapnia. *Neurology* 22:286, 1972.

148. Ponte J, Purves MJ: The role of the carotid body chemoreceptors and carotid sinus baroreceptors in the control of cerebral blood vessels. *J Physiol (Lond)* 237:315, 1974.

149. Thomas D, Crockard A: Cerebral metabolism and blood flow. In Crockard A, Hayward R, Hoff JT (eds): *Neurosurgery. The Scientific Basis of Clinical Practice.* Oxford/London/Edinburgh, Blackwell Scientific, 1985: 223–239.

150. Miller JD, Ledingham IMcA, Jennet WB: Effects of hyperbaric oxygen on intracranial pressure and cerebral blood flow in experimental cerebral oedema. *J Neurol Neurosurg Psychiatry* 33:745, 1970.

151. Artru AA: Cerebral metabolism and EEG during combination of hypocapnia and isoflurane-induced hypotension in dogs. *Anesthesiology* 65:602, 1986.

152. Artru AA: Partial preservation of cerebral vascular responsiveness to hypocapnia during isoflurane-induced hypotension in dogs. *Anesth Analg* 65:660, 1986.

153. Artru AA: Cerebral metabolism and the electroencephalogram during hypocapnia plus hypotension induced by sodium nitroprusside or trimethaphan in dogs. *Neurosurgery* 18:36, 1986.

154. Artru AA, Wright K, Colley PS: Cerebral effects of hypocapnia plus nitroglycerin-induced hypotension in dogs. *J Neurosurg* 64:924, 1986.

155. Artru AA, Colley PS: Cerebral blood flow responses to hypocapnia during hypotension. *Stroke* 15:878, 1984.

156. Artru AA: Cerebral vascular responses to hypocapnia during nitroglycerin-induced hypotension. *Neurosurgery* 16:468, 1985.

157. Rudehill A, Lindqvist C, Lundberg JM: Elevated plasma levels of neuropeptide Y upon electrical stimulation of sympathetic chain in humans. *J Neurosurg Anesth* 4:21, 1992.

158. Szabò C, Emilsson K, Hardebo JE, et al: Uptake and release of serotonin in rat cerebrovascular nerves after subarachnoid hemorrhage. *Stroke* 23:54, 1992.

159. Kawai K, Nitecka L, Ruetzler CA, et al: Global cerebral ischemia associated with cardiac arrest in the rat. I. Dynamics of early neuronal changes. *J Cereb Blood Flow Metab* 12:238, 1992.

160. Mans A, Kukulka KM, McAvoy KJ, et al: Regional distribution and kinetics of three sites on the $GABA_A$ receptor: Lack of effect of protacaval shunting. *J Cereb Blood Flow Metab* 12:334, 1992.

161. Diemer NH, Johansen FF, Jørgensen MB: N-methyl-D-aspartate and non-N-methyl-D-aspartate antagonists in global cerebral ischemia. *Stroke* 21:III-39, 1990.

162. Artru AA, Nugent M, Michenfelder JD: Anesthetics affect the cerebral metabolic response to circulatory catecholamines. *J Neurochem* 36:1941, 1981.

163. Matsui Y, Kumagae Y: Monoamine oxidase inhibitors prevent striated neuronal necrosis induced by transient forebrain ischemia. *Neurosci Lett* 126:175, 1991.

164. Maiese K, Pek L, Berger SB, et al: Reduction in focal cerebral ischemia by agents acting at imidazole receptors. *J Cereb Blood Flow Metab* 12:53, 1992.

165. Johansen FF, Diemer NH: Enhancement of GABA neurotransmission after cerebral ischemia in the rat reduces loss of hippocampal CA1 pyramidal cells. *Acta Neurol Scand* 84:1, 1991.

166. Erdö SL, Michler A, Wolff JR: GABA accelerates excitotoxic cell death in

cortical cultures: Protection by blockers of GABA-gated chloride channels. *Brain Res* 542:254, 1991.

167. Löscher W, Hönack D, Fassbender C-P: Regional alterations in brain amino acids after administration of the *N*-methyl-D-aspartate receptor antagonists MK-801 and CGP 39551 in rats. *Neurosci Lett* 124:115, 1991.

168. Suyama K: Changes of neuronal transmission in the hippocampus after transient ischemia in spontaneously hypertensive rats and the protective effects of MK-801. *Stroke* 23:260, 1992.

169. Lauritzen M, Hansen AJ: The effect of glutamate receptor blockade on anoxic depolarization and cortical spreading depression. *J Cereb Blood Flow Metab* 12:223, 1992.

170. Nellgård B, Gustafson I, Wieloch T: Lack of protection by the *N*-methyl-D-aspartate receptor blocker dizocilpine (MK-801) after transient severe cerebral ischemia in the rat. *Anesthesiology* 75:279, 1991.

171. Steinberg GK, Kunis D, Saleh J, et al: Protection after transient focal cerebral ischemia by the *N*-methyl-D-aspartate antagonist dextrorphan is dependent upon plasma and brain levels. *J Cereb Blood Flow Metab* 11:1015, 1991.

172. Lo EH, Steinberg GK: Effects of dextromethorphan on regional cerebral blood flow in focal cerebral ischemia. *J Cereb Blood Flow Metab* 11:803, 1991.

173. Lysko PG, Gagnon RC, Yue T-L, et al: Neuroprotective effects of SKF 10,047 in cultured rat cerebellar neurons and in gerbil global brain ischemia. *Stroke* 23:414, 1992.

174. Takizawa S, Hogan M, Hakim AM: The effects of a competitive NMDA receptor antagonist (CGS-19755) on cerebral blood flow and pH in focal ischemia. *J Cereb Blood Flow Metab* 11:786, 1991.

175. Warner MA, Neill KH, Nadler JV, et al: Regionally selective effects of NMDA receptor antagonist against ischemic brain damage in the gerbil. *J Cereb Blood Flow Metab* 11:600, 1991.

176. Chen M, Bullock R, Graham DI, et al: Evaluation of a competitive NMDA antagonist (D-CPPene) in feline focal cerebral ischemia. *Ann Neurol* 30:62, 1991.

177. Chen M-H, Bullock R, Graham DI, et al: Ischemic neuronal damage after acute subdural hematoma in the rat: Effects of pretreatment with a glutamate antagonist. *J Neurosurg* 74:944, 1991.

178. Nellgård B, Wieloch T: Postischemic blockade of AMPA but not NMDA receptors mitigates neuronal damage in the rat brain following transient severe cerebral ischemia. *J Cereb Blood Flow Metab* 12:2, 1992.

179. Pickard JD: Ionic and eicosanoid regulation of cerebrovascular smooth muscle contraction. In Wood JH (ed): *Cerebral Blood Flow*. New York, McGraw-Hill, 1987: 131–144.

180. Simeone FA, Vinall PE, Pickard JD: Response of extraparenchymal cerebral

arteries to biochemical environment of cerebrospinal fluid, In Wood JH (ed): *Neurobiology of Cerebrospinal Fluid, Vol I*. New York, Plenum, 1980: 303–311.

181. Wahl M, Kuschinsky W, Bosse O, Thurau K: Dependency of pial arterial and arteriolar diameter on perivascular osmolarity in the cat: A microapplication study. *Circ Res* 32:162, 1973.

182. Edvinsson L, McCulloch J, Uddman R: Substance P: Immunohistochemical localization and effect upon cat pial arteries in vitro and in situ. *J Physiol* 318:251, 1981.

183. Edvinsson L, Emson P, McCulloch J, et al: Neuropeptide Y: Cerebrovascular innervation and vasomotor effects in the cat. *Neurosci Lett* 43:79, 1983.

184. Griffith SG, Lincoln J, Burnstock G: Serotonin as a neurotransmitter in cerebral arteries. *Brain Res* 247:388, 1982.

185. Hendry SHC, Jones EG, Beinfeld MC: Cholecystokinin-immunoreactive neurons in rat and monkey cerebral cortex make symmetric synapses and have intimate associations with blood vessels. *Proc Natl Acad Sci U S A* 80:2400, 1983.

186. Sano Y, Takeuchi Y, Yamada H, et al: Immunohistochemical studies on the serotonergic innervation of the pia mater. *Histochemistry* 76:277, 1982.

187. Bolton TB: Mechanisms of action of transmitters and other substances on smooth muscle. *Physiol Rev* 59:606, 1979.

188. Hogestatt ED, Andersson KE: Mechanisms behind the biphasic contractile response to potassium depolarization in isolated rat cerebral arteries. *J Pharmacol Exp Ther* 228:187, 1984.

189. McCalden TA, Bevan JA: Sources of activator calcium in rabbit basilar artery. *Am J Physiol* 241:H129, 1981.

CHAPTER 8

Anesthetic Management of Patients with Traumatic Head Injury

Arthur M. Lam and Teresa S. Mayberg

Patients who have suffered traumatic head injuries may come under the care of the anesthesiologist for a variety of reasons. They may require acute resuscitation in the emergency room (see Chap. 5), treatment of a primary neurologic lesion (e.g., evacuation of a subdural hematoma) or treatment of an unrelated injury (e.g., laparotomy for a ruptured spleen). The purpose of this chapter is to review the pathophysiology of head injury and illustrate the applications of basic anesthetic principles to the management of patients with traumatic head injury.

NORMAL PHYSIOLOGY

Normal Values

Normal cerebral blood flow (CBF) is approximately 50 ml/100 g per min, or 700 ml/min in a 70 kg person. The cerebral metabolic rate for oxygen ($CMRO_2$) is 3.2 ml/100 g per min, or about 45 ml/min. Thus, the brain receives approximately 15 percent of the cardiac output but consumes 20 percent of the oxygen.

Regulation of Cerebral Blood Flow

The various factors that influence CBF are summarized in Fig. 8-1.

Autoregulation

Within the range of mean systemic blood pressure from 60 to 160 mmHg (or 50 to 150 mmHg of cerebral perfusion pressure), there is little variation in cerebral blood flow, and this homeostatic mechanism is termed "autoregulation." This maintenance of flow is effected through direct variation of cerebral vascular resistance with perfusion pressure. The process is extremely efficient, and although classically thought to occur in minutes, recent evidence suggests that it occurs in seconds,[1,2] and the process is accelerated during hypocapnia but delayed during hypercapnia. The purported mechanisms include both metabolic and mechanical causes.

Arterial CO_2 and O_2

Within the range of 25 to 55 mmHg, cerebral blood flow varies almost linearly with Pa_{CO_2}, changing by about 3 percent per mmHg. High arterial oxygen tension has a minimal vasoconstrictive effect on CBF whereas Pa_{O_2} less than 50 mmHg will cause vasodilation.

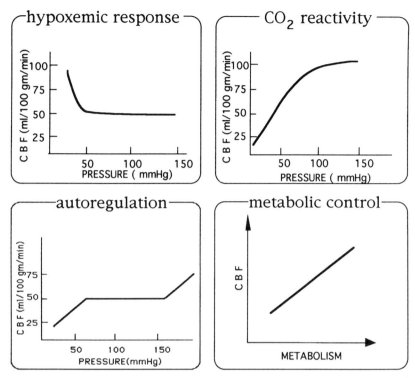

Figure 8-1 Normal regulatory control of cerebral blood flow. Pa_{CO_2} is by far the most influential determinant of cerebral blood flow under physiological conditions.

Flow-Metabolism Coupling

Normally cerebral blood flow and metabolism are tightly coupled on a regional basis. An increase in cortical activity will lead to a corresponding increase in cerebral blood flow. Thus, CBF usually increases in response to stimulation, and comatose patients have reduced CBF due to reduced metabolism.

Sympathetic Innervation

Although the cerebral blood vessels are supplied abundantly with sympathetic innervation, CBF is not affected appreciably by the sympathetic tone. Sympathetic stimulation, however, may shift the autoregulatory curve to the right, causing the cerebral circulation to fail at a higher blood pressure.

PATHOPHYSIOLOGY

The Concept of Secondary Injury

The main pathophysiology of head injury has been discussed in Chap. 2 and will not be repeated here. However, it is important to reiterate the concept of secondary injury, because primary injury is not treatable and can only be prevented. Secondary injury refers to the additional insults imposed on the damaged neuronal tissue following the primary impact and is the major focus of treatment regimens. This is particularly important in view of the common occurrence of patients with head injury admitted to hospitals in a conscious state only to die later.[3,4] The common denominator of secondary injury is cerebral ischemia, both global and focal. Contributing factors include hypoxia, hypercapnia, decreased cerebral perfusion from overly aggressive hyperventilation, systemic hypotension, intracranial hypertension, posttraumatic cerebral arterial spasm, and transtentorial and cerebellar herniation (Table 8-1).

The Role of Ischemia in Head Injury

Despite repeated demonstration in autopsy studies that 85 to 90 percent of patients who died of head injury had lesions compatible with ischemia,[5,6] clinical studies of cerebral blood flow and metabolism in severe head injury have failed to demonstrate significant ischemia.[7,8] Although cerebral blood

Table 8-1 Contributing factors to secondary injury

Systemic factors
  Hypoxemia
  Hypotension
  Hyperglycemia

Decreased cerebral perfusion
  Intracranial hypertension
    Hypercapnia
    Hypoxemia
    Systemic hypotension
    Venous obstruction
  Systemic hypotension
    Hypovolemia/associated injuries
  Overaggressive hyperventilation
  Posttraumatic cerebral arterial vasospasm

Transtentorial and cerebellar herniation

flows are frequently reduced, comatose patients also have reduced metabolism, and Obrist and coworkers[7] demonstrated that in 55 percent of the head-injured patients with Glasgow Coma Scale (GCS) score < 8 actually had relative hyperemia (high flow relative to metabolism). This apparent paradox has been resolved by recent studies that were able to investigate the patients within 8 h of injury. Both Marion and coworkers and Bouma and coworkers demonstrated that CBF was initially severely reduced, with a high arteriovenous oxygen content difference (AVD_{O_2}) reflecting a flow less than metabolism; however, the CBF gradually increased with time and could be in excess of metabolism over the next 24 h.[9–11] This hyperemia is more likely to occur in children. Both extremely low and high levels of CBF have been associated with poor prognosis.

A recent study by Bouma and coworkers measured CBF by stable xenon at the time of initial CT scan (approximate time from injury was 3 h) and demonstrated a significant reduction in CBF in more than 30 percent of the patients.[12] Furthermore, patients with the lowest CBF also had the worst prognosis. Jaggi and coworkers had previously reported that a low CMR_{O_2} is associated with a poor prognosis.[13] On the other hand, Weber and coworkers and Martin and coworkers have demonstrated that CBF can also decline following the initial hyperemic phase in 20 to 40 percent of the patients as a result of vasospasm,[14,15] and the occurrence of vasospasm is associated with a higher incidence of noncontusion-related cerebral infarction.[16] Thus, the change in $CBF/CMRO_2$ is by no means uniform in head-injured patients. The majority of the severely injured patients will suffer an initial decline in CBF, followed by a return to normal flow or relative hyperemia, and the flow may then decline again, particularly if vasospasm occurs.

The cause of the initial low CBF is not clear but systemic hypotension may be a significant contributory factor. The importance of maintenance of systemic perfusion has recently been confirmed by the results from the National Traumatic Coma Data Bank (NTCDB), which demonstrated that systolic blood pressure < 80 mmHg is a significant contributing factor to poor outcome, just as is elevated intracranial pressure (ICP).[17] The combination of increased ICP and systemic hypotension leads to a reduced cerebral perfusion pressure (CPP) and reduced CBF.

The autoregulatory mechanism may be impaired following a severe head injury. On the other hand, CO_2 reactivity is frequently preserved, but the magnitude may be reduced.[18] The complete absence of CO_2 reactivity has been shown to correlate with lack of vasoconstrictor response to barbiturates and is indicative of a poor prognosis.[19] In patients with impaired autoregulation, systemic hypotension will further aggravate cerebral perfusion. In contrast, in patients with intact autoregulation, hypotension will lead to cerebral vasodilation with resultant increase in ICP, and this may eventually lead to a decrease in CBF.[20] In patients who are severely injured, false autoregulation may occur, i.e., CBF fails to change with changes in blood pressure as the

ICP changes by the same magnitude as systemic blood pressure, an effect that leads to a constant cerebral perfusion pressure.[21]

On a biochemical basis, the ischemia may cause secondary injury by allowing accumulation of excitotoxic amino acids (glutamates), the interaction of which with NMDA (N-methyl-D-aspartate) receptors leading to intracellular accumulation of calcium ions. Subsequent activation of phospholipase, breakdown of arachidonic acid, generation of free radicals, and lipid peroxidation contribute to eventual neuronal death. The release of excitatory amino acids into cerebrospinal fluid in patients with severe head injury has been recently reported by Baker and coworkers.[22]

Intracranial Contents and ICP

The components that make up the intracranial contents are the brain bulk (80 percent), blood volume (5 percent), and cerebrospinal fluid (CSF) (15 percent). As the skull is a rigid box, an increase in volume in any of the components will lead to a rise in the ICP. This pressure-volume relationship is commonly referred to as the intracranial compliance curve (Fig. 8-2) although elastance curve is a more accurate description. A small increase in intracranial volume can be partially compensated by translocation of CSF into the spinal subarachnoid space and compression of the venous blood volume, but this compensatory mechanism is very limited, and once exhausted, any further increase in intracranial content will lead to an inordinate rise in ICP. The steepness of the increase depends on both the rate of increase in the volume and the nature of the compartment involved and cannot be predicted by the current ICP reading. To allow a better assessment of this compliance, Marmarou introduced the pressure-volume index (PVI)[23] which is defined mathematically as

$$PVI = \frac{\Delta V}{\log \frac{P_f}{P_o}}$$

where ΔV = volume of saline injected or withdrawn, P_f = final pressure, P_o = initial pressure. Conceptually, it is the volume whose addition or withdrawal from the intracranial vault will cause a tenfold change in intracranial pressure. Practically, this is determined by injecting or withdrawing 2 to 5 ml of fluid into the ventriculostomy catheter. The normal value is 25 ml, and a decrease to 18 ml is indicative of significant decrease in compliance (increase in elastance), and a value of 13 ml is considered to be a critical threshold, which carries a bad prognosis.[24] The PVI has been shown to be frequently decreased in patients with head injury.[10,24] Although potentially useful and conceptually sound, the PVI, nevertheless, has never achieved clinical utility.

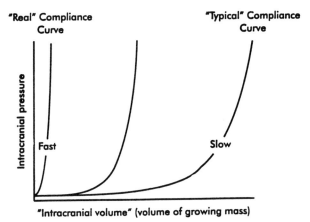

"Intracranial volume" (volume of growing mass)

Figure 8-2 Intracranial pressure "compliance curves." If intracranial contents are noncompressible and the skull were truly rigid, then the injection of any "extra" volume into the system would produce a very rapid increase in pressure (left curve, labeled *real*). However, this is not the pattern typically seen with a slowly growing mass lesion, which is shown on the right curve (labeled *typical*). Note, however, that the x axis is often mislabeled. This should note read "intracranial volume" but rather "volume of growing mass." As a mass grows, total volume remains almost constant because of compensatory mechanisms. Only when these are exhausted does pressure rise precipitously. Note also that the faster volume is added, the more quickly are compensatory mechanisms exhausted. (*From Todd MM, Warner DS: Principles and Practices of Anesthesiology, Vol. 2, Mosby Year Book, 1993, Chap. 71, with permission.*)

Significance of ICP in Head Trauma

Cerebral perfusion pressure (CPP) is determined by the difference between mean arterial blood pressure (MAP) and ICP. Thus, a high ICP can impede cerebral perfusion and lead to cerebral ischemia. In addition to ischemia, a high ICP can also cause uncal or cerebellar herniation. ICP is frequently increased in head-injured patients, and the causes are multifactorial (see control of ICP in a later section). A high ICP has been positively correlated with poor prognosis, and although this correlation has been suggested to be merely a reflection of the underlying pathology, more recent evidence confirmed that increased ICP contributes to the poor outcome and that aggressive treatment of patients with increased ICP will improve outcome.[25-27] An elevated ICP, despite aggressive therapy, was usually predictive of poor outcome and a prompt response to therapy was associated with a better outcome.[28] The recent data from the NTCDB further substantiate this contention.

Many of the techniques and drug therapies that are undertaken in the treatment of head-injured patients are aimed at influencing both CPP and ICP.

Obviously, many other factors may impact on the survival and/or recovery of a traumatized patient. In a study that attempted to isolate ICP and the influence of other factors on outcome, Marmarou and coworkers analyzed information from 428 patients as part of the NTCDB study.[17] They found that age, admission motor score, and pupillary response were predictive of outcome. In addition to those factors, they also found that an average ICP > 20 mmHg and a systemic arterial blood pressure < 80 mmHg were both independently predictive of a poor outcome. Interestingly, CPP alone was not found to be predictive of outcome because some hypotensive patients maintained a seemingly adequate CPP despite MAPs that were, presumably, insufficient to maintain adequate perfusion. However, the combination of hypotension and increased ICP were very predictive of poor outcome (Fig. 8-3). The authors of this report postulated that, although CPP per se may have been maintained in hypotensive patients with low ICPs, the overall perfusion was inadequate and led to cerebral ischemia.[17]

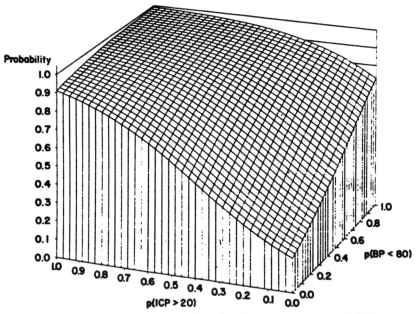

Figure 8-3 Three-dimensional surface of estimated outcome probability versus the proportion of intracranial pressure (ICP) measurements greater than 20 mmHg [p(ICP > 20)] and the proportion of blood pressure measurements less than 80 mmHg [p(BP < 80)] for the vegetative/dead outcome group. To simplify the presentation, the other modeled factors were fixed at the following values: age = 30 years, admission motor score = 3 (flexion), and abnormal pupils = 1. The substantial effect of hypotension is readily evident from the front-to-back upward sloping of the surface. The impact of ICP elevation is apparent from the right-to-left upward sloping of the surface.[17] (*From Marmarou et al.[17] With permission.*)

Measurement of ICP

ICP can be measured in a number of ways. The gold standard is via a ventriculostomy with an intraventricular catheter. With this method, treatment of high ICP can be accomplished with drainage of CSF, but this is also the most invasive method and is associated with a significant risk of infection. Other methods include epidural catheter (mechanical or fiberoptic), hollow subarachnoid bolt, and the recently introduced Camino fiberoptic catheter that can be placed extradurally, subdurally, or intraparenchymally (Fig. 8-4).[29] With the exception of the ventriculostomy, most ICP monitors can be placed on the bedside under local anesthesia via a small burr hole and the rate of infection is much lower than that associated with intraventricular placement. The noninvasive transcranial Doppler waveform can also provide valuable information regarding ICP, and the pulsatility has been correlated

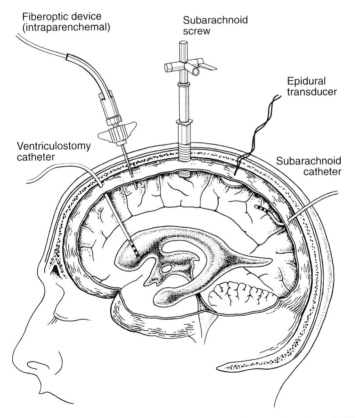

Figure 8-4 Different modalities available for monitoring of ICP. One of the most commonly used fiberoptic devices (Camino Catheter, Camino Laboratories, San Diego, CA) can be placed epidurally, subarachnoidally, or intraparenchymally.

with ICP although it probably reflects the CPP more than the ICP.[30,31] This may be useful in patients where ICP monitoring has not been instituted.

Indications of ICP Monitoring

All patients with GCS score of less than 8 should have routine ICP monitoring. Patients whose neurologic status could not be assessed because of either administration of sedative drugs or neuromuscular blocking agents should also be monitored. In patients with GCS score of 9 to 12 who require a major surgical procedure necessitating vigorous fluid therapy, the need for ICP monitoring may also arise, and a joint decision should be made between the anesthesiologist and the neurosurgeon. It is, however, recognized that ICP monitoring facilities may not be available in many centers and may not be considered routine monitoring in others.[32]

Control of ICP

The causes of increased ICP in head-injured patients are multifactorial and any of the three intracranial components may be involved. In addition, mass lesions following head injury are common. Treatment of ICP will be discussed in the context of each of these components.

Brain Bulk

Edema can develop quickly following a closed head injury, although this is unlikely to be the major cause of increased ICP in the immediate phase. Twenty percent mannitol (0.25 to 1.0 g/kg) is routinely given to reduce ICP, and the classic explanation for its mechanism is osmotic dehydration and, therefore, reduction in brain bulk (osmolality for 20 percent mannitol is 1098 compared to the normal serum osmolality of 290). However, the dehydration effect tends to occur late, is not sustained[33] and does not explain the rapid onset of action of mannitol.[34] Recent evidence suggests that mannitol may act on all three intracranial components via different mechanisms.

Mannitol decreases both cerebrovascular and systemic vascular resistance and may cause transient systemic hypotension followed by hypertension as the intravascular volume expands. Patients with poor cardiac function may develop congestive heart failure and pulmonary edema. The use of mannitol for increased ICP has been advocated for an ICP of 15 mmHg or more.[35] There is evidence that early initiation of treatment at an ICP of 15 mmHg as opposed to 20 or 25 mmHg may improve outcome.[27] Loop diuretics, such as furosemide, are commonly used during elective neurosurgery and may also be useful in the head-injured patient. They potentiate the action of mannitol without causing significant hemodynamic effects. The use of osmotic and loop diuretics can lead to electrolyte imbalance, and replacement therapy should be guided by periodic electrolyte and osmolality measurements. In patients resistant to the action of mannitol, use of hypertonic saline has been advocated although its action is transient in limited clinical studies.[36,37]

In cases of severe brain swelling, craniectomy with or without lobectomy may become necessary, with obvious undesirable impact on patient outcome.

Blood Volume

The increase in blood volume is considered to be the most important cause of increased ICP after head trauma. Both hypoxemia and hypercapnia will cause cerebral vasodilation and increase blood volume. In addition, systemic hypotension will provide further vasodilatory stimuli.[20] Hyperventilation is one of the most effective mechanisms in controlling cerebral blood volume (CBV). Although not well documented in humans, studies in cats suggest that the reduction of CBV is approximately 1 percent/mmHg as opposed to 3 percent/mmHg in CBF with change in Pa_{CO_2}.[38] However, it must be mentioned that although the desirable reduction in CBV occurs as a result of an increase in cerebral vascular resistance, the simultaneous reduction in CBF should be regarded as an unavoidable side effect rather than as a primary therapeutic goal. This is particularly important with the recent recognition that ischemia may be a significant contributory factor to poor outcome in severe head injury.

Besides the potential of causing cerebral ischemia, other disadvantages of hyperventilation include (1) left shift of the hemoglobin-oxygen dissociation curve, thus decreasing oxygen availability to the tissues; and (2) normalization of CBF and, thus, CBV with prolonged hyperventilation. A recent randomized trial of the use of prolonged hyperventilation in a small series of severely head-injured patients suggests that it has an adverse effect on patient outcome.[39] However, used properly, hyperventilation is a quick and effective tool for reducing CBV, can be life-saving in acute intracranial hypertension, and should not be withheld because of these concerns. A rational approach is to recognize that hyperventilation is a temporizing tool and not definitive treatment and that the level of hyperventilation should only be implemented to the extent necessary to reduce ICP. In the absence of ICP monitoring, Pa_{CO_2} should not be reduced to less than 25 mmHg unless there is other objective evidence of uncontrollable brain swelling. Monitoring of jugular bulb venous oxygen saturation may help to minimize the occurrence of global cerebral ischemia from hyperventilation (see more on monitoring in a later section). Recently, tromethamine (THAM), a buffering agent that may counteract tissue acidosis, was reported to have beneficial effects on ICP, although the overall patient outcome remained unchanged.[40]

Cerebral blood volume can also be reduced pharmacologically. Recent studies suggest that mannitol may also exert its ICP reduction action via reduction in CBV. Muizelaar proposed that cerebral autoregulation may be regulated by viscosity; thus, reduction in viscosity will lead to an increase in

CBF, which in turn, leads to vasoconstriction to maintain CBF constant.[41,42] Because mannitol reduces viscosity and increases CBF, it may cause viscosity-mediated vasoconstriction and, therefore, reduction in CBV. Although this vasoactive action was demonstrated in feline pial vessels[41] and corroborated in a clinical study,[42] it is not certain to what extent this accounts for mannitol's action.

Other studies have also reported that administration of mannitol is associated with a transient increase in blood flow and blood volume and may lead to an initial increase in ICP.[43] Paradoxically, in patients with intracranial hypertension, ICP did not increase following the administration of mannitol.[44] Thus, this transient increase in blood flow/volume with mannitol does not appear to be a clinically relevant problem.

Other cerebral vasoconstrictive agents include the intravenous anesthetic agents: barbiturates, etomidate, and propofol. All of these agents decrease CBF as well as cerebral metabolism, and the classical explanation of their action is predicated on flow-metabolism coupling; i.e., as metabolism decreases, blood flow and, consequently, blood volume decreases. However, because of the concurrent reduction in systemic blood pressure, the reduction in CBF may sometimes be in excess of metabolism. Of these agents, etomidate has the least cardiovascular depressant action and may be preferable in hemodynamically unstable patients.[45] Intravenous lidocaine is also a useful adjunct, but it only reduces CBF marginally as compared to the other drugs.[46] There is evidence that patients who have lost cerebrovascular reactivity to CO_2 also do not respond to barbiturate therapy.[19] Similarly, since the cerebrovasoconstrictive action is secondary to reduction of cerebral metabolism, patients with absent cortical electrical activity will not respond to barbiturate therapy.[47] Despite the initial enthusiasm for therapeutic barbiturate coma, this modality is now seldom used for the treatment of severe head injury. The reasons include the increased risk of nosocomial infection and pneumonia, lack of efficacy in improvement of outcome despite control of ICP,[48] and the cost of extended intensive care. Data from the NTCDB indicates that a small subset of patients with severe head injury may benefit from barbiturate therapy, but there are no consistent predictors of this subset prior to treatment.[49]

Hypothermia reduces the cerebral metabolic rate, decreases CBF and CBV, and, therefore, can reduce ICP. Although severe hypothermia is no longer employed, the recent discovery that mild hypothermia can significantly reduce neuronal injury in experimental head injury,[50,51] presumably be reducing the amount of glutamates released,[52] has revived the interest in the use of mild to moderate hypothermia in the treatment of head injury.[53] Preliminary clinical trials appear to be promising.[54–56]

Most of the clinical maneuvers used to reduce CBV are effected through the arterial and capillary blood volume compartments by changing the cerebral vascular resistance. Although the cerebral venous blood volume is the predominant blood volume compartment (75 percent), it tends to follow the arterial component passively and, therefore, is seldom considered separately. Failure to ensure adequate cerebral venous drainage, however, may lead to venous engorgement and uncontrollable increase in ICP. Thus, it is extremely important to maintain a slightly head-up position to improve venous drainage[57] (provided systemic hypotension does not occur with the head-up tilt), to ascertain that neck position does not cause kinking or compression of the internal jugular veins (which may occur with extreme neck flexion or extension, particularly when combined with head rotation), and to check all extraneous attachments to rule out accidental compression of venous drainage (collars, tracheal ties, and tracheostomy ties have all been known to cause cerebral venous compression with resultant increase in ICP).

Cerebrospinal Fluid Volume

It is estimated that this component may account for one-third of the increase in ICP following head injury. Although some inhalation anesthetics, such as halothane and enflurane, may increase the CSF compartment by increasing formation or reducing absorption,[58] this is not a major consideration in the acute treatment of increased ICP. If necessary, removal of CSF can be accomplished via a ventriculostomy. Recent studies suggest that administration of hypertonic saline reduces the production of CSF.[59] Thus, part of the action of mannitol, particularly the immediate action, may also be via inhibition of CSF production.[60]

Mass Lesions

Intracranial masses, such as epidural or subdural hematoma or foreign bodies causing brain compression, should be removed promptly. Surgical removal of intracerebral hematoma does not necessarily improve outcome but may be necessary to control intractable intracranial hypertension.

PRINCIPLES OF OPTIMAL ANESTHETIC MANAGEMENT FOLLOWING HEAD INJURY

The basic principles of anesthetic management in head injury are (1) to optimize cerebral perfusion, (2) to avoid cerebral ischemia, and (3) to avoid drugs or techniques that may cause an increase in ICP.

The systemic effects and associated injuries of head injury have been described in Chap. 3. The areas that bear direct influence on the anesthetic management are highlighted in the following section.

Maintenance of Systemic Hemodynamics

As mentioned above, systemic hypotension (systolic blood pressure <90 mmHg for 30 min) affects outcome negatively in patients with severe head injury.[61] The causes of hypotension are usually multifactorial. Young children may have sufficient blood loss from an intracranial hemorrhage and/ or scalp wound to be hypovolemic and hypotensive. This is usually not the case in adults, and hypotension should prompt an investigation of other sites of blood loss.

Because of the intense sympathetic stimulation associated with head injury, most patients present with hypertension and tachycardia. But these clinical signs are modified by the presence of other injuries as well as the state of the intracranial circulation. Most adults with an isolated head injury and significantly increased ICP will present with hypertension, and often with bradycardia particularly if there is brainstem compression. This has been described as the Cushing reflex, as reported by Cushing in his original study of the systemic response of raised ICP.[62] Because the increase in blood pressure is a compensatory response to maintain cerebral perfusion, moderate levels of hypertension should not be treated. Extreme hypertension (blood pressure well outside the range of autoregulation), however, should be treated because it will increase CBV and may further aggravate the increased ICP. The absence of hypertension and bradycardia does not necessarily rule out the presence of brainstem compression, because the development of systemic hypovolemia may prevent the occurrence of hypertension, and the sympathetic stimulation may prevent the development of bradycardia. The maintenance of an adequate urine output is a poor indicator of the volume status, particularly if mannitol had been administered recently. During surgical evacuation of an acute subdural or epidural hematoma with significant brain compression, it is fairly common to see an abrupt decrease in the blood pressure at the time of decompression. If the patient was hypertensive before injury, the decrease may return the blood pressure to a normal level. In patients who were normotensive but tachycardic, and with hypovolemia concealed by increased systemic vascular resistance, the decompression may result in a precipitous fall in blood pressure or cardiovascular collapse. The clinical course of such a patient is illustrated in Table 8-2.

A high index of suspicion, early initiation of vigorous fluid therapy, meticulous attention to the blood pressure, and prompt treatment of hypotension with intravenous fluids at the time of decompression are keys to successful management. The capability to administer rapid intravenous infusion coupled with large-bore intravenous catheters must be present and ready with these patients. Pharmacologic support with vasopressors, such as phenylephrine or epinephrine, may be needed until adequate fluid resuscitation is achieved.

Maintenance of Adequate Oxygenation and Ventilation

Patients with severe head injury often suffer from hypoxemia and hypercapnia at the time of initial resuscitation,[63] both of which cause cerebral vasodilation and increase in ICP. Although in most urban centers the paramedical personnel are trained and equipped to establish airway and ventilation, this training

Table 8-2 Changes in systemic hemodynamics with evacuation of an epidural hematoma in a 30-year-old male during isoflurane (0.5%) and fentanyl anesthesia[a]

Time	Blood pressure	Heart rate	IV	EBL	U/O
0300	120/60	155	2.5	?	1.0
0400	100/50	115	4.5	?	2.0
0415	20/—	160	5.0	0.8	2.3

Fluid resuscitation plus intravenous administration of epinephrine (1 mg × 3)

Time	Blood pressure	Heart rate	IV	EBL	U/O
0430	120/80	130	10.0	1.2	2.5
0830	120/60	125	22.0	2.5	5.6

[a] Blood pressure = systolic/diastolic blood pressure in mmHg; heart rate = beats per min; IV = intravenous infusion of Plasmalyte in liters; EBL = estimated blood loss at the time of surgery; ? indicates the unknown quantity of preexisting blood loss; U/O = urine output in liters.

is by no means universal. Moreover, although ventilation can generally be controlled and hypercapnia corrected, oxygenation may remain a problem in patients with concomitant pulmonary contusion, aspiration, or neurogenic pulmonary edema. Treatment of hypoxemia with a high inspired-oxygen fraction and employment of positive end-expiratory pressure may be necessary.

Maintenance of Cerebral Perfusion

The purpose of this section is to reemphasize the interaction between systemic hemodynamics, control of intracranial pressure, and the use of hyperventilation on cerebral perfusion. As mentioned previously, CBF normally decreases in response to hyperventilation. This CO_2 reactivity is usually, but not always, preserved following head injury.[12,18,21,64-66] Moreover, there may be large interpatient variability. In patients with normal CO_2 reactivity and preexisting low CBF following head trauma, hyperventilation may decrease regional CBF to less than ischemic levels.[67] Arteriovenous oxygen content difference correspondingly widens beyond the normal range.[7,9] Cerebral perfusion would be further aggravated by the presence of systemic hypotension. Thus, one should always be mindful of the potentially negative impact of extreme hyperventilation on cerebral perfusion. Other methods to improve cerebral perfusion by lowering the ICP have been discussed previously under the section headed Control of ICP.

Optimal Use of Anesthetic Agents

Anesthetic agents exert independent action on cerebral blood flow and metabolism, which may or may not be beneficial to the injured brain. The overall results depend not only on the intrinsic action of the anesthetics on cerebral blood flow and metabolism, but also the interaction with systemic hemodynamics, intracranial pressure, CO_2 reactivity, cerebrospinal fluid production/absorption, and surgical stimulation.

CBF and CMRO_2

This topic has been discussed in Chap. 7 and will only be briefly summarized here.

INTRAVENOUS AGENTS Intravenous agents including barbiturates, etomidate and propofol decrease cerebral blood flow and metabolism. The decrease in CBF is mediated by a decrease in $CMRO_2$.[68] All of these drugs, including propofol,[69-71] can, therefore, decrease ICP. Although the reduction in flow has been shown to be secondary to the reduction in metabolism (flow-metabolism coupling), this coupling is not perfect. The decrease in CBF sometimes exceeds the corresponding decrease in $CMRO_2$, leading to widening of cerebral arteriovenous oxygen content difference.[71,72] To what extent this is due to the simultaneous change in systemic hemodynamics is not known. Because the reduction in CBF is secondary to a decrease in $CMRO_2$, there agents will have no effect on CBF or ICP in patients without cerebral metabolism as seen by EEG activity. Lidocaine causes a small reduction in $CMRO_2$ as well as CBF[46] and is a useful adjunct in attenuating the cerebrovascular response to laryngoscopy and tracheal intubation.[73-75]

Use of ketamine is traditionally avoided in the anesthetic management of patients at risk of intracranial hypertension because of early studies that suggest increases in $CMRO_2$, CBF, and ICP.[76-79] The increase in CBF, however, may be partly mediated by a sympathetically induced increase in blood pressure, and partly by a concomitant increase in Pa_{CO_2} in spontaneously breathing subjects. More recent studies report no increase in ICP or flow when ventilation is controlled[80,81] or diazepam is concurrently administered.[82] When given in a background of isoflurane-nitrous oxide anesthesia, no increase in flow velocity is seen.[83] There is renewed interest in ketamine because it blocks excitatory amino acid receptors in the brain.[84] Ketamine is chemically related to MK-801, which has been shown to block stimulation of N-methyl-D-aspartate (NMDA) receptors. Activation of these receptors opens receptor-gated calcium channels which allows intracellular accumulation of calcium ions leading to neuronal injury and death. Shapira and coworkers recently demonstrated the cerebral protection effect of ketamine in experimental head injury in rats.[85] However, until clinical studies establish that ketamine can be safely used in patients with intracranial hypertension, its routine use in these patients cannot yet be recommended.

OPIOIDS Opioids generally have negligible effects on CBF and $CMRO_2$. However, synthetic opioids including fentanyl, sufentanil, and alfentanil have recently been reported to cause an increase in ICP in patients with various intracranial lesions including tumors and head trauma.[86,87] This increase was assumed to be secondary to an increase in CBF; however, blood flow studies in healthy volunteers were unable to demonstrate any increase in CBF with sufentanil administration.[88] Although a recent flow velocity study demonstrated increases with high-dose sufentanil as well as fentanyl, Pa_{CO_2} was not carefully controlled in this investigation.[89] Moreover, in the majority of the studies that demonstrate an increase in ICP, the systemic arterial blood pressure was allowed to fall following the administration of the opioid,[86,90] thus providing a potent impetus for cerebral vasodilation and increase in ICP.[20] When blood pressure was carefully supported, there was no clinically relevant increase in ICP or flow velocity with intravenous administration of alfentanil or sufentanil.[91-93] Similar observations have been made by Weinstabl and coworkers.[94,95] This underscores the importance of giving these agents judiciously and avoiding systemic hypotension. Clinically, no difference in operating conditions between these opioids has been observed, suggesting that their cerebrovascular effects are likely to be similar.[96]

Although controversy persists regarding the effect of synthetic opioids on ICP, there is no evidence that they are direct cerebral vasodilators. More importantly, if not used correctly, they may lead to hypotension and potential cerebral ischemia.

INHALATION AGENTS These agents are generally thought to be cerebral vasodilators. Halothane consistently causes cerebral vasodilation in experimental studies and probably should not be used in patients with increased ICP. In contrast, isoflurane does not cause increase in CBF at a dose range between 1.0 and 1.5 MAC although the effects on CBV are less clear. The recently introduced inhaled agent, desflurane, appears to have cerebrovascular properties similar to isoflurane.[97,98] CO_2 reactivity is well preserved with both agents, thus, it is safe to use them in patients with head injury provided that moderate hyperventilation can be implemented. However, in patients with high ICP, it would be prudent to avoid these agents or at least use low doses and supplement with an intravenous anesthetic, such as thiopental or propofol.

CO_2 Reactivity

Both intravenous and inhaled agents preserve the cerebrovascular response to CO_2.[98-100] Because CBF is generally decreased by the intravenous agents, the CO_2 reactivity as calculated by the flow-CO_2 regression slope is lower with intravenous agents compared to inhalation agents. The normal slope averages about 1.5 ml/100 g per min per mmHg change in Pa_{CO_2}. This value is slightly reduced during thiopental anesthesia and maintained during isoflurane or desflurane anesthesia. Irrespective of the agents used, because near maximal cerebrovasoconstriction occurs at about 25 mmHg, at this level of hyperventilation, CBF is comparable independent of what anesthetic agent is being used.

CSF Formation and Absorption

Anesthetic agents can alter the rate of CSF absorption and formation, leading to a change in CSF volume, and ultimately a change in ICP.[58] Increasing the resistance to CSF absorption and/or increasing the formation of CSF will lead to an expansion of the CSF volume and an increase in ICP while a reduction in resistance and/or decrease in formation will have a salutary effect on ICP. Relative to the total intracranial volume, these changes are small, and therefore are clinically unimportant in acute situations but may assume increasing importance after 2 to 4 h of anesthesia. With the exception of ketamine, which has been shown to increase the resistance to CSF absorption, other intravenous anesthetic agents appear to have minimal effects on CSF absorption and production. Of the inhaled anesthetic agents, enflurane has the least desirable effect, with a simultaneous increase in CSF absorption resistance and CSF formation, while isoflurane has the most favorable profile, with decreased CSF absorption resistance and an unchanged rate of CSF formation. Nitrous oxide appears to have no effect on either parameter. The effects of desflurane and sevoflurane have not been clarified. Although the magnitude of these changes is small and clinical relevance not well established, it is prudent to consider these factors when faced with persistent cerebral swelling unresponsive to usual therapeutic maneuvers.

Intravenous Fluid Therapy

The fluid management of patients with head injuries can be complicated. One should keep in mind that concurrent multisystem injury may render the patient hypovolemic and that every effort should be made to restore normal blood volume. With the exception of children, isolated head injury generally does not cause systemic hypotension. Therefore, adequate venous access must be established in all patients with head injuries who are hypotensive. In addition, hypovolemia may be masked by systemic hypertension secondary to sympathetic stimulation or the reflex response to increased ICP. Evacuation of a space-occupying lesion and decompression may lead to a catastrophic fall in systemic blood pressure as sympathetic tone is suddenly decreased (see previous sections). Rapid fluid infusion may be required. Uncorrected hypovolemia will cause hypotension and aggravate cerebral ischemia. However, with overzealous fluid therapy, not only pulmonary edema but also cerebral swelling may occur. Venous congestion can also impede cerebral venous drainage and raise ICP. Fluid replacement, therefore, should be guided by blood pressure, pulse rate, urine output, and the central venous pressure and/or pulmonary artery occlusion pressure. To optimize oxygen delivery to the brain, the level of hematocrit should not be allowed to decrease below 30 percent, and blood should be replaced accordingly. Glucose-containing solutions should be avoided in all situations where cerebral ischemia may occur because an abundant supply of substrate during ischemia will promote anaerobic metabolism, which will result in the production of pyruvate and lactate, leading to acidosis, vasoparalysis and increased cerebral injury.[101,102] Hyperglycemia is consistently found in head-injured patients within 12 h after injury.[103] Furthermore, hyperglycemia may be a predictor of outcome[104] as patients with high serum glucose have a worse prognosis than those patients with low glucose levels.[105,106] Thus, blood serum glucose levels exceeding 200 mg/dl should probably be treated judiciously with insulin.

The maintenance of osmotic pressure appears to be more important than the maintenance of oncotic pressure. In experimental studies, an acute drop in osmolality affects ICP more than an acute drop in oncotic pressure.[107,108] Thus hypotonic solutions may cause more cerebral edema and should be avoided. The use of crystalloid versus colloid solutions remains controversial. Colloids can expand the intravascular volume more efficiently, but should the blood-brain barrier become disrupted, more cerebral edema can occur. Hetastarch has been reported to cause coagulation abnormalities and should be used with care.[109] In contrast, hypertonic saline has been found to be useful in maintaining systemic perfusion without raising ICP during resuscitation of hemorrhagic shock associated with experimental head injury.[37,110–112] However, clinical studies assessing the use of hypertonic saline in humans remain limited.[36]

Coagulation

Coagulation abnormalities can be seen following head trauma. Release of tissue thromboplastin may activate the extrinsic pathway, and disruption of endothelial surfaces may activate the intrinsic pathway. Increases in fibrinogen degradation products as well as frank disseminated intravascular coagulation (DIC) may ensue.[113] Hypothermia and massive blood transfusions may also lead to clotting abnormalities.[114] The incidence of coagulopathy in head injured patients has been reported to be between 19[61] and 24 percent.[115] Severe clotting abnormalities are indicative of a poor outcome,[116] and head-injured patients with coagulation abnormalities are much more likely to develop delayed brain injury then those with normal studies.[117] Therefore, coagulation studies should be performed routinely, and aggressive replacement of clotting factors is advised in the face of abnormalities. However, in a retrospective study, early administration of fresh frozen plasma was not shown to be effective.[118]

Preoperative Assessment and Initial Resuscitation

Most head-injured patients present in the operating room on an emergency basis. Consequently there is often insufficient time, or at a minimum, the anesthesiologist feels rushed regarding the preoperative assessment. The importance of a quick, yet reasonably thorough preoperative check, cannot be overemphasized. The systemic effects of severe head injury have been outlined in detail in Chap. 3. The initial examination of a traumatized patient involves a thorough but expeditious search for other serious injuries. The Glasgow Coma Scale (GCS)[119] is universally accepted for the evaluation of the level of consciousness in patients with head injury. The score, ranging from 3 to 15, not only allows a quick assessment of the patient's neurologic status without delaying resuscitation efforts, but is also useful in following the patient's clinical course and prognostication (Table 8-3). Patients with substantial head injuries may have associated cervical spine injuries.[120] Therefore, a radiologic examination should be completed ideally prior to the induction of anesthesia. However, the patient's injuries may necessitate urgent tracheal intubation prior to obtaining cervical films. Moreover, a negative plain film does not completely rule out a spinal cord injury, particularly in young children. In most situations, therefore, manual axial traction should be applied during anesthetic induction and tracheal intubation.[121,122] Because all trauma patients should be considered to have a full stomach, cricoid pressure should also be used. Following tracheal intubation, the patient's neck should be immobilized. The choice of induction agents depends largely on the patient's hemodynamic and intracranial status.

INTRAOPERATIVE MANAGEMENT

Intracranial Procedures

Induction of Anesthesia

In patients who have a normal airway and are hemodynamically stable, a rapid sequence induction of anesthesia with thiopental 3 to 4 mg/kg, lidocaine 1 to 1.5 mg/kg, and a muscle relaxant is indicated. Either a high dose of a nondepolarizing muscle relaxant or succinylcholine 1 mg/kg is appropriate.

Table 8-3 Glasgow coma scale

Eye opening		Best verbal response		Best motor response	
Spontaneous	4	Oriented	5	Obeys commands	6
To speech	3	Confused	4	Localizes to pain	5
To pain	2	Inappropriate	3	Withdraws from pain	4
None	1	Incomprehensible	2	Flexes to pain	3
		None	1	Extends to pain	2
				None	1

The use of succinylcholine is controversial. The disadvantages include a potential increase in ICP from increased CO_2 production and/or cerebral stimulation via afferent muscle activity,[123–125] and potassium release.[126] In a recent study in animals with space-occupying lesions, only a minimal increase in ICP (2.8 mmHg) and decrease in CPP (6.3 mmHg) were reported following succinylcholine administration.[127] Pretreatment with metocurine[128] has been reported to ablate increases in ICP with succinylcholine. In patients with moderate to severe brain injury, no clinically significant increase in ICP or change in flow velocity was observed.[129] The increase in serum potassium is an important consideration, but only at later stages (> 48 h after the initial injury), and not in the initial setting. Therefore, the minimal risks associated with the use of succinylcholine must be balanced against the potentially damaging effects of hypoxemia and hypercapnia as well as the additional effect of straining and coughing on the brain, which can cause far more damage than the transient effects of succinylcholine. Thiopental and lidocaine decrease ICP, and their simultaneous use with succinylcholine further minimizes any adverse effect of succinylcholine.[74,130] In hemodynamically unstable patients, etomidate, 0.2 to 0.3 mg/kg,[45] and a reduced dose of lidocaine in addition to succinylcholine should be given. Alternatively, vecuronium, 0.1 mg/kg, or pancuronium, 0.08 mg/kg, can be used to facilitate intubation although the onset time of paralysis will be slightly longer. Atracurium should probably be avoided because of its hypotensive effects.

Thiopental and propofol are relatively contraindicated in hypovolemic patients. Although, in general, ketamine is the induction agent of choice in hypovolemic patients, concerns about its effect on ICP have contraindicated its use in patients with head trauma. There is no ideal method for treating a head-injured patient with an airway that is anticipated to be difficult. Hypnotics and muscle relaxants should be used cautiously or avoided altogether in situations where the ability to ventilate the patient is in doubt. In a stable cooperative patient, the airway can be anesthetized topically using local anesthetics and direct or fiberoptic laryngoscopy undertaken. Retrograde intubation of the trachea is also an option. Patients with basilar skull fracture are at added risk from nasal tracheal intubations. Bacteria and even the endotracheal tube may pass into the brain through the skull defect.[131] Therefore, if a nasal intubation is attempted, a fiberoptic endoscope should be used to facilitate navigating past the nasopharynx. Long-term nasal intubation cannot be recommended in patients with basilar skull fractures because it may contribute to ascending infections.

Maintenance of Anesthesia

ANESTHETIC REQUIREMENT Although there is a general perception that head-injured patients have reduced anesthetic requirements, this belief has never been substantiated. Archer and coworkers reported that rats subjected to cryogenic injury demonstrated a reduced need for phenobarbital to prevent movement in response to tail clamping.[132] However, Todd and coworkers could not demonstrate a similar reduction in halothane requirement using an identical model.[133] Similarly, Shapira and coworkers could not demonstrate any reduction in halothane requirement in experimental head injury in rats until near-fatal injury had been inflicted.[134] Because inadequate anesthesia in a head-injured patient may cause increased cerebral stimulation and resultant increased $CMRO_2$, CBF, and possibly ICP, the anesthesiologist must always be on guard against such occurrences. However, there is presently no satisfactory method of assessing the depth of anesthesia in head-injured patients, in whom the cardiovascular signs are at best unreliable, and muscle movements are usually prevented with neuromuscular blockade.

ANESTHETIC AGENTS AND TECHNIQUE The choice will partly depend on the patient's preoperative neurologic status and the presence of associated injuries. The goal is to optimize cerebral perfusion and prevent increase in ICP. In general, intravenous agents (except ketamine) decrease $CMRO_2$ and CBF and are the most appropriate for use in patients with severe head injury. In hemodynamically stable patients not expected to be awakened at the end of the procedure, a continuous thiopental infusion in the dose of 4 to 5 mg/kg per h constitutes an excellent anesthetic.

Inhalation agents can also be used in most head-injured patients. Low-dose isoflurane is appropriate in patients with mild injury expected to be awakened at the end of the procedure. It can also be used to control systemic hypertension. Isoflurane is preferred to enflurane and halothane because it does not cause an increase in ICP during hypocapnia.[135] In addition, in prolonged cases, CSF production and absorption become important considerations, and isoflurane neither increases the rate of formation nor the resistance to absorption of CSF.[136] On the other hand, although nitrous oxide can be safely used during elective neurosurgery,[137] it can expand the volume of intracranial air and should not be used prior to dural opening if there is a possibility of preexisting intracranial air. Nitrous oxide can also cause an increase in CBF and ICP.[138,139] Therefore, although the use of nitrous oxide in neurosurgical anesthesia remains controversial,[140] it is best avoided in the management of patients with an acute head injury. The use of opioids and other adjuncts such as lidocaine have already been discussed previously.

TREATMENT OF INTRACRANIAL HYPERTENSION The principles of management of intracranial hypertension have already been outlined in a previous section headed Control of ICP. It is useful and practical to always think of all three intracranial components in planning the anesthetic approach. Essentially, hyperventilation to maintain Pa_{CO_2} between 25 to 33 mmHg should be initiated in patients with intracranial hypertension. If available, cerebral venous oxygen saturation measurements may allow optimal determination of the level of hyperventilation because inadequate CBF (global) will result in a widened AVD_{O_2} and, therefore, a low cerebral venous oxygen saturation, provided that there is an absence of arterial hypoxemia or anemia (see below). Mannitol and furosemide should be given early to reduce the risk of herniation as well as ischemia.

The importance of cerebral venous congestion has already been mentioned, but this topic is often neglected in anesthetic management and, therefore, should be reemphasized. In addition to making sure that the neck veins are not compressed, venous drainage should also be promoted by placing the patient in a slightly head-up position. Certainly, placement of a patient with high ICP in a steep Trendelenburg position for insertion of a central venous catheter should be discouraged. Excessive rotation of the head should also be curtailed to prevent compression of the internal jugular veins. On the other hand, it is possible that a moderate head-up position to reduce ICP may cause systemic hypotension, with an overall decrease in CPP.[20,141] Feldman and coworkers observed that, although MAP decreased when the head was elevated, ICP also decreased, and there was no significant change in CPP or CBF.[51] As long as MAP is kept above acceptable levels (> 80 mmHg), elevation of the patient's head by 30° to treat increased ICP is appropriate, although this may not be possible because of surgical requirements. In addition, the head-up position also increases the risk of intraoperative venous air embolism.

Neuromuscular blockade should be maintained in all patients intraoperatively to prevent coughing or straining. Excessive airway pressure should be avoided because the intrathoracic pressure is transmitted to the internal jugular vein, and a high pressure may interfere with cerebral venous drainage. Similarly, the advantages of positive end-expiratory pressure (PEEP) must be balanced against this potential risk and should be used with caution and limited to < 10 mmHg. Vecuronium is the preferred muscle relaxant because pancuronium may cause hypertension and tachycardia, and atracurium may cause hypotension. Atracurium, however, offers an advantage in patients on chronic dilantin therapy because its action is not antagonized.[142] Laudanosine, a metabolite of atracurium, has been reported to be a central nervous system stimulant, but its clinical signifiance is unknown.

CSF drainage through a ventricular catheter can quickly reduce ICP and should be considered if one has been placed.

If acute brain swelling develops intraoperatively, correctable causes including hypercapnia, hypoxemia, hypertension, and venous obstruction should be immediately ruled out. If the swelling does not respond to hyperventilation and the administration of osmotic and/or loop diuretic, a trial dose of thiopental, 150 to 200 mg, should be given, and if effective, a continuous infusion implemented. In contrast, steroids, though routinely given to neurosurgical patients, have not been shown to be useful in head-injured patients.[143–145] There is, however, interest in the use of the 21-aminosteroids which are potent lipid antioxidants devoid of glucocorticoid action.[146] Its definitive use, however, must await the results of clinical trials.

MONITORING Basic monitoring should include electrocardiography, esophageal stethoscope, temperature, urine output, pulse oximetry, and noninvasive systemic blood pressure measurements. Special emphasis should be placed on end-tidal CO_2 monitoring as a means of continuously assessing the level of hyperventilation. We routinely monitor invasive arterial blood pressure and measure frequent arterial samples. Additionally, levels of hematocrit, electrolytes and coagulation should also be measured. Central venous pressure monitoring allows a more rational approach to fluid replacement, particularly when osmotic diuretics are used. Pulmonary artery pressure is monitored in the elderly or in those with known cardiac history. However, central venous pressure monitoring is often not possible because of time constraints. Precordial Doppler should be used if venous air embolism is considered to be a risk.

Advanced techniques of monitoring neurosurgical patients include ICP monitor, the use of jugular bulb catheters to monitor the cerebral venous oxygen saturation (Sjv_{O_2}), and the transcranial Doppler (TCD).

ICP Monitoring If a patient requires urgent surgical care for an extracranial problem (e.g., splenectomy) before a thorough radiologic examination of the central nervous system is complete, an ICP monitor should be placed. This allows continous assessment of intracranial hemodynamics and can be extremely useful in the perioperative management. Nonsurgical techniques can be used to treat increases in ICP until such time as the cause can be investigated or surgically addressed. If the patient's most threatening problem is neurosurgical, then an ICP monitor should not be placed and the patient should proceed directly to the operating room as soon as possible.

Sjv_{O_2} Monitoring A jugular bulb catheter to monitor Sjv_{O_2} can usually be placed within a matter of minutes.[147] In head-injured patients we do not use the Trendelenburg position to place the catheter as this position may aggravate intracranial hypertension. When a cervical spine injury has not been ruled out, the patient's neck should be placed in a neutral position. Successful cannulation of the jugular bulb in this position has been well documented by Goetting and coworkers.[148] Sjv_{O_2} monitoring can be used to guide the level of hyperventilation. We have documented instances of excessive hyperventilation (Pa_{CO_2} = 20 to 25 mm Hg) leading to potential cerebral ischemia (Sjv_{O_2} < 50 percent) in some traumatized patients with increased ICPs. In these patients, decreasing the hyperventilation has, in some cases, improved cerebral perfusion and decreased ICP.

Sheinberg and coworkers reported that the use of continuous Sjv_{O_2} monitoring with a fiberoptic catheter enabled them to detect episodes of cerebral desaturation associated with intracranial hypertension, hypocapnia, systemic hypotension, and cerebral vasospasm in ICU patients.[149] Cruz has also recently reported his experience with the use of Sjv_{O_2} monitoring in the management of head-injured patients in the intensive care unit.[150] However, as many as half of the episodes identified as cerebral desaturation (Sjv_{O_2} < 50 percent) were false positives in Sheinberg's study.[149] This is consistent with our preliminary experience using the fiberoptic catheter in the operating room. In this setting, we have found that intermittent blood sampling through a 5.25-inch, 16-gauge catheter to be reliable and useful.[147]

TCD Monitoring The transcranial Doppler is a noninvasive monitor that measures cerebral blood flow velocity. Blood flow velocity is calculated by measuring the shift in frequency spectra of the Doppler signal. Although many of the intracranial arteries may be insonated, the middle cerebral artery is easy to detect and receives most of the blood flow from the internal carotid artery. The role of TCD monitoring in the head-injured patient has been the subject of many recent studies.[30,151,152] Flow velocity waveform patterns have been correlated with various pathologic states. A normal TCD flow velocity waveform pattern resembles a normal arterial pressure waveform. As ICP increases, there is a characteristic loss of the diastolic component of the waveform. If the ICP continues to increase there will be a reversal of flow during diastole. This pattern has been termed "to-and-fro flow" or "oscillating flow." This pattern is consistent with ICPs that will lead to cessation of cerebral blood flow and death if not corrected (Fig. 8-5).[153–156] The pulsatility index (PI) is one way of mathematically describing the waveform pattern. It is calculated by dividing the systolic-diastolic velocity difference by the mean velocity. A very large PI has been associated with spike and oscillating patterns. It has been used to noninvasively predict increased ICP.[16] However, when we examined the ability of the TCD to predict intracranial hypertension we found that it correlated better with CPP than with ICP.[30] The pulsatility index also has limitations. The PI will increase when there is "extrinsic" compression as seen with an increased ICP. However, an increase in the "intrinsic" resistance of a vessel (e.g., vasoconstriction from hyperventilation) will also cause the PI to increase. Interpretation of the PI is easier in extreme cases. For instance, in severe intracranial hypertension, not only will the PI be increased but an oscillating flow pattern will also develop if the MAP is not adequate. Reversal of flow, i.e., retrograde flow during diastole, is indicative of intracranial circulatory arrest and has been associated with brain death.[155,157,158] The diagnosis of vasospasm usually requires very high velocities and an elevated ratio of MCA (middle cerebral artery) velocity to extracranial ICA (internal carotid artery) velocity.[14,15] The TCD has been useful in detecting hyperemic states indicated by high flow velocities with normal to low PI values.

OTHER CONSIDERATIONS
Brain Temperature Brain temperature has increasingly been shown to affect the extent of brain injury during ischemia. In experimental models, hypothermia has been shown to decrease[50] and hyperthermia to increase the infarct size during ischemia.[51,159] Brain temperature often exceeds systemic temperature, although the gradient may be small.[160] Patients are likely to be hypothermic at the time of initial presentation. It may be prudent not to actively rewarm

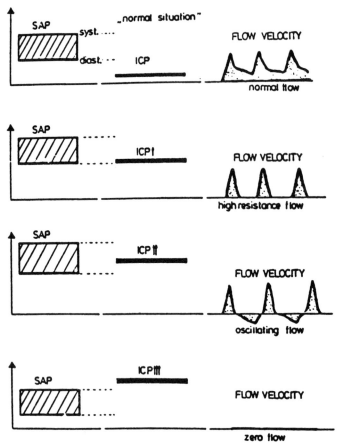

Figure 8-5 Relationship between systemic arterial blood pressure (SAP), intracranial pressure (ICP), and flow velocity as measured in the middle cerebral artery by transcranial Doppler ultrasonography (TCD). In all displayed TCD spectra, upward deflections indicate blood flow toward the Doppler probe, whereas downward deflections appear with flow directions away from the probe. (*From Hassler et al.*[155] *With permission.*)

patients unless their temperature is low enough to pose additional risks from dysrhythmias or coagulopathy. Preliminary clinical trials of mild to moderate hypothermia therapy for the treatment of head injury have demonstrated efficacy in the treatment of intracranial hypertension and potential improvement in outcome.[54,55]

Intraoperative Hypotension   Intraoperative hypotension should be treated vigorously with fluid therapy. At the same time, a noncranial cause must be sought. Vasopressors may be necessary if a prompt response to fluid infusion therapy is not evident. The risk of sudden significant hypotension immediately following release of intracranial pressure from a subdural or an epidural hematoma has already been mentioned.

Intraoperative Hypertension Mild to moderate intraoperative hypertension requires no treatment, although severe hypertension (mean arterial pressure > 130 to 140 mmHg) should be treated to prevent the development of brain edema. Low dose isoflurane can be used as an adjunct to intravenous agents to control blood pressure response to surgical stimulation provided that the patient is being hyperventilated. If necessary, esmolol (500 μg/kg in divided doses), labetalol (5 to 10 mg-boluses) or propranolol (0.5 to 1.0 mg-boluses) can be used safely because none of these agents has any direct influence on intracranial hemodynamics. Vasodilators, such as sodium nitroprusside and nitroglycerin, can cause an increase in ICP and probably should not be used unless ICP is being monitored.[161,162]

Emergence and Recovery

Patients with severe head injury requiring surgery usually need continuing postoperative care in the neurointensive care unit, and their trachea cannot be extubated at the end of the procedure. Therapy that has begun should be continued; muscle paralysis should initially be maintained to allow optimal ventilation and prevent coughing and movement during transport to radiology suites for CT scanning. Hyperventilation should be continued but gradually tapered provided that ICP can be controlled. Systemic blood pressure should be maintained at greater than a mean of 90 mmHg, and any coagulation defect should be treated. For optimal treatment, continuous ICP monitoring is essential. Continuous jugular bulb oximetry monitoring has been advocated by some investigators, although the high false-positive rate dictates that actual confirmation with laboratory determination of blood gases is necessary before definitive action can be taken based on the oximetry readings.

In patients with mild to moderate head injury (GCS score 12 to 15) undergoing evacuation of an epidural or subdural hematoma, it is not unreasonable to allow the patient to wake up at the end of the procedure. Care must be taken to avoid excessive coughing and bucking, which may cause not only a transient increase in ICP, but more importantly, an increased risk of venous bleeding. Judicious use of narcotics is essential as oversedation will lead to respiratory depression, retention of CO_2, and consequent increase in ICP. Intravenous lidocaine, given up to 3 mg/kg in divided doses during emergence, has a negligible effect on ventilation and causes minimal sedation, but it suppresses coughing effectively, and is a useful adjunct during this difficult period. A practical anesthetic approach to the patient with a severe head injury is outlined in Fig. 8-6.

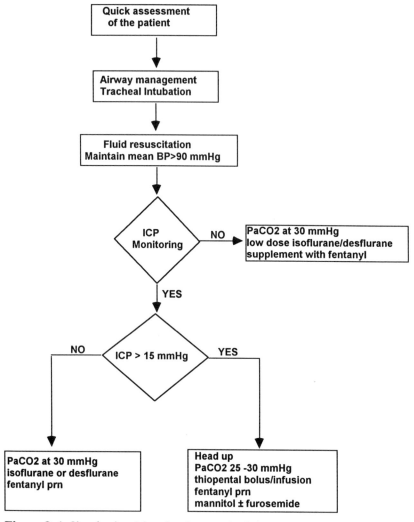

Figure 8-6 Simple algorithm for the anesthetic management of an acutely head-injured patient.

EXTRACRANIAL PROCEDURES

As briefly alluded to in the preceding section, it is not uncommon that a severely head-injured patient undergoes emergency surgery for a nonneurosurgical procedure. Depending on the urgency of the extracranial procedure, the patient may or may not be harboring a surgically treatable intracranial lesion. Patients with mild to moderate head injury may also present for unrelated surgical procedures, such as reduction and fixation of a fractured femur, on a semielective basis when the patient's condition has stabilized. Although the basic principles of neuroresuscitation remain the same, the treatment of these two situations are different and will be discussed separately. Several important points that are often forgotten when dealing with these patients are (1) both the brain injury and systemic injury are continuously evolving, (2) a preoperative normal or seminormal CT scan does not preclude development of edema or delayed hemorrhage, (3) the systemic circulation does not reflect the state of the cerebral circulation, and (4) fluid resuscitation that is essential for the systemic circulation may be detrimental to the brain. The preoperatvie assessment of a head-injured patient scheduled for nonneuro-surgical procedures is the same as the assessment of an acutely injured patient scheduled for a craniotomy procedure.

Emergency Procedures

The principles governing emergency procedures are the same as outlined previously under the section headed Intracranial Procedures. Because of the emergent nature, the patient often arrives with his or her trachea already intubated with muscle paralysis effected by the use of neuromuscular blockade. Thus, the level of consciousness cannot be assessed. The neurologic status can only be inferred from the GCS score at the time of initial resuscitation. Occasionally there is not even enough time to obtain a CT scan. All these patients should have ICP monitoring placed as soon as possible. Vigorous fluid resuscitation is often necessary, but may aggravate cerebral edema. Without ICP monitoring, it is difficult to gauge optimal thereapy. If not interfering with the surgical procedure, and tolerated by the patient hemodynamically, a slight head-up position is advocated. In centers where ICP monitoring is not routinely used, the use of the noninvasive TCD may reveal additional useful information regarding the intracranial circulation.[30] Certainly, in patients with elevated ICP approaching the systemic blood pressure, the diagnosis of intracranial circulatory arrest can be made readily with TCD.[155–157,163] If not quickly reversed, the presence of this oscillating flow pattern on TCD inevitably results in death.

   Colloid may be preferable to crystalloid if a large amount of fluid therapy is required. Fluid overload must be avoided, however, because elevation of central venous pressure may impede cerebral venous drainage and cause a further increase in ICP and cerebral edema.

Elective Procedures

The difficulty with elective procedures is the problem of monitoring. As the neurologic status can be monitored in patients with mild to moderate head injury (GCS score > 12), they usually do not require ICP monitoring. However, they may still have physiologic disturbances including increased intracranial elastance and impaired autoregulation. Moreoever, the imposition of general anesthesia removes the ability to monitor the neurologic status, and preoperative placement of ICP monitoring may be required. This is particularly important in patients with a fluctuating level of consciousness and applies also during surgical procedures where large intraoperative fluid shift is anticipated. This caution would also apply to patients with abnormal CT scans who are functionally alert. The anesthetic management should be based on the assumption that these patients, although awake, have decreased intracranial compliance (increased elastance) and are prone to develop cerebral edema and increased ICP.

Induced hypotension is sometimes requested by orthopedic surgeons during spine-stabilizing procedures in patients with intact spinal cord function or fixed spinal cord injury. Many of these patients suffer concomitant head injury, and the cerebral circulation may behave abnormally. Certainly induced hypotension is contraindicated in patients with a known head injury. But even in patients who have only suffered a brief concussion, the use of this technique remains hazardous because the autoregulatory capacity may still be imparied.[164]

SUMMARY

The acutely head-injured patient represents an anesthetic challenge with potential multiple system involvement. Adherence to basic principles and adoption of a systematic approach would allow the anesthesiologist to implement a rational therapy with optimal patient outcome.

REFERENCES

1. Aaslid R, Lindegaard K-F, Sorteberg W, et al: Cerebral autoregulation dynamics in humans. *Stroke* 20:45, 1989.

2. Aaslid R, Newell DW, Stooss R, et al: Simultaneous arterial and venous transcranial Doppler assessment of cerebral autoregulation dynamics. *Stroke* 22:1148, 1991.

3. Lobato RD, Rivas JJ, Gomez PA, et al: Head-injured patients who talk and deteriorate into coma: Analysis of 211 cases studied with computerized tomography. *J Neurosurg* 75:256, 1991.

4. Rockswold GI, Leonard PR, Nagib MG: Analysis of management in thirty-three closed head injury patients who "talked and deteriorated." *Neurosurgery* 21:51, 1987.

5. Graham DI, Adams JH, Doyle D: Ischaemic brain damage in fatal nonmissile head injuries. *J Neurol Sci 39:213, 1978.*

6. Graham DI, Ford I, Adams JH, et al: Ischemic brain damage is still common in fatal nonmissile head injury. *J Neurol Neurosurg Psychiatry* 52:346, 1989.

7. Obrist WD, Langfitt TW, Jaggi JL, et al: Cerebral blood flow and metabolism in comatose patients with acute head injury. *J Neurosurg* 61:241, 1984.

8. Roberston CS, Contant CF, Gokaslan ZL, et al: Cerebral blood flow, arteriovenous oxygen difference, and outcome in head-injured patients. *J Neurol Neurosurg Psychiatry* 55:594, 1992.

9. Bouma GJ, Muizelaar JP, Choi SC, et al: Cerebral circulation and metabolism after severe traumatic brain injury: The elusive role of ischemia. *J Neurosurg* 75:685, 1991.

10. Bouma GJ, Muizelaar JP: Cerebral blood flow, cerebral blood volume, and cerebrovascular reactivity after severe head injury. *J Neurotrauma* 9:S333, 1992.

11. Marion DW, Darby J, Yonas H: Acute regional cerebral blood flow changes caused by severe head injuries. *J Neurosurg* 74:407, 1991.

12. Bouma GJ, Muizelaar JP, Stringer WA, et al: Ultraearly evaluation of regional cerebral blood flow in severely head-injured patients using xenon-enhanced computerized tomography. *J Neurosurg* 77:360, 1992.

13. Jaggi JL, Obrist WD, Gennarelli TA, et al: Relationship of early cerebral blood flow and metabolism to outcome in acute head injury. *J Neurosurg* 72:176, 1990.

14. Weber M, Grolimund P, Seiler RW: Evaluation of posttraumatic cerebral blood flow velocities by transcranial Doppler ultrasonography. *Neurosurgery* 27:106, 1990.

15. Martin NA, Doberstein C, Zane C, et al: Posttraumatic cerebral arterial spasm: transcranial Doppler ultrasound, cerebral blood flow, and angiographic findings. *J Neurosurg* 77:575, 1992.

16. Chan KH, Dearden NM, Miller JD: The significance of posttraumatic increase in cerebral blood flow velocity: A transcranial Doppler ultrasound study. *Neurosurgery* 30:697, 1992.

17. Marmarou A, Anderson RL, Ward JD, et al: Impact of ICP instability and hypotension on outcome in patients with severe head trauma. *J Neurosurg* 75:S59, 1991.

18. Cold GE: Cerebral blood flow in acute head injury. The regulation of cerebral blood flow and metabolism during the acute phase of head injury, and its significance for therapy. *Acta Neurochir Suppl (Wien)* 49:1, 1990.

19. Schalen W, Messeter K, Nordstrom CH: Cerebral vasoreactivity and the prediction of outcome in severe traumatic brain lesions. *Acta Anaesthesiol Scand* 35:113, 1991.

20. Rosner MJ, Daughton S: Cerebral perfusion pressure management in head injury. *J Trauma* 30:933, 1990.

21. Enevoldsen EM, Jensen FT: Autoregulation and CO_2 responses of cerebral blood flow in patients with acute severe head injury. *J Neurosurg* 48:689, 1978.

22. Baker AJ, Moulton RJ, Macmillan VH, et al: Excitatory amino acids in cerebrospinal fluid following traumatic brain injury in humans. *J Neurosurg* 79:369, 1993.

23. Marmarou A, Shulman K, Lamorgese J: Compartmental analysis of compliance and outflow resistance of the cerebrospinal fluid system. *J Neurosurg* 43:523, 1976.

24. Maset AL, Marmarou A, Ward JD, et al: Pressure-volume index in head injury. *J Neurosurg* 67:832, 1987.

25. Miller JD, Becker DP, Ward JD, et al: Significance of intracranial hypertension in severe head injury. *J Neurosurg* 47:503, 1977.

26. Miller JD, Butterworth JF, Gudeman SK, et al: Further experience in the management of severe head injury. *J Neurosurg* 54:289, 1981.

27. Saul TG, Ducker TB: Effect of intracranial pressure monitoring and aggressive treatment on mortality in severe head injury. *J Neurosurg* 56:498, 1982.

28. Marshall LF, Smith RW, Shapiro HM: The outcome with aggressive treatment in severe head injuries. II. Acute and chronic barbiturate administration in the management of head injury. *J Neurosurg* 50:26, 1979.

29. Crutchfield JS, Narayan RK, Robertson CS, et al: Evaluation of a fiberoptic intracranial pressure monitor. *J Neurosurg* 72:482, 1990.

30. Mayberg TS, Lam AM: Perioperative use of transcranial doppler in patients with head injury. *Anesth Analg* 74:S197, 1992.

31. Chan K, Miller JD, Dearden NM, et al: The effect of changes in cerebral perfusion pressure upon middle cerebral artery blood flow velocity and jugular bulb venous oxygen saturation after severe brain injury. *J Neurosurg* 77:55, 1992.

32. Stuart GG, Merry GS, Smith JA, et al: Severe head injury managed without intracranial pressure monitoring. *J Neurosurg* 59:601, 1983.

33. McManus ML, Strange K: Acute volume regulation of brain cells in response to hypertonic challenge. *Anesthesiology* 78:1132, 1993.

34. Hartwell RC, Sutton LN: Mannitol, intracranial pressure, and vasogenic edema. *Neurosurgery* 32:444, 1993.

35. Smith HP, Kelly DL, McWhorter JM, et al: Comparison of mannitol regimens in patients with severe head injury undergoing intracranial monitoring. *J Neurosurg* 65:820, 1986.

36. Fisher B, Thomas D, Peterson B: Hypertonic saline lowers raised intracranial pressure in children after head trauma. *J Neurosurg Anesthesiol* 4:4, 1992.

37. Battistella FD, Wisner DH: Combined hemorrhagic shock and head injury: Effects of hypertonic saline [7.5%] resuscitation. *J Trauma* 31:182, 1991.

38. Grubb RL, Raichle ME, Eichling JO, et al: The effects of changes in Pa_{CO_2} on cerebral blood volume, blood flow, and vascular mean transit time. *Stroke* 5:630, 1974.

39. Muizelaar JP, Marmarou A, Ward JD, et al: Adverse effects of prolonged hyperventilation in patients with severe head injury: A randomized clinical trial. *J Neurosurg* 75:731, 1991.

40. Wolf AL, Lion L, Marmarou A, et al: Effect of THAM upon outcome in severe head injury. *J Neurosurg* 78:54, 1993.

41. Muizelaar JP, Wei EP, Kontos HA, et al: Mannitol causes compensatory cerebral vasoconstriction and vasodilatation in response to blood viscosity changes. *J Neurosurg* 59:822, 1983.

42. Muizelaar JP, Lutz HH III, Becker DP. Effect of mannitol on ICP and CBF and correlation with pressure autoregulation in severely head-injured patients. *J Neurosurg* 61:700, 1984.

43. Ravussin P, Archer DP, Tyler JL, et al: Effects of rapid mannitol infusion on cerebral blood volume. A positron emission tomography study in dogs and man. *J Neurosurg* 64:104, 1986.

44. Ravussin P, Abou-Madi M, Archer D, et al: Changes in CSF pressure after mannitol in patients with and without elevated CSF pressure. *J Neurosurg* 69:869, 1988.

45. Moss E, Powell D, Gibson RM, et al: Effect of etomidate on intracranial pressure and cerebral perfusion pressure. *Br J Anaesth* 51:347, 1979.

46. Kastrup J, Petersen P, Dejgard A: Intravenous lidocaine and cerebral blood flow: impaired microvascular reactivity in diabetic patients. *J Clin Pharmacol* 30:318, 1990.

47. Michenfelder JD, Theye RA: The interdependency of cerebral functional and metabolic effects following massive doses of thiopental in the dog. *Anesthesiology* 41:231, 1974.

48. Ward JD, Becker DP, Miller JD, et al: Failure of prophylactic barbiturate coma in the treatment of severe head injury. *J Neurosurg* 62:383, 1985.

49. Eisenberg HM, Frankowski RF, Contant CF, et al: High-dose barbiturate control of elevated intracranial pressure in patients with severe head injury. *J Neurosurg* 69:15, 1988.

50. Xue D, Huang ZG, Smith KE, et al: Immediate or delayed mild hypothermia prevents focal cerebral infarction. *Brain Res* 587:66, 1992.

51. Ginsberg MD, Sternau LL, Globus MY, et al: Therapeutic modulation of brain temperature: Relevance to ischemic brain injury. *Cerebrovasc Brain Metab Rev* 4:189, 1992.

52. Busto R, Globus MY-T, Dietrich WD, et al: Effect of mild hypothermia on ischemia-induced release of neurotransmitters and free fatty acids in rat brain. *Stroke* 20:904, 1989.

53. Clifton GI, Jiang JY, Lyeth BG: Marked protection by moderate hypothermia after experimental traumatic brain injury. *J Cereb Blood Flow Metab* 11:114, 1991.

54. Marion DW, Obrist WD, Carlier PM, et al: The use of moderate therapeutic hypothermia for patients with severe head injuries: A preliminary report. *J Neurosurg* 79:354, 1993.

55. Shiozaki T, Sugimoto H, Taneda M, et al: Effect of mild hypothermia on uncontrollable intracranial hypertension after severe head injury. *J Neurosurg* 79:363, 1993.

56. Clifton GL, Allen S, Berry J, et al: Systemic hypothermia in treatment of brain injury. *J Neurotrauma* 9:S487, 1992.

57. Feldman Z, Kanter MJ, Robertson CS, et al: Effect of head elevation on intracranial pressure, cerebral perfusion pressure, and cerebral blood flow in head-injured patients. *J Neurosurg* 76:207, 1992.

58. Artru AA: New concepts concerning anesthetic effects on intracranial dynamics: Cerebral spinal fluid and cerebral blood volume. *ASA Annual Refresher Course Lecture* 133, 1987.

59. Foxworthy JC, Artru AA: Cerebrospinal fluid dynamics and brain tissue composition following intravenous infusions of hypertonic saline in anesthetized rabbits. *J Neurosurg Anesthesiol* 2:256, 1990.

60. Sahar A, Tsipstein E: Effects of mannitol and furosemide on the rate of formation of cerebrospinal fluid. *Exp Neurol* 60:584, 1978.

61. Piek J, Chesnut RM, Marshall LF, et al: Extracranial complications of head injury. *J Neurosurgery* 77:901, 1992.

62. Cushing H: Concerning a definite regulatory mechanism of the vaso-motor centre which controls blood pressure during cerebral compression. *Johns Hopkins Hospital Bulletin* 126:290, 1901.

63. Pfenniger EG, Lindner KH: Arterial blood gases in patients with acute head injury at the accident site and upon hospital admission. *Acta Anaesthesiol Scand* 35:148, 1991.

64. Fieschi C, Battistini N, Deduschi A, et al: Regional cerebral blood flow and intraventricular pressure in acute head injuries. *J Neurol Neurosurg Psychiatry* 37:1378, 1974.

65. Hoyer S, Piscol K, Stoeckel H, et al: CBF and metabolism in patients wtih acute brain injury with regard to autoregulation. *Eur Neurol* 8:174, 1972.

66. Overgaard J, Tweed WA: Cerebral circulation after head injury. I. Cerebral blood flow and its regulation after closed head injury with emphasis on clinical correlations. *J Neurosurg* 41:531, 1974.

67. Cold GE: Does acute hyperventilation provoke cerebral oligaemia in comatose patients after acute head injury? *Acta Neurochir (Wien)* 96:100, 1989.

68. Steen PA, Milde JH, Michenfelder JD: Cerebral metabolic and vascular effects

of barbiturate therapy following complete global ischemia. *J Neurochemistry* 31:1317, 1978.

69. Herregods L, Verbeke J, Rolly G, et al: Effect of propofol on elevated intracranial pressure. Preliminary results. *Anaesthesia* 43:107, 1990.

70. Pinaud M, Lelausque J-N, Chetanneau A, et al: Effects of Propofol on cerebral hemodynamics and metabolism in patients with brain trauma. *Anesthesiology* 73:404, 1990.

71. Van Hemelrijck J, Fitch W, Mattheussen M, et al: Effect of propofol on cerebral circulation and autoregulation in the baboon. *Anesth Analg* 71:49, 1988.

72. Vandesteene A, Trempont V, Engelman E, et al: Effect of propofol on cerebral blood flow and metabolism in man. *Anaesthesia* 43:42, 1988.

73. Bedford RF, Winn HR, Tyson G, et al: Lidocaine prevents increased ICP after endotracheal intubation. In Shulman K (ed): *Intracranial Pressure IV,* Berlin, Springer-Verlag, 1980:595.

74. Hamill JF, Bedford RF, Weaver DC, et al: Lidocaine before endotracheal intubation: Intravenous or laryngotracheal? *Anesthesiology* 55:578, 1981.

75. Wojciechowski ZJ, Lam AM, Eng CC, et al: Effect of intravenous lidocaine on cerebral blood flow velocity during endotracheal intubation. *Anesthesiology* 77:A194, 1992.

76. Gibbs JM: The effect of intravenous ketamine on cerebrospinal fluid pressure. *Br J Anaesth* 44:1298, 1972.

77. Shapiro HM, Wyte SR, Harris AB: Ketamine anaesthesia in patients with intracranial pathology. *Br J Anaesth* 44:1200, 1972.

78. Dawson B, Michenfelder JD, Theye RA: Effect of ketamine on canine cerebral blood flow and metabolism: Modification by prior administration of thiopental. *Anesth Analg* 50:443, 1971.

79. Takeshita H, Okuda Y, Sari A: The effects of ketamine on cerebral circulation and metabolism in man. *Anesthesiology* 36:69, 1972.

80. Pfenninger E, Dick W, Ahnefeld FW: The influence of ketamine on both normal and raised intracranial pressure of artifically ventilated animals. *Eur J Anaesthesiol* 2:297, 1985.

81. Schwedler M, Miletich DJ, Albrecht RF: Cerebral blood flow and metabolism following ketamine administration. *Can Anaesth Soc J* 29:222, 1982.

82. Thorsen T, Gran L: Ketamine/diazepam infusion anaesthesia with special attention to the effect on cerebrospinal fluid pressure and arterial blood pressure. *Acta Anaesth Scand* 24:1, 1980.

83. Mayberg TS, Lam AM, Winn HR, et al: The effect of ketamine on cerebral blood flow velocity and intracranial pressure during isoflurane-nitrous oxide anesthesia in humans. *Anesthesiology* 79:A204, 1993.

84. Rothman SM, Olney JW: Glutamate and the pathophysiology of hypoxic-ischemic brain damage. *Ann Neurol* 19:105, 1986.

85. Shapira Y, Artru AA, Lam AM: Ketamine decreases cerebral infarct volume and improves neurological outcome following experimental head trauma in rats. *J Neurosurg Anesthesiol* 4:231, 1992.

86. Sperry RJ, Bailey PL, Reichman MV, et al: Fentanyl and sufentanil increase intracranial pressure in head trauma patients. *Anesthesiology* 77:416, 1992.

87. Marx W, Shah N, Long C, et al: Sufentanil, alfentanil and fentanyl: Impact on cerebrospinal fluid pressure in patients with brain tumors. *J Neurosurg Anesth* 1:3, 1989.

88. Mayer N, Weinstabl C, Podreka I, et al: Sufentanil does not increase cerebral blood flow in healthy human volunteers. *Anesthesiology* 73:240, 1990.

89. Trindle MR, Dodson BA, Rampil IJ: Effects of fentanyl versus sufentanil in equianesthetic doses on middle cerebral artery blood flow velocity. *Anesthesiology* 78:454, 1993.

90. Jacques A, Durbec O, Viviand X, et al: Sufentanil increases intracranial pressure in patients with head trauma. *Anesthesiology* 79:493, 1993.

91. Mayberg TS, Lam Am, Eng CC, et al: The effect of alfentanil on cerebral blood flow velocity and intracranial pressure during isoflurane-nitrous oxide anesthesia in humans. *Anesthesiology* 78:288, 1993.

92. Slee TA, Lam AM, Winn HR: Cerebral blood flow velocity and intracranial pressure response to sufentanil—a dose response study. *Anesthesiology* 73:A176, 1990.

93. Markovitz BP, Duhaime A, Sutton LS, et al: Effects of alfentanil on intracranial pressure in children undergoing ventriculoperitoneal shunt revisions. *Anesthesiology* 76:71, 1992.

94. Weinstabl C, Mayer N, Richling B, et al: Effect of sufentanil on intracranial pressure in neurosurgical patients. *Anaesthesia* 46:837, 1991.

95. Weinstabl C, Mayer N, Spiss CK: Sufentanil decreases cerebral blood flow velocity in patients with elevated intracranial pressure. *Eur J Anaesthesiol* 9:481, 1992.

96. From RP, Warner DS, Todd MM, et al: Anesthesia for craniotomy: A double-blind comparisons of alfentanil, fentanyl, and sufentanil. *Anesthesiology* 73:896, 1990.

97. Young WL: Effects of desflurane on the central nervous system. *Anesth Analg* 75:S32, 1992.

98. Ornstein E, Young WL, Fleischer L, et al: Desflurane and isoflurane have similar effects on cerebral blood flow in patients with intracranial mass lesions. *Anesthesiology* 79:498, 1993.

99. Eng C, Lam AM, Mayberg TS, et al: The influence of propofol with and without nitrous oxide on cerebral blood flow velocity and CO_2 reactivity in humans. *Anesthesiology* 77:872, 1992.

100. Fox J, Gelb AW, Enns J, et al: The responsiveness of cerebral blood flow to changes in arterial carbon dioxide is maintained during propofol-nitrous oxide anesthesia in humans. *Anesthesiology* 77:453, 1992.

101. Lanier WL, Stangland KJ, Scheithauer BW, et al: The effects of dextrose infusion and head position on neurologic outcome after complete cerebral ischemia in primates: Examination of a model. *Anesthesiology* 66:39, 1987.

102. Pulsinelli WA, Levy DE, Sigsbee B, et al: Increased damage after ischemic stroke in patients with hyperglycemia with or without established diabetes mellitus. *Am J Med* 74:540, 1983.

103. De Salles AAF, Muizelaar JP, Young HF: Hyperglycemia, cerebrospinal fluid lactic acidosis, and cerebral blood flow in severely head-injured patients. *Neurosurgery* 21:45, 1987.

104. Young B, Ott L, Dempsey R, et al: Relationship between admission hyperglycemia and neurologic outcome of severely brain-injured patients. *Ann Surg* 210:466, 1989.

105. Lam AM, Winn HR, Cullen BF, et al: Hyperglycemia and neurological outcome in patients with head injury. *J Neurosurg* 75:545, 1991.

106. Michaud LJ, Rivara FP, Longstreth WT Jr, et al: Elevated initial blood glucose levels and poor outcome following severe brain injuries in children. *J Trauma* 31:1356, 1991.

107. Zornow MH, Todd MM, Moore SS: The acute cerebral effects of changes in plasma osmolality and oncotic pressure. *Anesthesiology* 67:936, 1987.

108. Kaieda R, Todd MM, Cook LN, et al: Acute effects of changing plasma osmolality and colloid osmotic pressure on brain edema formation after cryogenic injury in the rabbit. *Neurosurgery* 24:671, 1989.

109. Cully MD, Larson CP, Silverberg GD: Hetastarch coagulopathy in a neurosurgical patient. *Anesthesiology* 66:706, 1987.

110. Gunnar W, Kane J, Barrett J: Cerebral blood flow following hypertonic saline resuscitation in an experimental model of hemorrhagic shock and head injury. *Braz J Med Biol Res* 22:287, 1989.

111. Prough DS, Johnson JC, Stump DA, et al: Effects of hypertonic saline versus lactated Ringer's solution on cerebral oxygen transport during resuscitation from hemorrhagic shock. *J Neurosurg* 64:627, 1986.

112. Prough DS, Whitley JM, Taylor CL, et al: Regional cerebral blood flow following resuscitation from hemorrhagic shock with hypertonic saline. Influence of a subdural mass. *Anesthesiology* 75:319, 1991.

113. van der Sande JJ, Veltkamp JJ, Boekhout-Mussert RJ, et al: Head injury and coagulation disorders. *J Neurosurg* 49:357, 1978.

114. Ferrara A, MacArthur JD, Wright HK, et al: Hypothermia and acidosis worsen coagulopathy in the patient requiring massive transfusion. *Am J Surg* 160:515, 1990.

115. Kumura E, Sato M, Fukuda A, et al: Coagulation disorders following acute head injury. *Acta Neurochir (Wien)* 85:23, 1987.

116. Olson JD, Kaufman HH, Moake J, et al: The incidence and significance of hemostatic abnormalities in patients with head injuries. *Neurosurgery* 24:825, 1989.

117. Stein SC, Young GS, Talucci RC, et al: Delayed brain injury after head trauma: Significance of coagulopathy. *Neurosurgery* 30:160, 1992.

118. Winter JP, Plummer D, Bottini A, et al: Early fresh frozen plasma prophylaxis of abnormal coagluation parameters in the severely head-injured patient is not effective. *Ann Emerg Med* 18:553, 1989.

119. Teasdale G, Jennett B: Assessment of coma and impaired consciousness. A practical scale. *Lancet* 2:81, 1974.

120. Crosby ET, Lui A: The adult cervical spine: Implications for airway management. *Can J Anaesth* 37:77, 1990.

121. Lam AM: Spinal cord injury and management. *Curr Opin Anesthesiol* 5:632, 1992.

122. Lanier WL, Milde JH, Michenfelder JD: Cerebral stimulation following succinylcholine in dogs. *Anesthesiology* 64:551, 1986.

123. Wright SW, Robinson GG, Wright MB: Cervical spine injuries in blunt trauma patients requiring emergent endotracheal intubation. *Am J Emerg Med* 10:104, 1992.

124. Lanier WL, Iaizzo PA, Milde JH: Cerebral function and muscle afferent activity following intravenous succinylcholine in dogs anesthetized with halothane: The effects of pretreatment with a defasciculating dose of pancuronium. *Anesthesiology* 71:87, 1989.

125. Cottrell JE, Hartung J, Giffin JP, et al: Intracranial and hemodynamic changes after succinylcholine adminstration in cats. *Anesth Analg* 62:1006, 1983.

126. Frankville DD, Drummond JC: Hyperkalemia after succinylcholine administration in a patient with closed head injury without paresis. *Anesthesiology* 67:264, 1987.

127. Ducey JP, Deppe SA, Foley KT: A comparison of the effects of suxamethonium, atracurium and vecuromium on intracranial haemodynamics in swine. *Anaesth Intensive Care* 17:448, 1989.

128. Stirt JA, Grosslight KR, Bedford RF, et al: "Defasciculation" with metocurine prevents succinylcholine-induced increases in intracranial pressure. *Anesthesiology* 67:50, 1987.

129. Kovarik WD, Lam AM, Slee TA, et al: The effect of succinylcholine on intracranial pressure, cerebral blood flow velocity and electroencephalogram in patients with neurologic disorders. *J Neurosurg Anesth* 3:245, 1991.

130. Marsh ML, Dunclop BJ, Shapiro HM, et al: Succinylcholine-intracranial pressure in neurosurgical patients. *Anesth Analg* 59:550, 1980.

131. Grande CM, Barton CR, Stene JK: Appropriate techniques for airway management of emergency patients with suspected spinal cord injury. *Anesth Analg* 67:714, 1988.

132. Archer DP, Priddy RE, Tang TKK, et al: The influence of cryogenic brain injury on the pharmacodynamics of pentobarbital: evidence for a serotonergic mechanism. *Anesthesiology* 75:634, 1991.

133. Todd MM, Weeks JB, Warner DS: A focal cryogenic brain lesion does not reduce the minimum alveolar concentration for halothane in rats. *Anesthesiology* 79:139, 1993.

134. Shapira Y, Paez A, Lam AM, et al: Influence of traumatic head injury on halothane MAC in rats. *Anesth Analg* 74:S282, 1992.

135. Adams RW, Cucchiara RF, Gronert GA, et al: Isoflurane and cerebrospinal fluid pressure in neurosurgical patients. *Anesthesiology* 54:97, 1981.

136. Artru A: Isoflurane does not increase the rate of CSF production in the dog. *Anesthesiology* 60:193, 1984.

137. Domino KB, Hemstad JR, Lam AM, et al: Effect of nitrous oxide on intracranial pressure after cranial-dural closure in patients undergoing craniotomy. *Anesthesiology* 77:421, 1992.

138. Laitinen LV, Johansson GG, Trakkanen L, et al: The effect of nitrous oxide on pulsatile cerebral impedance and cerebral blood flow. *Br J Anesth* 39:781, 1967.

139. Misfeldt BB, Jorgensen PB, Rishoj M: The effect of nitrous oxide and halothane upon the intracranial pressure in hypocapnic patients with intracranial disorders. *Br J Anaesth* 46:853, 1974.

140. Lam AM, Mayberg TS: Use of nitrous oxide in neuroanesthesia, why bother! *J Neurosurg Anesth* 4:285, 1992.

141. Rosner MJ, Coley IB: Cerebral perfusion pressure, intracranial pressure, and head elevation. *J Neurosurg* 65:636, 1986.

142. Ornstein E, Matteo RS, Schwartz AE, et al: The effect of phenytoin on the magnitude and duration of neuromuscular block following atracurium or vecuronium. *Anesthesiology* 67:191, 1987.

143. Braakaman R, Schouten HJA, Blaauw-van Dishoeck M, et al: Megadose steroids in severe head injury. Results of a prospective double-blind clinical trial. *J Neurosurg* 58:326, 1983.

144. Dearden NM, Gibson JS, McDowall DG, et al: Effect of high-dose dexamethasone on outcome from severe head injury. *J Neurosurg* 64:81, 1986.

145. Cooper PR, Moody S, Clark WK, et al: Dexamethasone and severe head injury. *J Neurosurg* 51:307, 1979.

146. Hall ED, Yonkers PA, Andrus PK, et al: Biochemistry and pharmacology of lipid antioxidants in acute brain and spinal cord injury. *J Neurotrauma* 9(2):S425, 1992.

147. Matta BF, Mayberg TS, Lam AM, et al: Clinical experience in the intraoperative use of jugular venous bulb catheter during neurosurgical procedures. *Can J Anaesth* 79:A224, 1993.

148. Goetting MG, Preston G: Jugular bulb catheterization: Experience with 123 cases. *Crit Care Med* 18:1220, 1990.

149. Sheinberg M, Kanter MJ, Roberston CS, et al: Continuous monitoring of jugular venous oxygen saturation in head-injured patients. *J Neurosurg* 76:212, 1992.

150. Cruz J: On-line monitoring of global cerebral hypoxia in acute brain injury. Relationship to intracranial hypertension. *J Neurosurg* 79:228, 1993.

151. Sanker P, Richard KE, Weigl HC, et al: Transcranial Doppler sonography and intracranial pressure monitoring in children and juveniles with acute brain injuries or hydroencephalus. *Childs Nerv Syst* 7:391, 1991.

152. Saunders W, Cledgett R: Transcranial blood velocity in head injury: A transcranial ultrasound Doppler study. *Surg Neurol* 29:401, 1988.

153. Klingelhofer J, Conrad B, Benecke R, et al: Intracranial flow patterns at increasing intracranial pressure. *Klin Wochenschr* 65:542, 1987.

154. Giulioni M, Ursino M, Alvisi C: Correlations among intracranial pulsatility, intracranial hemodynamics, and transcranial Doppler wave form: Literature review and hypothesis for future studies. *Neurosurgery* 22:807, 1988.

155. Hassler W, Steinmetz H, Gawlowski J: Transcranial Doppler ultrasonography in raised intracranial pressure and in intracranial circulatory arrest. *Neurosurgery* 68:745, 1988.

156. Werner C, Kochs E, Rau M, et al: Transcranial Doppler sonography as a supplement in the detection of cerebral circulatory arrest. *J Neurosurg Anesthesiol* 2:159, 1990.

157. Powers AD, Graeber MC, Smith RR: Transcranial Doppler ultrasonography in the determination of brain death. *Neurosurgery* 24:884, 1989.

158. Ropper AH, Kehne SM, Wechsler L: Transcranial Doppler in brain death. *Neurology* 37:1733, 1987.

159. Minamisawa H, Nordstrom C-H, Smith M-L, et al: The influence of mild body and brain hypothermia on ischemic brain damage. *J Cereb Blood Flow Metab* 10:365, 1990.

160. Mellergard P, Nordstrom CH: Intracerebral temperature in neurosurgical patients. *Neurosurgery* 28:709, 1991.

161. Ghani GA, Sung YF, Weinstein MS, et al: Effects of intravenous nitroglycerine on the intracranial pressure and volume response. *J Neurosurg* 58:562, 1983.

162. Griswold WR, Reznik V, Mendoza SA: Nitroprusside-induced intracranial hypertension. *JAMA* 246:2679, 1981.

163. Newell DW, Grady S, Sirotta P, et al: Evaluation of brain death using transcranial Doppler. *Neurosurgery* 24:509, 1989.

164. Lam AM: Change in cerebral blood flow velocity pattern during induced hypotension—a non-invasive indicator of increased intracranial pressure? *Br J Anaesth* 68:424, 1992.

CHAPTER 9

Anesthesia for Pediatric Head Injury

Mark M. Harris

Pediatric head trauma is a major public health concern affecting thousands of individuals annually and costing millions of dollars in acute emergency and chronic convalescent care. The anatomic, physiologic, and psychologic differences of childhood create different types of injuries, offer different therapeutic options, and lead to different outcomes than are seen in adult head injury. Therefore, the principles of anesthetic management in pediatric head trauma represent a synthesis of neuropathophysiology, emergency trauma medicine, and pediatric anesthesia. The consulting anesthesiologist should be familiar with the basic principles of pediatric life support, and, in addition, be able to manage the suspected cervical spine injury, commence emergency care for massive extracranial injury, secure central or intraosseous venous access, and initiate ventilatory or medical therapy for elevated intracranial pressure. This chapter will acquaint the consulting anesthesiologist with the background necessary to understand and manage the head-injured child.

EPIDEMIOLOGY, COST, AND PUBLIC HEALTH IMPLICATIONS

Pediatric head trauma is a significant public health concern in the United States resulting in approximately 7000 deaths and 150,000 injuries per year.[1,2] The financial and social costs of these injuries are staggering. Annual direct hospital costs for all acute pediatric head trauma in the United States are estimated to be $270 million.[3] Chronic hospitalization is required for approximately 15,000 brain-injured children annually[4] with mean annual bed occupancy estimated at 247 days.[5] Based on average rehabilitative in-patient costs of $500 per day in central Virginia, long-term care probably exceeds $1.8 billion annually. Placing a cash value on lost income and productivity is extremely difficult, but the Centers for Disease Control estimates losses from all pediatric trauma to amount to approximately $8 billion annually.[2] Adjusting these figures to include death (7000) and severe disability (6000 to 7000), lost income and lost productivity resulting from pediatric head trauma are estimated at $4.5 billion annually.

The costs of pediatric head trauma must also be calculated in human terms. Our society places great value upon childhood health, and all pediatric tragedies disrupt family integrity. The human ramifications of childhood trauma are plainly visible after injury; for example, 66 percent of uninjured siblings are reported to have emotional disturbances, 32 percent of couples report worsening of their marital situation, and 20 percent of families have exhausted their life savings.[6]

Trauma physicians believe that the motor vehicle is the "most lethal component" of the child's environment.[7] Motor vehicle accidents (MVAs) account for 19 percent of all pediatric trauma hospitalizations, 24 percent of the total pediatric acute care budget,[3] 37 percent of pediatric brain injuries,[1] and the majority of pediatric head trauma fatalities.[7] The majority of MVAs involve automobile occupant injuries (51 percent), but motorcycle (21 percent), pedestrian-vehicle (16 percent), and bicycle-vehicle accidents (11 percent) are also usually included as "MVAs."[1] Pediatric MVA victims are more likely to sustain severe head injury (29 percent) than all other categories of childhood injury with the sole exception of assaults. (Thirty-four percent of assaulted children sustain brain injury.[1]) Among all age groups, infants aged <1 year appear to have the greatest risk of serious head injury following MVAs,[1] and this probably results from inadequate passive restraints.[8] Alcohol consumption is an important factor in teenage MVAs, because 40 percent of teenage drivers involved in MVAs are reported to have blood alcohol levels greater than 100 mg/dl.[1]

Nonaccidental head injury is increasing rapidly among American children and represents 10 percent of the total reportable head trauma.[9] The explanation for the rapid increase in pediatric violence in the United States is complex and includes weapon availability, gang-related violence, parental neglect, and risk-taking behavior. The "shaken baby" syndrome is one type of abusive head injury seen in emergency rooms and is characterized by retinal hemorrhages, subdural and/or subarachnoid hemorrhages, high cervical cord injury with minimal or absent signs of external craniofacial trauma.[10] It is differentiated from other abusive injuries, such as traumatic subarachnoid hemorrhage where the examining physician can usually document a demonic picture of wanton injury (malnourishment, dehydration, bruises, burns, or ulcerations).[11]

Preventing head injury is a major public health goal in this country and involves such diverse areas as furniture design, play areas, toys, bicycle safety, vehicle restraints, recreational supervision, and improved community awareness.[12] The results of many of these public health strategies are well known; for example, the introduction of mandatory child restraints has reduced motor vehicle head injury 25 percent and reduced hospitalizations 36 percent in some localities.[8] The use of bicycle helmets has been proved to reduce head injury 85 percent,[13] and community bicycle safety campaigns have been rewarded with increased helmet usage, greater public awareness, and reduced hospitalization.[13,14] Efforts to reduce abusive behavior and gang-related violence have met with variable success. Gun control, police deterrent, and peer-oriented programs offer some hope in locations where homicide rates among teenage populations have doubled over the past 25 years.[2,9] Alcohol awareness is another essential part of these strategies as is the encouragement of responsible alcohol consumption. Prosecuting drunk driving, designating drivers who will remain alcohol free, and discouraging public intoxication are important societal goals to reduce teenage head injuries.

OUTCOME AFTER HEAD INJURY

Age is often cited as a major predictor of outcome in head injury. Mortality among adults is approximately 4 times higher than children[15] and results from differences in the mechanisms of injury, the types of extracranial injuries, and the pathophysiologic responses to trauma. Based upon many studies, pediatric head injury mortality ranges from 2.5 to 12.5 percent for moderate injury[15,16] and 9 to 32 percent in severe head injury.[16-21] The relationship between age and outcome has been analyzed in a recent prospective longitudinal study of 8814 head-injured patients.[15] The pediatric cohort comprised 1906 children aged <14 years and exhibited a combined mortality of 2.5 percent; the adult group, aged >14 years, had a combined mortality of 10.4 percent (Fig. 9-1). Adults were more likely to present with lower Glasgow Coma Scale scores (12.1 percent versus 5.6 percent) (Fig. 9-2), the mechanism of adult injury was often MVAs, and outcome differences between groups were encountered for all levels of severity (greater mortality at most GCS scores was found in adults). Extracranial injury increased the mortality associated with head injury approximately twice as much in the adult population (Table 9-1), and differences between children and adults were observed in motor score (better survival for children at every score), blood pressure (children displayed 3 times the mortality if they presented in shock), type of intracranial injury (the percentage of subdural hematomas increased with age), and specific lesion types (the mortality associated with epidural hematomas was 4.3 percent in pediatrics versus 21.5 percent in adults).[15]

Although this study documents the relatively low mortality associated with pediatric head injury, the long-term outcome for survivors is not encouraging; for example, the mean acute care hospitalization is reported to be only 7 to 8 days, but the total hospitalization averages almost 250 days.[5] In addition, 28 percent are left permanently disabled or to exist in a persistent vegetative state, and 100 percent with severe injury have long-term neurologic sequelae

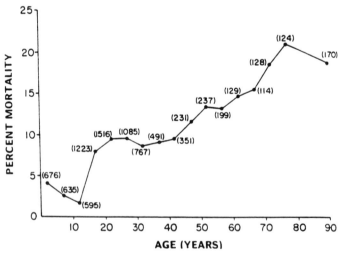

Figure 9-1 Age-related mortality for 8671 patients reported by Luerssen.[15]

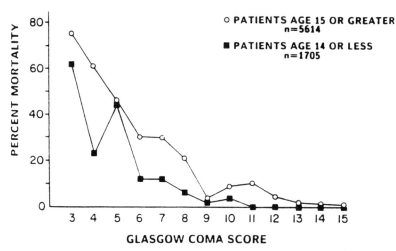

Figure 9-2 Age-related mortality as a function of injury severity after admission to hospital. (*From Luerssen,*[15] *with permission.*)

(94 percent with moderate head injury have permanent neurologic residual dysfunction).[1] Long-term outcome varies with degree of initial neurologic impairment and type of rehabilitative service provided. A 21-month additional study of head-injured children who had been in coma and undergone tracheostomies and gastrostomies suggested possible outcomes including normal (29 percent), mild behavioral or cognitive problems (53 percent), motor residual defects (9 percent), and severe intellectual and motor deficits (9 percent).[4] According to another study, 48 percent of the most severely injured survivors achieve functional independence after 2 years,[22] although recovery may be protracted if victims were too young to possess language skills.[23]

Table 9-1 Age-related mortality (%) associated with extracranial injury

Extracranial injury	Age 0–14 years (% mortality)	Age >14 years (% mortality)
Multiple trauma	6.4	13.8
Arm, leg, pelvic	6.0	15.0
Thoracic	17.5	21.6
Abdominal	16.7	26.6
Thoracic and abdominal	15.0	35.4

SOURCE: Modified from Luerssen.[15]

PATHOPHYSIOLOGY

Bruce and coworkers[18,19,24] presented the first comprehensive prospective studies in a group of 85 children (mean age = 7.1 years) with severe injury (GCS score <9) resulting from MVAs, falls, and child abuse. Of particular notice was the fact that surgically correctable mass lesions were found in only 12 children [included were epidural hematomas (n = 5), compound depressed skull fractures (n = 5), and acute subdural hematomas (n = 2)[17]] and that cerebral metabolic measurements (performed in 6 older children) revealed markedly increased cerebral blood flow and a reduction in CMR_{O_2}.[17,24]

Muizelaar and coworkers investigated severe pediatric head injury in two recent studies[25,26] where surgically correctable lesions were found in only 6 of 32 children (19 percent) including epidural (n = 2), subdural (n = 2), intracerebral (n = 1) and a combination of hematomas (n = 1). Using xenon washout techniques, CBF was evaluated in the group (mean age = 13.6 years; GCS score = 5.4). Initial CBF before 24 h was generally lower than that obtained after 24 h (survivors 48.8 ± 24.8 versus nonsurvivors 34.7 ± 9.9 ml/100 g per min, $p < .07$), however, there was no difference in late CBF between survivors and nonsurvivors (57.6 ± 24.3 versus 51.5 ± 22.9 ml/100 g per min). Jugular arteriovenous oxygen content difference (AVD_{O_2}) was low normal (4.5 to 4.8 O_2/dl) for all severity levels and there was no correlation between CMR_{O_2} and injury severity (Figure 9-3). Mean CMR_{O_2} in favorable outcome cases was 2.19 ± 0.82 ml/100 g per

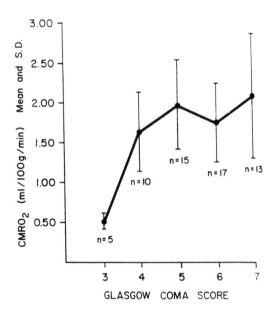

Figure 9-3 Relationship between cerebral metabolic rate of oxygen (CMR_{O_2}) and Glasgow Coma Scale Score. (*From Muizelaar,[25] with permission.*)

min and in unfavorable outcomes it averaged 1.52 ± 0.58 ml/100 g per min ($p < .001$). These findings suggest that uncoupling between CBF and CMR_{O_2} begins shortly after injury and lasts more than 24 h. The authors also examined cerebral autoregulation in a similar group of 26 patients (mean age = 13.2 years and GCS score = 5.5).[26] Autoregulation was found to be intact in 59 percent but did not correlate with GCS score, outcome, time after injury, or site of injury.[26]

These injury patterns are different from those which are seen in adults. In one study of 20 adult patients (mean age = 32 years, GCS score <7), 90 percent presented with surgically correctable lesions,[27] and injury resulted in overall reduced CBF. (One group averaged 37.4 ± 6.2 ml/100 g per min and a second group averaged 24.1 ± 3.4 ml/100 g per min). AVD_{O_2} was 2.6 ± 1.0 ml versus 4.2 ± 1.9 ml/dl in the "higher" and "lower" flow groups, while CMR_{O_2} was 0.98 ± 0.37 ml/100 g per min in the higher flow group versus 0.99 ± 0.41 ml/100 g per min in the lower flow group.

ANESTHETIC MANAGEMENT

Overview

According to a 7-year retrospective study of 25,134 pediatric deaths in the Northern Health Region of Great Britain, inadequate airway protection is the most important cause of avoidable head injury deaths[28](Table 9-2). The authors felt that approximately 22 percent of prehospital and 42 percent of in-hospital deaths were avoidable, and they recommended that regional health districts in Great Britain should ". . . revise urgently their guidelines for optimal management and indications for neurosurgical referral to include children with severe head injuries and audit their systems of care for all patients with head injuries."[28]

Table 9-2 Pediatric head-injury fatalities in northern Great Britain

	Before hospitalization (n = 125)	After hospitalization (n = 130)
Median age (years)	10	10
Age range	6 weeks–15 years	2 weeks–15 years
Median injury severity score	35	31.5
Injury severity score range	16.0–75.0	4.0–75.0
Number with injury score = 75	36	2

SOURCE: Modified from Sharples.[28]

The subsequent debate over this study appeared in the *British Medical Journal* and included the following representative comments:

1. ". . . there are great logistical problems in providing immediate care by personnel capable of anesthetizing and performing endotracheal intubation in seriously injured children at the roadside."[29]
2. ". . . exacerbation of minor primary injury by the secondary injuries of hypotension, hypoxia, hypercarbia, and raised intracranial pressure due to coughing, straining, and respiratory obstruction. Comatose patients with trauma are all too commonly erroneously transferred unintubated, breathing spontaneously through a small tube and accompanied only by a nurse or a senior house officer from the orthopaedic department. Published audits for head injury and trauma indicate avoidable factors in 35–54% of patients who die."[30]
3. ". . . the finding at necropsy of aspirated gastric contents after major trauma is not uncommon, particularly in victims of trauma without few evident injuries who may have been exposed to intensive resuscitative procedures before intubation and protection of the airway. It is potentially misleading to equate the presence of gastric contents in the airways at necropsy with appreciable hypoxia before death."[31]

Although prompt endotracheal intubation following serious trauma may reduce avoidable respiratory deaths, successful intubation requires advanced training not often available to general emergency medical personnel. Basic airway management in the United States includes administration of supplemental oxygen, manipulation of the head, use of artificial airways, provision of bag-mask ventilation, and stabilization of the cervical spine. Pediatric endotracheal intubation skills are taught only in advanced courses, and often little or no opportunity exists for the student to obtain practical airway management experience.[32,33] A recent study of 63 pediatric trauma victims concluded that iatrogenic airway complications could be expected in 25 percent of the victims.[34] The highest complication rates occurred when intubation was attempted at the scene of the accident. According to these data, prehospital personnel were unable to intubate the trachea in 6 of 14 attempts (42.8 percent); they also performed 2 unsuccessful needle cricothyroidotomies, and caused 6 other intubation-related complications including a right mainstem bronchus intubation, a massive subcutaneous emphysema, an esophageal intubation, a failed nasotracheal intubation through an open LeFort III fracture, and an inadvertent extubation during transportation.[34]

Airway complications are also likely to occur in pediatric head trauma victims after arrival in the hospital. According to the Northern Regional study, 31 head-injured children sustained unexpected respiratory arrest in hospital [radiology (n = 1), interhospital transfer (n = 8), on-the-ward (n = 22).[28] Failure to prevent death in this group of children resulted from an "appalling deficiency in resuscitation knowledge and skills among junior house staff."[30] Do similar deficiencies exist among hospital-based physicians and housestaff in the United States? The answer to this is unknown, but data from the University of Pittsburgh suggests that American emergency department management is superior. Among pediatric trauma victims requiring emergency endotracheal intubation, the success rate is reported to be 97 percent at community hospitals and 100 percent at a major children's hospital.[34]

A variety of nonrespiratory catastrophes should be anticipated in "stable" hospitalized head-injured victims, because examining physicians fail to diagnose and treat existing neurologic and extracranial injury. According to the Northern Regional study, fatal extracranial injury was misdiagnosed in 13 children. These injuries include ruptured spleens (n = 6), lacerated livers (n = 3), rupture of one or more abdominal viscus (n = 2), lacerated iliac artery (n = 1), and pneumothorax (n = 1).[28] Because management errors occur in all hospital settings, the consulting anesthesiologist must maintain a high index of suspicion, encourage exhaustive searches for extracranial injury, and remember that emergency burr holes or ventriculostomy occasionally can be life saving in pediatric traumatic head injury. Preventing avoidable deaths of children with multiple trauma and head injury requires careful, continuous assessment of neurologic status, communication among caregivers, prompt response to calls for assistance, and skill in pediatric airway management. All aspects of the process must operate optimally to minimize mortality.

Clinical Management of the Pediatric Airway

The need for pediatric airway management will depend upon the nature and severity of neurologic and extracranial injuries. Airway management for the apneic, comatose child without pulses or blood pressure is well known; i.e., the consulting physician administers oxygen, begins bag/mask ventilation, and prepares to intubate the trachea. Airway management in the conscious child is much more controversial and depends upon the neurologic findings, associated injuries, and the expertise of the treating physician. The child with a history of head trauma, minimal extracranial injury, no skull fracture, presenting with a normal neurologic examination (performed by a neurosurgeon or neurologist), and GCS score of 15 will predictably be discharged to home without airway support.[35] In contrast, the lucid child with a similar history and minor neurologic and/or physical findings may require definitive emergency airway management later in his/her hospital course (Fig. 9-4). Children who present with an initial lucid period followed by neurologic deterioration and death within 24 h display the "talk and die" syndrome.[36,37] The common pathophysiologic findings in this syndrome include diffuse hyperemia (39 percent), intradural mass lesions (32 percent), and epidural hematomas (29 percent).[38] Airway management in the lucid child with isolated head injury, stable neurologic status, and GCS score >8

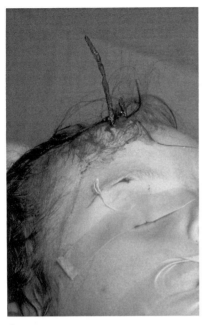
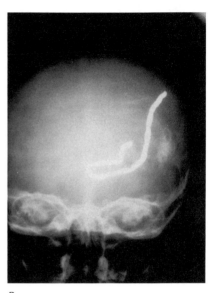

A   B

Figure 9-4 Projectile head injury that did not result in loss of consciousness or neurologic injury. The child arrived in the emergency room alert, did not require emergency airway management and made an uncomplicated recovery after craniotomy.

should be expectant. The child with isolated head injury but with vacillating neurologic status, seizures, protracted vomiting, symptomatic intracranial hypertension, or GCS score <9 requires immediate airway management; i.e., bag/mask ventilation and endotracheal intubation to secure the airway. Airway management is more difficult when neurologic evaluation is complicated by alcohol or drug intoxication. In all patients airway control must proceed in a calculated manner to minimize the risk of pulmonary aspiration.

Aspiration of gastric contents is a relatively common cause of morbidity in pediatric head trauma[28] and results from obtunded airway reflexes, delayed gastric emptying, and difficulty during endotracheal intubation. Both the head-injured patient who sustains a respiratory arrest on the wards and the acute trauma victim who is intubated in the field by emergency technicians are at greater risk for pulmonary aspiration than the child undergoing endotracheal intubation by an anesthesiologist in the operating room. A study of 110 pediatric trauma victims revealed aspiration to be extremely rare when they underwent endotracheal intubation with preoxygenation as tolerated, followed by thiopental, 5 mg/kg, cricoid pressure, and succinylcholine, 1 mg/kg.[39] Using a multiorifice tube, gastric volume and pH were recorded after induction of anesthesia. Children who fasted for 4 to 6 h, had significantly greater gastric volume than those who fasted 6 to 10 h; however, nearly half (49 percent) of children who fasted in excess of 8 h had gastric residual volumes greater than 0.4 ml/kg. Minor trauma (as compared with moderate or major trauma) and complaints of hunger were associated with significantly reduced gastric volume. (Eighty-seven percent of children complaining of hunger had empty stomachs.[39]) No child vomited on induction of general anesthesia (21 percent vomited—all during emergence), and not one aspirated. In view of these findings, the authors concluded that vomiting "appeared to bear no direct relationship to volume of gastric aspirate, fasting time, severity of injury, or the provision of analgesia."[39]

All children with severe head injury, normal airway anatomy, and spontaneous ventilation should be intubated using a rapid sequence induction technique consisting of preoxygenation as tolerated, an intravenous induction agent, a neuromuscular relaxant, and application of cricoid pressure. Securing adequate intravenous access and beginning appropriate volume resuscitation before endotracheal intubation is essential. Although the anesthesiologist must be sensitive to fears in the awake, traumatized, frightened child, oral, nasal, or rectal sedatives are unnecessary and securing an appropriate intravenous catheter should be accomplished without delay. Preoxygenation in the anxious child can be accomplished either by a mask applied to the face or by "blow-by" techniques. If the child objects to application of cricoid pressure, it can be applied immediately after loss of consciousness.

Choice of induction agents for rapid sequence intubation in the injured child will depend upon hemodynamic status, associated injuries, and ICP. Etomidate, 0.15 to 0.3 mg/kg, maintains cardiovascular stability without increasing ICP[40] and can be used safely in pediatrics. Intravenous thiopental, 3 to 5 mg/kg; methohexital, 1 to 2 mg/kg; or propofol, 1 to 2 mg/kg, can produce severe cardiovascular depression in hypovolemic patients. Intravenous ketamine, 1 to 3 mg/kg, will maintain blood pressure at the expense of increasing ICP, although prior hyperventilation will help to inhibit this rise. The choice of neuromuscular relaxants for rapid sequence techniques in children is usually a matter of personal preference. Intubation can be accomplished with either succinylcholine, 1 to 2 mg/kg, or several nondepolarizing relaxants including vecuronium, 0.25 mg/kg; pancuronium, 0.2 mg/kg; and atracurium, 0.5 to 1.0 mg/kg. Although succinylcholine is reported to cause a rise in ICP in dogs and in adult patients,[41,42] it produces rapid and reliable intubating conditions, and both hyperventilation and deep anesthesia may minimize any rise.

When the child's airway has been secured and after the patient is transported to the intensive care unit, the anesthesiologist may be consulted to assess extubation criteria. Prolonged endotracheal intubation is relatively benign, and its side effects (subglottic stenosis and postextubation stridor) can be prevented by loose-fitting endotracheal tubes.[43] It should be remembered that children intubated emergently in the field or in emergency departments may be at increased risk of postextubation difficulty due partly to the increased likelihood of airway injury at intubation.[34] In general, absence of an air leak at 30 cm of water pressure is the only positive predictor of postextubation stridor in pediatric trauma.[44]

The Suspected Cervical Spine Injury

The Handbook of Advanced Trauma Life Support (ATLS) states "Assume a cervical spine fracture in any patient with an injury above the clavicle. . . . Pediatric spinal cord injury is rare. Only 5 percent of all spinal cord injuries occur in the pediatric age group."[32] According to the National Highway Traffic Safety Administration analysis of 10,151 adult and pediatric patients with detailed medical records who were victims of tow-away passenger-car crashes, severe cervical spine injury is documented in only 131 (1.2 percent) and fatal neck injury is seen in 53 (0.5 percent).[45] Pediatric cervical spine injuries are rare (3.8 percent of the total) and are usually less severe than similar injuries observed among adults (aged 16 to 25 years).[45] However, cervical spinal injury in children with severe head injury following MVAs is characterized by devastating trauma to the upper cervical cord, apnea, absent vital signs, and 100 percent mortality.[46,47]

In general, cervical spine injuries in children can be divided into adult and juvenile types. Injuries in children aged less than 8 years are almost exclusively ligamental occurring at the atlanto-occipital, atlantoaxial, and C2-C3 levels, whereas older children and adults usually present with fractures at any point throughout the cervical spine.[48–50] Children with Down syndrome,[51,52] achondroplasia,[53] and those placed in forward-facing car seats[54] seem to be at increased risk for cervical spine injury after trauma.

Although there are no definitive data, the technique of endotracheal intubation appears to have little impact on cervical spine injury after severe head injury. Immediate, devastating cervical spine injury is relatively common in severe head injury, and to quote Bohn and coworkers, "Given the fact that intubation and hyperventilation provide the most important initial treatment in severe head injury, it is difficult to justify the use of the more difficult and potentially harmful technique of blind nasal intubation in children . . . oral intubation under direct laryngoscopy can be safely performed without causing damage to the cord."[47] When severe head injury mandates prompt endotracheal intubation, treatment by rapid sequence intravenous induction, oral intubation, and cervical spine stabilization offers speed and safety.

Intracranial Hypertension

Intracranial hypertension, like hypoxemia and hypotension, is a common treatable cause of secondary brain injury. Operative procedures are usually not necessary because of the low incidence of surgically correctable lesions. (Between 15 and 19 percent reported incidence of hematomas.[17,25]) Most centers use a combination of muscle paralysis and hyperventilation to a Pa_{CO_2} of 25 mmHg. Hypothermia to 32°C and pentobarbital coma have been advocated for refractory intracranial hypertension, but Bruce and coworkers have recommended not using mannitol because it "has been shown to increase CBF."[17] Writing 10 years later, Muizelaar and coworkers[25] found no positive correlation between cerebral blood flow and intracranial hypertension adding that "Mannitol administration reduces blood viscosity . . . it never leads to increased CBV or ICP. . . . We, therefore, do not agree with Bruce and coworkers who advised against the use of mannitol in children for fear of increasing hyperemia . . . ."[25] For refractory intracranial hypertension, Muizelaar and coworkers recommended manipulation of blood pressure. They wrote "In three cases in whom mannitol could not be continued . . . induced hypertension could control ICP until osmolarity had come down."[26]

Steroid therapy is a useful adjunct for the treatment of intracranial hypertension in Reye's syndrome,[55] and it has been recommended in pediatric severe head injury.[17] However, a randomized study of 82 children (GCS score <8, mean age = 9 years) suggests that barbiturate coma has no effect on outcome in head injury.[56] Extreme hyperventilation (<25 mmHg) may provide some advantages in specific refractory cases, and one pediatric textbook observes "There are children in whom ICP is uncontrollable at a Pa_{CO_2} of 15 to 16, and yet a reduction of their Pa_{CO_2} to 12 mmHg results in a stable, well-controlled ICP . . . a compromise is to monitor the child's jugular venous oxygen tension . . . when hyperventilation reduces the Pa_{CO_2} below 20 mmHg to control ICP."[57]

The effects of most general anesthetics on intracranial pressure in pediatric head injury are speculative. As mentioned previously, succinylcholine has been implicated in acute intracranial hypertension in some adults, but no controlled trials of the relaxant have been performed in children with head injury. There is little data available on the use of volatile anesthetics in pediatric head injury. Isoflurane, 1.5 percent expired concentration, has been studied in ventricular shunt dysfunction; ICP does not change, although cerebral perfusion pressure decreases 5 percent.[58] Agents with predictable effects upon CMR_{O_2} and ICP, such as thiopental, fentanyl, nondepolarizing relaxants, and low concentrations of isoflurane constitute our anesthetics of choice for infants and children with head trauma and suspected intracranial hypertension. When rapid intubating conditions are essential, we use succinylcholine and hyperventilation.

EXTRACRANIAL INJURY

Extracranial injury (multiple trauma, thoracic and abdominal injury) significantly increases the chance of adverse outcome in pediatric head injury.[15] Blunt, abdominal injury can result in splenic or hepatic laceration requiring significant blood replacement during initial resuscitation. Hemodynamically stable children with abdominal injury may be observed without surgery if they have no other operative injuries and display only modest transfusion requirements (16 to 21 mg/kg after resuscitation).[59] Children with head injury who were restrained by lap type safety belts are at risk for flexion spinal injuries (chance-type fractures) and visceral, hepatic, splenic, and renal injury.[60,61] Abdominal ecchymoses from lap belts should alert the anesthesiologist of additional occult abdominal injury that may have been overlooked in this era of increased nonoperative treatment.[62]

Thoracic injury in children is different from similar injury in adults, because chest wall elasticity and resilience reduce the likelihood of flail chest and rib fractures and increase the likelihood of great vessel disruption, airway injury, pneumothorax, and pulmonary contusion. The mortality of children with major thoracic injury is 26 percent while the presence of hemothorax or injury to the heart or great vessels increases that rate to 50 percent.[63] The incidence of direct myocardial injury in blunt thoracic trauma is unknown, but the lack of autopsy evidence suggests that direct cardiac injury is rare.[64]

VASCULAR ACCESS AND FLUID RESUSCITATION

Volume resuscitation of head-injured children with severe extracranial injury demands rapid intravenous cannulation and immediate transfusion of blood products or balanced salt solutions. Intraosseous access has become a popular alternative to intravenous cannulation in neonates and small infants. The tibial intramedullary cavity can be entered from the anteromedial surface several centimeters below the tibial tuberosity with either a specially designed intraosseous needle or adult epidural needle.[65,66] This technique gives rapid access to the central circulation for administration of fluid volumes or medications.

Transfusion with type-specific blood, colloid or crystalloid, is the first priority for the child with hemorrhagic shock, head trauma, and massive extracranial injury. When blood is unavailable, hypertonic saline, hydroxyethyl starch, or other colloids may be administered[67,68] although whether they are better than balanced saline solutions is controversial. The use of small-volume resuscitation with hypertonic, hyperoncotic solutions will expand extracellular fluid volume, increase central venous pressure, and improve cardiac output without significantly raising mean arterial blood pressure.[69] The principal cerebral effect of small-volume hypertonic saline resuscitation is a transiently increased cerebral blood flow. In contrast, small-volume resuscitation with hydroxyethyl starch caused no cerebrovascular changes in normal dog models.[69] Balanced salt solution has been compared with hypertonic saline in a recent study of head-injured children.[70] Balanced salt solution or hypertonic saline was administered in a blinded, randomized fashion for persistent intra-cranial hypertension after initial volume resuscitation and stabilization using vasopressors. Administration of hypertonic saline resulted in a significant reduction of ICP, whereas isotonic saline produced no change. Although the results were positive, the accompanying editorial[71] discussed the adverse hypotensive effects of hypertonic saline and concluded that further work was necessary to "define the optimum speed of administration of hypertonic solutions."[71] Until questions about doses and rate of administration have been resolved, balanced saline resuscitation, i.e., 20 ml/kg repeated until blood pressure increases, peripheral perfusion improves, and cross-matched blood becomes available, will continue to be the method of choice in the hypotensive head-injured child.

SUMMARY AND CONCLUSIONS

The anesthetic management of pediatric head trauma is based on many of the principles of adult neuroanesthesia; however, children present with their own unique responses to injury, including cerebral hyperemia, cervical spine disruption, and specific extracranial injuries. To manage head injury success-fully, the consultant anesthesiologist must understand pediatric anatomy and physiology, be able to secure the airway, establish intravenous access, initiate fluid resuscitation, and begin therapy for intracranial hypertension. The consul-tant must also have a high index of suspicion for occult extracranial and intracranial injury in the child with a "stable" head injury.

REFERENCES

1. Kraus JF, Rock A, Hemyari P: Brain injuries among infants, children, adolescents, and young adults in the United States. *Am J Dis Child* 144:684, 1990.

2. Division of Injury Control, Centers for Disease Control: Childhood injuries in the United States. *Am J Dis Child* 144:627, 1990.

3. MacKenzie EJ, Morris JA, Lissovoy GV, et al: Acute hospital costs of pediatric trauma in the United States: How much and who pays. *J Pediatr Surg* 25:970, 1990.

4. Mahoney WJ, D'Souza BJ, Haller JA, et al: Long-term outcome of children with severe head trauma and prolonged coma. *Pediatrics* 71:756, 1983.

5. Grosswasser Z, Costeff H, Tamir A: Survivors of severe traumatic brain injury in childhood. *Scand J Rehabil Med Suppl* 12:6, 1985.

6. Harris BH, Schwaitzberg SD, Seman TM, et al: The hidden morbidity of pediatric trauma. *J Pediatr Surg* 24:103, 1989.

7. Tepas JJ, DiScala C, Ramenofsky ML, et al: Mortality and head injury: The pediatric perspective. *J Pediatr Surg* 25:92, 1990.

8. Margolis LH, Wagenaar AC, Liu W: The effects of a mandatory child restraint law on injuries requiring hospitalization. *Am J Dis Child* 142:1099, 1988.

9. Christoffel KK: Violent death and injury in U.S. children and adolescents. *Am J Dis Child* 144:697, 1990.

10. Hadley MN, Sonntagh VKH, Rekate HL, et al: The infant whiplash-shake syndrome: A clinical and pathological study. *Neurosurgery* 24:536, 1989.

11. Sivaloganathan S: Traumatic subarachnoid haemorrhage as part of the NAI syndrome. *Med Sci Law* 30:138, 1990.

12. MacKellar A: Head injuries in children and implications for their prevention. *J Pediatr Surg* 24:577, 1989.

13. Thompson RS, Rivara FP, Thompson DC: A case-control study of the effectiveness of bicycle safety helmets. *N Engl J Med* 320:1361, 1989.

14. Bergman AB, Rivara FP, Richards D, et al: The Seattle children's bicycle helmet campaign. *Am J Dis Child* 144:727, 1990.

15. Luerssen TG, Klauber MR, Marshall LF: Outcome from head injury related to patient's age. *J Neurosurg* 68:409, 1988.

16. Kalff R, Kocks W, Pospiech J, et al: Clinical outcome after head injury in children. *Child's Nerv Syst* 5:156, 1989.

17. Bruce DA, Raphaely RC, Goldberg AI, et al: Pathophysiology, treatment, and outcome following severe head injury in children. *Child's Brain* 5:174, 1979.

18. Bruce DA, Schut L, Bruno LA, et al: Outcome following severe head injuries in children. *J Neurosurg* 48:679, 1978.

19. Pfenniger J, Kaiser G, Lutschg J, et al: Treatment and outcome of the severely head-injured child. *Intensive Care Med* 9:13, 1983.

20. Esparza Z, Portillo JM, Sarabia M, et al: Outcome in children with severe head injuries. *Child's Nerv Syst* 1:109, 1985.

21. Zuccarello M, Facco E, Zampieri P, et al: Severe head injury in children: Early prognosis and outcome. *Child's Nerv Syst* 1:158, 1985.

22. Splaingard ML, Gaebler D, Havens P, et al: Brain injury: Functional outcome in children with tracheostomies and gastrostomies. *Arch Phys Med Rehabil* 70:318, 1989.

23. Costeff H, Groswasser Z, Landman Y, et al: Survivors of severe traumatic brain injury in childhood. I: late residual disability. *Scand J Rehabil Med Suppl* 12:10, 1985.

24. Bruce DA, Alavi A, Bilaniuk L, et al: Diffuse cerebral swelling following head injuries in children: The syndrome of "malignant brain edema." *J Neurosurg* 54:170, 1981.

25. Muizelaar JP, Marmarou A, DeSalles AA, et al: Cerebral blood flow and metabolism in severely head-injured children. I. Relationship with GCS scores, outcome, ICP, and PVI. *J Neurosurg* 71:63, 1989.

26. Muizelaar JP, Ward JD, Marmarou A, et al: Cerebral blood flow and metabolism in severely head-injured children. II. Autoregulation. *J Neurosurg* 71:72, 1989.

27. Cold GE: The relationship between cerebral metabolic rate of oxygen and cerebral blood flow in the acute phase of head injury. *Acta Anaesthesiol Scand* 30:453, 1986.

28. Sharples PM, Storey A, Aynsley-Green A, et al: Avoidable factors contributing to death of children with head injury. *BMJ* 300:87, 1990.

29. Wardrope J: Death of children with head injury (letter). *BMJ* 300:534, 1990.

30. McQuill PJ: Death of children with head injury (letter). *BMJ* 300:534, 1990.

31. Pigott TJD, Lowe JS: Death of children with head injury (letter). *BMJ* 300:534, 1990.

32. Advanced Trauma Life Support. American College of Surgeons, Chicago, 1989.

33. Chameides L (ed): *Textbook of Pediatric Advanced Life Support*. Dallas, American Heart Association, 1988.

34. Nakayama DK, Gardner MJ, Rowe MI: Emergency endotracheal intubation in pediatric trauma. *Ann Surg* 211:218, 1990.

35. Rosenthal BW, Bergman I: Intracranial injury after moderate head trauma in children. *J Pediatr* 115:346, 1989.

36. Humphries RP, Hendrick EB, Hoffman HJ: The head-injured child who "talks and dies." *Child's Nerv Syst* 6:139, 1990.

37. Snoek JW, Minderhoud JM, Wilmink JT: Delayed deterioration following mild head injury in children. *Brain* 107:15, 1984.

38. Lobato RD, Rivas JJ, Gomez PA, et al: Head-injured patients who talk and deteriorate into coma. *J Neurosurg* 75:256, 1991.

39. Bricker SRW, McLuckie A, Nightingale DA: Gastric aspirates after trauma in children. *Anaesthesia* 44:721, 1989.

40. Glass PS, Leiman BC, Reves JG: Etomidate: What is its present role in anesthesia. *Semin Anesth* 7:143, 1988.

41. Lanier WL, Milde JH, Michenfelder JD: Cerebral stimulation following succinylcholine in dogs. *Anesthesiology* 64:551, 1986.

42. Minton MD, Grosslight KR, Stirt JA, et al: Increases in intracranial pressure from succinylcholine. Prevention by prior nondepolarizing blockade. *Anesthesiology* 65:165, 1986.

43. Battersby EF, Hatch DJ, Towey RM: The effects of prolonged nasoendotracheal intubation in children. *Anaesthesia* 32:154, 1977.

44. Kemper KJ, Benson MS, Bishop MJ: Predictors of postextubation stridor in pediatric trauma patients. *Crit Care Med* 19:352, 1991.

45. Huelke DF, O'Day J, Mendlesohn RA: Cervical injuries suffered in automobile crashes. *J Neurosurg* 54:316, 1981.

46. Bohn D, Swan P, Sides C, et al: High cervical spine injuries associated with severe head injury in children: An unrecognized cause of cardiorespiratory arrest. *Crit Care Med* 17:S117, 1989.

47. Bohn D, Armstrong D, Becker L, et al: Cervical spine injury in children. *J Trauma* 30:463, 1990.

48. Hill SA, Miller CA, Kosnik EJ, et al: Pediatric neck injuries. *J Neurosurg* 60:700, 1984.

49. Hadley MN, Zabramski JM, Browner CM, et al: Pediatric spinal trauma. *J Neurosurg* 68:18, 1988.

50. Ruge JR, Sinson GP, McLone DG, et al: Pediatric spinal injury: The very young. *J Neurosurg* 68:25–30, 1988.

51. Pueschel SM, Scola FH: Atlantoaxial instability in individuals with Down syndrome: Epidemiologic, radiographic, and clinical studies. *Pediatrics* 80:555, 1987.

52. Davidson RG: Atlantoaxial instability in individuals with Down syndrome: A fresh look at the evidence. *Pediatrics* 81:857, 1988.

53. Reid CS, Pyeritz RE, Kopits SE, et al: Cervicomedullary compression in young patients with achondroplasia: Value of comprehensive neurologic and respiratory evaluation. *J Pediatr* 110:522, 1987.

54. Fuchs S, Barthel MJ, Flannery AM, et al: Cervical spine fractures sustained by young children in forward-facing car seats. *Pediatrics* 84:348, 1989.

55. Frewen TC, Swedlow DB, Watcha M, et al: Outcome in severe Reye syndrome with early pentobarbital coma and hypothermia. *J Pediatr* 100:663, 1982.

56. Bohn D, Swan S, Sides C: High-dose barbiturate in the management of severe pediatric head injury: A randomized controlled trail. *Crit Care Med* 17:S118, 1989.

57. Swedlow DB: Anesthesia for neurosurgical procedures. *In* Gregory GA (ed): *Pediatric Anesthesia*, 2d ed. New York, Churchill Livingstone, 1990.

58. Aloy A, Dirnberger H, Kalinowsky R, et al: Characteristics of isoflurane in hydrocephalic children with ventricular shunt dysfunction. *Anesthesiology* 63:A348, 1985.

59. Cosentino CM, Luck SR, Barthel MJ, et al: Transfusion requirements in conservative nonoperative management of blunt splenic and hepatic injuries during childhood. *J Pediatr Surg* 25:950, 1990.

60. Reid AB, Letts RM, Black GB: Pediatric Chance fractures: Association with intraabdominal injuries and seatbelt use. *J Trauma* 30:384, 1990.

61. Anderson PA, Rivara FP, Maier RV, et al: The epidemiology of seatbelt-associated injuries. *J Trauma* 31:60, 1991.

62. Cobb LM, Vinocur CD, Wagner CW, et al: Intestinal perforation due to blunt trauma in children in an era of increased nonoperative treatment. *J Trauma* 26:461, 1986.

63. Peclet MH, Newman KD, Eichelberger MR, et al: Thoracic trauma in children: An indicator of increased mortality. *J Pediatr Surg* 25:961, 1990.

64. Langer JC, Winthrop AI, Wesson DE, et al: Diagnosis and incidence of cardiac injury in children with blunt thoracic trauma. *J Pediatr Surg* 24:1091, 1989.

65. Harte FA, Chalmers PC, Walsh RF, et al: Intraosseous fluid administration: A parenteral alternative in pediatric resuscitation. *Anesth Analg* 66:687, 1987.

66. Rosetti VA, Thompson BM, Miller J, et al: Intraosseous infusions: An alternative route of pediatric intravascular access. *Ann Emerg Med* 14:885, 1985.

67. Mermel GW, Boyle WA: Hypertonic saline resuscitation following prolonged hemorrhage in the awake dog. *Anesthesiology* 65:A91, 1986.

68. Rockow EC, Falk JL, Fein IA, et al: Fluid resuscitation in circulatory shock: A comparison of the cardiorespiratory effects of albumin, hetastarch, and saline solutions in patients with hypovolemic and septic shock. *Crit Care Med* 11:839, 1983.

69. Prough DS, Whitley JM, Olympio MA, et al: Hypertonic/hyperoncotic fluid resuscitation after hemorrhagic shock in dogs. *Anesth Analg* 73:738, 1991.

70. Fisher B, Thomas D, Peterson B: Hypertonic saline lowers raised intracranial pressure in children after head trauma. *J Neurosurg Anesthesiol* 4:4, 1992.

71. Smerling A: Hypertonic saline in head trauma: A new recipe for drying and salting. *J Neurosurg Anesthesiol* 4:1, 1992.

Intensive Care Management and Monitoring

David W. Newell and Arthur M. Lam

Previous chapters have discussed much of the pathology and pathophysiology of acute head injury and the immediate objectives of its management. Equally important is the intensive care unit (ICU) management of those patients who did not require surgery and the postoperative management of those who had mass lesions removed. One should always remember the objectives of prevention of secondary injury and provision of optimal conditions for the recovery from primary brain injury. Intensive care management is geared toward providing optimal systemic support for cerebral energy metabolism and adequate cerebral perfusion for the injured brain. Many of the factors leading to recovery of primary brain injury are poorly understood, but it is evident that a significant component of the neurologic dysfunction that occurs after primary brain injury is reversible given the right conditions for recovery. Secondary brain injury can occur in the ICU in the form of hypoxia and ischemia from pulmonary complications, hypotension, or high intracranial pressure (ICP) from a variety of causes. The prompt recognition and treatment of these complications are essential in head injury managment. This chapter will discuss the theoretical and practical aspects of intracranial pressure and its management as well as other aspects of monitoring and treatment of the head-injured patient.

MONITORING AND MANAGEMENT OF INTRACRANIAL PRESSURE

Concepts of Intracranial Pressure

The idea that abnormal intracranial pressure may occur and contribute to the pathogenesis of brain injury can be traced to the Monro-Kellie doctrine.[1] This doctrine states that, because the brain and spinal cord are surrounded by inelastic coverings, changes in the volume of the contents would result in changes in the intracranial pressure. The volume of the intracranial contents consists of the brain tissue, blood, and cerebrospinal fluid. All of these components are relatively incompressible; therefore, an increase in one of the components or introduction of an expanding mass lesion will result in a decrease in the others so that the total volume is fixed. Increases in intracranial pressure as a result of increases in volume can occur according to the compliance of the system (see also Chap. 5).

The intracranial compliance can be defined as the change in intracranial volume divided by the change in intracranial pressure,[2] or more appropriately, the intracranial elastance can be defined as the change in intracranial pressure divided by the change in intracranial volume. The intracranial compliance, or the ability of the system to absorb a change in volume, will be reduced as mass lesions enlarge, thereby reducing the amount of blood and CSF available to "buffer" the system. The intracranial compliance or elastance can be determined in patients with ventricular catheters in place. The slope of the CSF volume versus pressure curve can be obtained by adding a known amount of fluid to the CSF through a ventricular catheter and noting the rise in pressure.[2,3] Knowledge of the intracranial compliance can be helpful in head-injured patients by warning the physician of impending dangerous increases in ICP. The intracranial pressure wave form can also yield some information about the intracranial compliance. Although it is influenced by many factors including the recording method, the cardiac contractility, and the arterial pulse pressure, it usually has a higher pulse wave amplitude at a lower intracranial compliance[2] (see Figs. 10-1 and 10-2).

ICP Monitoring

Continuous monitoring of intracranial pressure has become a standard practice in caring for patients with severe head injury. Various methods of monitoring are available and include epidural systems, subarachnoid bolts, and more recently, fiber-optic catheters that can be used in a subarachnoid bolt system or in a ventricular catheter (see Chap. 5). Ventriculostomy has always been considered the gold standard for ICP monitoring; however, fiber optic subarachnoid bolts compare very favorably.[4] Computerized recording of the ICP wave forms with the capability for trend analysis has become standard in most modern intensive care units (see Fig. 10-1). Information gained from intracranial pressure monitoring can be used to guide ICP management as

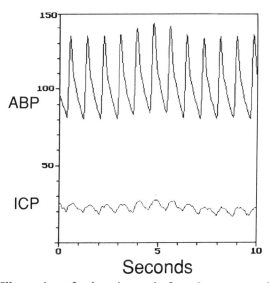

Figure 10-1 Illustration of a short interval of continuous recording of ICP and arterial blood pressure. Notice the transmitted pulse wave in the ICP wave form due to transient cerebral blood volume changes (Scale = mmHg).

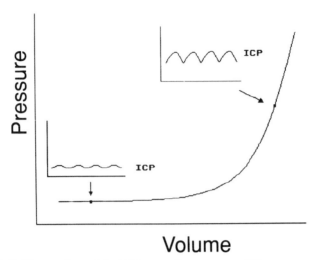

Figure 10-2 Illustration of the ICP wave form at two different pressures illustrating the effect of intracranial compliance differences on the ICP wave amplitude.

well as management of the cerebral perfusion pressure (CPP), which is the arterial blood pressure minus the intracranial pressure. Monitoring of ICP can also give early warning of expansion of mass lesions.

Characteristics of ICP Tracings

Measurements of intracranial pressure were first accomplished using the lumbar puncture and ventricular puncture methods. Continuous monitoring and recording of ICP was first reported by Guillaume and Janny[5] and later by Lundberg.[6] Lundberg published an extensive description of his findings during ICP monitoring in neurosurgical patients[6] and carefully described the characteristics of the recordings as well as the influence of various pathologic conditions on the measurements. Lundberg observed various waves in the ICP tracings which he termed A-waves, B-waves, and C-waves.

A-waves or plateau waves, named because of their characteristic shape on the ICP tracing, are characterized by a sudden sharp increase in ICP to levels of 60 to 80 mmHg with a variable duration usually from 5 to 20 min. These waves often occurred in patients with large intracranial mass lesions, and their increasing frequency was a poor prognostic sign (see Fig. 10-3). Subsequently, it has been confirmed that an increase in cerebral blood volume and a decrease in cerebral blood flow (CBF) occurs during these waves.[7,8] Rosner and coworkers[9] have demonstrated in an experimental model that A-waves represent vasodilatation in response to a decrease in cerebral perfusion pressure. With reduced intracranial compliance this vasodilatation leads to increases in ICP, which then further increases vasodilatation and a positive feedback mechanism is thus established. Treatment of A-waves includes increasing intracranial compliance, increasing cerebral perfusion pressure, and avoiding sudden stimuli that increase ICP or lower blood pressure.

B-waves described by Lundberg consist of repeating waves of variable amplitude in the ICP tracing, but usually between 10 and 20 mmHg.[6] The frequency is also variable but is usually between 0.5 and 2 per minute. B-waves have been described in states of reduced intracranial compliance and are also believed to be due to fluctuations of intracranial blood volume.[10] Figure 10-4 illustrates typical B-waves. Lundberg commented in his original description that they were associated with respiratory changes, and this has led to the widespread belief that they are due to CO_2 changes. He also observed the waves in ventilated patients, however, and stated that this observation permitted no definite conclusion as to their origins. Newell and coworkers[11] demonstrated that continuous B-waves occurred in ventilated patients while recording end tidal CO_2. They clearly demonstrated that B-waves can occur despite a constant end tidal CO_2 concentration. They also demonstrated that the middle cerebral and extracranial internal carotid artery velocity, when measured using Doppler ultrasound, fluctuated synchronously with B-waves, and the amplitude of the waves was related to the ICP and the degree of velocity fluctuation. Velocity fluctuations at this frequency in the middle cerebral artery (MCA) were also demonstrated in normal volunteers. Therefore, there is a high probability that vasomotor waves causing fluctuations in cerebral blood flow can occur spontaneously at this frequency with concomi-

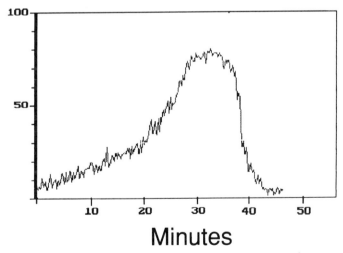

Minutes

Figure 10-3 Example of a plateau wave or Lundberg A-wave[6] in the intracranial pressure tracing. These waves are due to sudden increases in cerebral blood volume and cause decreased cerebral blood flow. Scale = mmHg

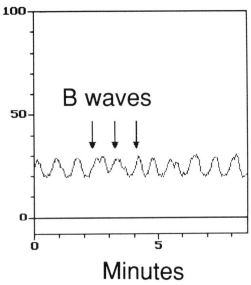

Figure 10-4 Typical B-waves in the ICP tracing described by Lundberg.[6] These waves reflect periodic fluctuation in cerebral blood volume due to vasomotor waves of the regulating vessels and usually indicate decreased intracranial compliance. Scale = mmHg

tant fluctuations in cerebral blood volume. These become amplified in the ICP tracing when the intracranial compliance is reduced. The mechanism that controls the CBF fluctuations is unknown, but some authors suggest that a brainstem pacemaker may be responsible.[12,13]

Lundberg[6] also described C-waves, which also may be due to reduced intracranial compliance reflecting small changes in intracranial blood volume in the ICP tracing. Lundberg suggested that these waves reflect arterial Traube-Hering waves and that their significance may be the indication of reduced intracranial compliance in some instances. Waves in the ICP tracing related to artificial respiration can also be seen, particularly if patients are hypovolemic. Figure 10-5 illustrates ICP waves produced by artificial respiration.

Indications for ICP Monitoring

Since the advent of continuous ICP monitoring, its most frequent use has been in head-injured patients. The true prevalence of high intracranial pressure after head injury and the pathophysiologic significance of this condition was not known until more experience was accumulated with the technique. ICP management has now been established as a critical component of the care of severely head-injured patients and it is useful to ensure an adequate CPP as well as an early warning of the expansion of mass lesions. Studies have demonstrated a high prevalence of increased ICP after head injury in patients who have abnormal CT scans on admission to the hospital or in patients who are not following commands.[14] ICP monitoring may also be indicated in patients with mild or moderate head injuries who require immediate general anesthesia for surgical treatment of systemic injuries.

Utility of ICP Measurements

Continuous monitoring of ICP following head injury has provided the essential information for guiding much of the therapy used to prevent secondary brain injury. It has also provided a rational basis to evaluate the effects of various modalities used to decrease ICP. Normally ICP should remain less than 10 mmHg,[15] and usually treatment is initiated to decrease ICP following head injury when it is consistently more than 14 to 20 mmHg.[16]

Increased ICP may produce secondary brain injury by several mechanisms. Increased pressure and pressure gradients caused by mass lesions may cause shifts in the position of brain subcomponents resulting in herniation. The classic herniations which have been described include (1) subfalcine, (2) uncal, (3) transtentorial, and (4) tonsillar. Each has specific clinical correlates and also specific patterns of pathologic damage that can occur as a result. A particular intracranial pressure that causes each of these entities cannot be specified, but more importantly, pressure gradients can occur that can result in herniation, even when the overall ICP is not extremely high. Brain herniation is often reversible after prompt recognition and treatment but may leave permanent injury to particular brain structures. For example, temporal lobe

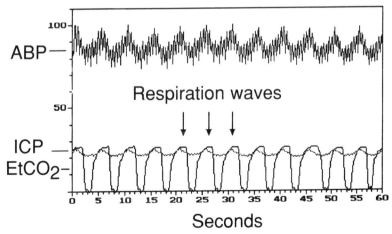

Figure 10-5 Waves in the ICP tracing produced by secondary effects from artificial respiration. Scale = mmHg

masses can cause uncal herniation without markedly elevated ICP and should be treated if clinical signs exist.

Another major role of ICP monitoring is in helping to define the CPP and, thus, guide the therapy designed to ensure adequate cerebral perfusion. Autoregulation (the ability to maintain constant cerebral blood flow despite changing cerebral perfusion pressure) can be lost following head injury, and therefore, the brain is less protected from ischemia due to blood pressure fluctuations and increases in ICP.[17,18] Decreases in arterial blood pressure can be as harmful as increased ICP in causing secondary brain ischemia. It is generally agreed that the cerebral perfusion pressure is optimal at a level greater than 70 mmHg; however, the exact optimal limits of CPP are controversial. A recent study has supported the concept that maintaining an adequate CPP is beneficial after head injury.[19]

Continuous monitoring of ICP is also useful in providing early diagnosis of increases in the size of mass lesions. In patients who are unconscious, sedated or given paralytic agents, subtle changes in neurologic function are not always a sensitive indication of progressing brain injury. Progressive increases in ICP in these patients can prompt repeat CT scanning to detect surgically removable lesions that may be responsible for secondary deterioration in brain function.

Data are now available that clearly indicate that sustained elevation of ICP after head injury is associated with a poor prognosis.[20,21] Marmarou and coworkers[21] have recently reported data from the Traumatic Coma Data Bank that determined the relationship among increased ICP, hypotension, and outcome in patients with severe head injury. They demonstrated that the proportion of hourly ICP readings greater than 20 mmHg was highly significant in association with a poor outcome. The proportion of hourly blood pressure readings less than 60 mmHg was also highly significant in association with a poor outcome. Figure 10-6 illustrates these results.

Monitoring of ICP is now an integral part of head injury management and, despite some of the pitfalls that may be encountered, it provides valuable information for providing optimal care in the treatment of patients with head injury.

TREATMENT OF INCREASED ICP

There can be a variety of causes of increased intracranial pressure, and a number of treatments can be instituted depending on the cause. When ICP control becomes necessary, one must ensure that no new surgically correctable mass lesion has developed causing a progressive increase in ICP. Consideration must also be given to the maintenance of optimal conditions for ICP control and the accurate diagnosis of the causes of increased ICP to allow for rational treatment. Monitoring ICP using a ventricular catheter permits

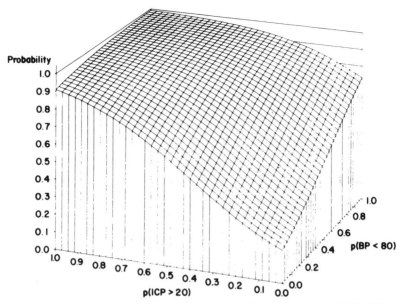

Figure 10-6 Relationship between outcome and hypotension and ICP. Three-dimensional surface of estimated outcome probability versus the proportion of intracranial pressure (ICP) measurements greater than 20 mmHg [p(ICP > 20)] and the proportion of blood pressure measurements less than 80 mmHg [p(BP < 80)] for the vegetative/dead outcome group. To simplify the presentation, the other modeled factors were fixed at the following values: age = 30 years; admission motor score = 3 (flexion); and abnormal pupils = 1. The substantial effect of hypotension is readily evident from the front-to-back upward sloping of the surface. The impact of ICP elevation is apparent from the right-to-left upward sloping of the surface.

CSF drainage, which can be effective in controlling elevated ICP. Other strategies for ICP control are listed below.

Head Elevation

In order to maintain optimal conditions for cerebral venous return, the head of the bed should be elevated to 20 to 30° and one must ensure that a cervical collar or head rotation does not cause venous obstruction. The effect of head elevation on ICP has been well documented; however, there has been controversy as to the best head position for maintenance of optimal CPP.[22–24] In some patients, particularly those who may be hypovolemic, raising the head of the bed can reduce the cerebral perfusion pressure.[24] A recent study measured ICP, CPP, mean carotid pressure, and CBF at 0° and 30° angles in 22 head-injured patients. The results indicated that when the head of the bed was elevated from 0 to 30°, no significant change in CPP or CBF occurred, but there was a significant reduction in ICP.[23]

Paralysis and Sedation

Excess agitation and movement can occur, especially in ventilated patients, making necessary the use of sedation and neuromuscular paralysis to help control ICP. Excess muscular activity, such as coughing or posturing and straining against the ventilator, can cause ICP to rise to abnormally high levels in patients who would otherwise have an acceptable ICP. Pancuronium bromide, or other shorter-acting agents, such as vecuronium and atracurium, can be given in moderate repeated doses to allow intermittent neurologic assessment. Intravenous lidocaine is also useful in suppression of cough and prevention of an increase in ICP associated with tracheal suctioning. Analgesics or narcotics can also be combined if paralysis alone is ineffective in decreasing ICP in agitated patients. Morphine given in small doses or a slow infusion can be useful and is also relatively rapidly reversible for neurologic assessment.

Hyperventilation

Hyperventilation can be a very effective way to rapidly reduce ICP. It is useful in acute situations and is routinely used in the initial stages of resuscitation of head-injured patients. The mechanism of action of hyperventilation is to cause generalized vasoconstriction primarily in the small regulatory arteries in the brain, which reduces the cerebral blood volume and reduces ICP. In patients with sudden increases in ICP due to expanding mass lesions, hyperventilation should be used to temporarily decrease ICP until more definitive therapy can be initiated. There are two aspects of the use of hyperventilation that are controversial: (1) The degree of hyperventilation that should be used, and (2) The importance of prolonged or chronic hyperventilation in head injury. One of the concerns over using vigorous hyperventilation is whether it can result in cerebral ischemia.[25,26] It is recognized that autoregulation can be impaired or lost both focally and globally after head injury. Some authors suggest that hyperventilation can cause a "steal" of blood from poorly regulating brain areas and worsen focal ischemia. Moreover, vigorous manual "bagging" may also cause more generalized ischemia in certain patients.[25–27]

Concerns over prolonged or chronic hyperventilation stem from experimental observations that the vasoconstriction caused by decreasing Pa_{CO_2} is not sustained for long periods. Muizelaar[28] demonstrated in rabbits that the observed pial artery vasoconstriction that occurs in response to hyperventilation begins to reverse after several hours and is gone at 24 h. If these experiments accurately reflect the situation in humans, they may indicate that there is a good rationale to use hyperventilation for short-term ICP control but not for prolonged periods. A recent prospective randomized trial of hyperventilation in patients with severe head injury was completed and concluded that hyperventilation for 5 days was deleterious in those patients with motor scores on the Glasgow Coma Scale of 4 to 5.[29] The outcome in these patients was significantly worse at 3 and 6 months, but no difference was observed at 12 months after injury. A third arm of the study by Muizelaar and coworkers included patients treated with hyperventilation and the buffer tromethamine (THAM). The addition of THAM reversed the deleterious effect of hyperventilation. The mechanism responsible for the poorer outcome at 3 and 6 months is unclear. There was no evidence of increased cerebral ischemia in the hyperventilated group. One possible factor may have been a rebound in ICP in the hyperventilated group. We try therefore, to keep the Pa_{CO_2} between 35 to 40 mmHg and to begin mannitol therapy as the next step for ICP control. Hyperventilation is used to cause a short-term decrease of ICP, e.g., during transport of the patient or CT scanning or during other situations when ICP can become transiently elevated. Efforts should be made to avoid prolonged continuous hyperventilation.

Diuretic Therapy

Reduction of ICP in head-injured patients can be accomplished effectively using osmotic diuretics. Mannitol has become the most commonly administered agent and is usually administered intravenously as a 20% or 25% solution. Doses commonly used range between 0.25 and 1.0 g/kg body weight. Mannitol may be used on a repeated schedule, but the serum osmolarity must be followed to ensure that systemic dehydration does not take place. Serum osmolarity should not be allowed to increase to more than 320 mosmol/kg. The mechanism of ICP reduction by mannitol may be related to its osmotic effect in shifting fluid from the brain tissue compartment to the intravascular compartment[30,31] as well as its ability to improve blood rheology by decreasing blood viscosity. The latter effect causes vasoconstriction, which keeps blood flow constant when autoregulation is present, and can, therefore, reduce blood volume and ICP.[32]

Barbiturate Therapy for ICP Control

On the basis of reports by Shapiro and coworkers[33,34] indicating that barbiturates can lower ICP, barbiturate therapy has been used extensively in head-injured patients when other therapies, mostly hyperventilation and mannitol, failed to decrease ICP adequately. The mechanism of action of barbiturates is believed to be due to their ability to inhibit synaptic transmission, thereby decreasing the cerebral metabolic rate of oxygen consumption (CMR_{O_2}). In patients where metabolism and cerebral blood flow is coupled, decreased CMR_{O_2} causes vasoconstriction, reducing blood volume and, thereby, decreasing ICP.[35] Subsequent to the use of barbiturate therapy in head-injured patients, it was observed that some patients responded well with effective ICP control while others had a poor response.[35,36] There are two major reasons why some patients may not respond to barbiturate therapy: One is because their CMR_{O_2} may be already low because of their head injury and is not further decreased to any significant extent by barbiturates; the other is that cerebral blood flow and metabolism may be uncoupled. In this situation, even though CMR_{O_2} can be decreased, vasoconstriction does not occur.[35]

Several studies evaluating the effect of barbiturates on ICP control and outcome in head injury have been published.[36–38] An improvement in the outcome could not be demonstrated in several early studies, and a significant prevalence of hypotension was seen.[37,38] In these initial studies, barbiturates were given prophylactically to patients, and one study compared mannitol therapy with barbiturate therapy. Subsequently, a multicenter prospective study was performed in which those patients who failed conventional therapy to control ICP were to receive barbiturates or to continue conventional therapy.[36] There was a $2:1$ benefit in the barbiturate-treated group with respect to ICP control. This benefit was extended to $4:1$ when patients were stratified by cardiac complications before random selection. In the treatment group, approximately one-third of the patients had their ICP controlled with barbiturates. An improvement in the outcome was also noted in those patients who responded as compared with the nonresponders.

Treatment with barbiturates requires a significant commitment of resources and personnel and is associated with a significant risk of complications. The most significant complication has been cardiac depression and instability, and therefore, it is generally accepted that patients with significant preexisting cardiac abnormality or instability should not undergo this therapy. Intensive monitoring is required including arterial blood pressure monitoring, pulmonary artery catheter monitoring, EEG monitoring, and frequent blood chemistries monitoring for barbiturate levels. In addition, intensive nursing assessment for pulmonary and thrombotic complications is required.[39] Patients must be normovolemic, and hypovolemia and hypotension must be avoided. Barbiturate treatment is usually started with a slow intravenous infusion of pentobarbital, 5 to 10 mg/kg over 10 to 30 min while carefully observing the blood pressure. EEG monitoring is helpful to define the limits of therapy as indicated by the occurrence of burst suppression. Once burst suppression is achieved, then a constant infusion may be maintained. Serum levels should range between 30 and 50 mg/dl, and controlled burst suppression should be present on EEG.[40]

Decompressive Craniectomy

In patients with refractory ICP increases, surgical decompressive craniectomy has been another treatment option. The practice of surgical decompression of the bony covering of the brain and opening of the dura was practiced by Cushing,[41] who performed subtemporal decompression for intracranial hypertension. Craniectomy for head injury has been performed using several different methods. The majority of the reports, however, have been in the pre-CT era. Kjellberg[42] reported the technique of bifrontal craniectomy in patients with refractory intracranial hypertension from a variety of causes. Another method of circumferential craniectomy was reported on a small number of patients with poor results.[43] The most common procedure used for cranial decompression has been hemicraniectomy or large unilateral cranial flaps with dural patching. Several series of patients undergoing hemicraniectomy for the treatment of hemispheric swelling associated with acute subdural hematoma have been reported.[44-48] Reports indicate that this procedure can be effective in reducing ICP,[49,50] but the exact role of the procedure has been controversial. We have used this procedure in patients with secondary deterioration and midline shift with high ICP, not controlled by medical therapy, and for intraoperative brain swelling after the removal of subdural hematomas[48] (see Chap. 6).

Other Agents Used to Lower ICP

THAM

The buffer THAM has been used in experimental head injury as well as in several recent human trials.[51-53] The mechanisms of action include correcting intracellular as well as CSF acidosis and causing vasoconstriction with reduction of cerebral blood volume. THAM has been shown to be effective in reducing ICP in two human studies.[52,53] Wolf and coworkers[53] demonstrated in a prospective randomized trial that there was no difference in outcome in the THAM-treated group; however, THAM was effective in decreasing ICP, and the THAM-treated group required less aggressive ICP treatment by other methods than the control group.

THE USE OF STEROIDS IN HEAD INJURY

High doses of steroids, mostly dexamethasone, have proven very effective in the treatment of brain swelling associated with tumors. Dexamethasone was also used frequently in the past to reduce brain edema and ICP in head-injured patients. Several large studies have now been performed indicating that steroids are not effective in reducing ICP and do not improve outcome in head-injured patients.[54-57] Moreover, in patients with severe head injury who often have associated polytrauma, an increased risk of infections has been associated with steroid use.[58] More recently, newer steroids, including methylprednisolone and 21-aminosteroids, which have a much lower glucocorticoid effect than dexamethasone, have been effective in experimental brain and spinal cord injury and may act as antioxidants inhibiting free radical formation.[59] Trials are currently underway to evaluate the use of these compounds following head injury. The 21-aminosteroid, Tirilazad, does not influence cerebral blood flow and the cerebrovascular response to CO_2 in healthy humans.[60]

MONITORING OF CEREBRAL BLOOD FLOW

Cerebral blood flow measurements have yielded much important information about the pathophysiology of head injury. The exact involvement of CBF measurements in head-injured patients, however, remains controversial. The first practical method of obtaining CBF measurements was the Kety-Schmidt method using nitrous oxide washin. Subsequently, the xenon washout method became the most common technique, initially using intracarotid xenon injections, and subsequently using an intravenous delivery method.[61] Portable systems are available that can be used in the intensive care unit. Other methods for evaluating cerebral blood flow in head-injured patients include thermal dilution probes,[62] laser Doppler probes,[63] transcranial Doppler,[64] single photon emission computed tomography (SPECT), positron emission tomography (PET), and xenon-CT.[65]

Most of the data on CBF after head injury have been gathered using the xenon washout method.[61] This method can provide repeated single measurements of flow values in the vicinity of externally placed detectors. Langfitt and Obrist[66] have determined several clinical uses of CBF measurements using this method in head-injured patients. These include (1) ensuring adequate CBF; (2) assessing outcome prediction; (3) evaluation of cerebrovascular responses, such as autoregulation and CO_2 reactivity, and (4) assessing the effects of treatments on CBF. It has been demonstrated that CBF can be normal, increased, or reduced after head injury. Obrist and coworkers[61] have shown that increased CBF values usually indicate cerebral hyperemia and occur when there is uncoupling of CBF from cerebral metabolism. This condition is associated with high ICP. Low CBF after head injury has been associated with poor outcome.[66]

Recently xenon-CT has been used to measure CBF much earlier during the hospitalization of head-injured patients than had previously been done using the external detector system.[65] In order to evaluate the time interval in which cerebral ischemia can occur, the measurements in the study were made at the time of the admission CT scans. Bouma and coworkers[65] reported that a significant number of patients demonstrated low CBF at this point in time, thus indicating early ischemia. In a group of 35 comatose head-injured patients, 31.4 percent demonstrated global or regional ischemia. Patients with diffuse swelling were especially prone to ischemia, which was associated with early mortality.

Laser Doppler and thermodilution probes have been used in neurosurgical patients to measure blood flow continuously.[62,63] Continuous monitoring offers advantages over the single measurement methods; however, the probes must be implanted surgically and can only measure CBF in a very focal region. These drawbacks have limited the use of these techniques in head injury.

Transcranial Doppler has also been used to evaluate cerebral circulatory changes after head injury. By observing relative changes in blood flow velocity, blood flow changes can be evaluated under certain circumstances, and information about autoregulation and CO_2 reactivity can be collected.[64,68–70] Chan and coworkers[71] have reported a relationship between middle cerebral artery blood flow velocity and outcome in head-injured patients. Low blood flow velocity, probably indicating low CBF, correctly predicted 80 percent of the deaths. Low blood flow velocity with reversal of flow in diastole has also been demonstrated to indicate progressive impairment and arrest of the cerebral circulation (see Chaps. 5 and 11). Transcranial Doppler has also been useful in indicating posttraumatic vasospasm.[72–74] Recent studies indicate that vasospasm has been underrecognized in head injury and may be associated with cerebral infarction.[64,72–75] Weber and coworkers[73] reported a 40 percent prevalence of vasospasm in head-injured patients using transcranial Doppler criteria. Martin and coworkers[74] have also reported a high prevalence of cerebral vasospasm using transcranial Doppler in head injured-patients. In a series of 30 head-injured patients, 27 percent developed vasospasm as confirmed by Doppler criteria. Three patients developed severe vasospasm confirmed by angiography, and one patient developed a cerebral infarction. Both of these studies discovered an association between posttraumatic vasospasm and subarachnoid hemorrhage. Posttraumatic vasospasm, which can easily be diagnosed with transcranial Doppler, must be considered as a cause of secondary deterioration in head-injured patients, especially in those with subarachnoid hemorrhage (see Figure 10-7).

MONITORING OF JUGULAR VENOUS OXYGEN SATURATION

Sampling of venous blood from the jugular bulb by using a retrograde jugular catheter can be performed to determine the jugular venous oxygen saturation (Sjv_{O_2}). More recently, fiberoptic catheters have been used to continously monitor the Sjv_{O_2} in head-injured patients. Initial experience with this technique indicates that it can be performed with minimal complications and can provide useful information.[76–79] One difficulty which has been encountered is interruption of the signal due to catheter movement. A strong positive correlation has been established between Sjv_{O_2} measurements derived from the cooximeter catheter and Sjv_{O_2} measurements derived from blood sampling.[78] Sheinberg and coworkers[78] reported the results of continuous Sjv_{O_2} monitoring in 45 head-injured patients. They associated episodes of desaturation,

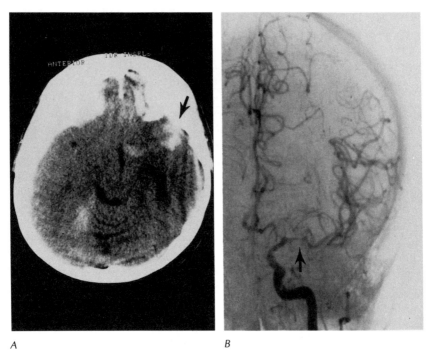

A   B

Figure 10-7 Illustration of posttraumatic vasospasm. *A.* CT scan indicating subarachnoid blood in the left sylvian fissure in a patient with a right sided subdural hematoma (arrow). *B.* Severe spasm of the left middle cerebral artery indicated by transcranial Doppler and confirmed by cerebral angiography (arrow). This patient developed two small watershed infarctions as a result of the vasospasm.

which they defined as decreases in Sjv_{O_2} to less than 50 percent, with intracranial hypertension, hypoxemia, systemic hypotension, and vasospasm. Other uses for fiberoptic catheters include avoidance of ischemia from hyperventilation,[25,27] calculation of CMR_{O_2} and estimation of CBF.[61,79]

MONITORING OF EEG AND MULTIMODALITY-EVOKED POTENTIALS

Monitoring of Electroencephalogram

With the advent of modern imaging techniques, the electroencephalogram (EEG) no longer has any value as a diagnostic tool in patients suffering from head injury. Although various patterns (alpha coma, spindle coma, delta coma, burst suppression, electric silence, etc.) have been described,[80] EEG monitoring does not materially alter the management of these patients.

Monitoring of Somatosensory-Evoked Potential

Monitoring of somatosensory-evoked potential (SSEP) in comatose patients for prognostic purposes was first introduced into clinical practice by Hume and Cant.[81] They reported that the central conduction time (the time required for the impulse generated in response to a peripheral stimulus to travel from the brainstem to the primary sensory cortex; i.e., the difference in latency between the brainstem component and the cortical component) correctly predicted outcome in approximately 78 percent of patients suffering from traumatic coma.[82] In contrast, monitoring of brainstem auditory-evoked potential (BAEP) was less sensitive but more specific; i.e., significant changes in BAEP represented rostral-caudal deterioration and inevitably led to death, whereas the presence of a normal BAEP did not necessarily result in good outcome.[83] Houlden and coworkers reported that in 51 patients with head injuries, SSEP grades had a higher positive correlation with the Glasgow Outcome Score than GCS scores did.[84] Conversely, Lindsay and coworkers reported that SSEP monitoring increased only slightly the predictive accuracy when compared with the clinical data alone. These authors concluded that evoked potential monitoring may be useful in paralyzed or sedated patients, but is not justified in patients where neurologic examination is feasible.[85]

In some centers, multimodality-evoked potential monitoring including visual, somatosensory, and brainstem auditory potentials is used for prognostic purposes.[86] In general, SSEP monitoring has the optimal correlation with outcome, and the addition of the other modalities improves the prognostic accuracy only marginally. More recently, motor-evoked potential (MEP) monitoring has been investigated as a prediction of outcome[87,88]; however, the results are inconclusive. Although Facco and coworkers reported that the addition of MEP to SSEP monitoring improved the outcome prediction and decreased the rate of false negatives,[87] Zentner and Rohde determined that MEP, in comparison with SSEP had no prognostic value.[88] The value of evoked potential monitoring as a predictor of outcome in patients in coma and with severe head trauma was recently reviewed.[89,90]

Few studies have addressed the use of evoked potential monitoring in actual patient care management despite its demonstrated utility as a predictor of outcome. Moulten and coworkers performed automated continuous computerized monitoring of SSEP in 36 patients in posttraumatic coma and reported that, in addition to its use for outcome prediction, the management of three patients was altered as a result of SSEP monitoring.[91] The authors conclude that continuous monitoring of SSEPs is a useful adjunct in the management of comatose head-injured patients. SSEP and BAEP usually resist the influence of intravenous anesthetic agents and remain recordable in patients treated with sedative agents, such as benzodiazepines and barbiturates, although the latencies may be increased and the amplitudes of the waveforms reduced.[92] Of particular importance is the fact that SSEP and BAEP can be recorded in patients managed with therapeutic barbiturate coma in electrocortical silence.[92] Evoked potential monitoring in these patients is valuable in providing the only physiological assessment of brain/brainstem function.

To summarize the literature, SSEP monitoring provides useful prediction in posttraumatic coma; the addition of BAEP monitoring provides only marginal benefit, and the use of MEP remains unproved. The use of evoked potential monitoring is not justified in patients where neurologic examination is feasible and, because of its technical complexity, its efficiency in improving patient management must also be considered unproved. It is, however, useful in the management of patients in therapeutic barbiturate coma. We currently do not use evoked potential monitoring routinely in the intensive care unit.

EXTRACRANIAL COMPLICATIONS IN HEAD-INJURED PATIENTS

Secondary injury to the brain can occur as a result of extracranial complications as well as from intracranial causes. Extracranial factors can interact and lead to cerebral damage as a result of infection, hypoxia, hypotension, coagulopathy, and other harmful conditions that can disturb overall homeostasis. The Traumatic Coma Data Bank[93] analyzed the role of extracranial complications in determining the outcome in 734 severely head-injured patients. The most frequent complication was electrolyte disturbance (59 percent), but this did not appear to alter the outcome. Hypotension, pneumonia, coagulopathy, and sepsis were significant contributors to poor outcome and occurred frequently. Figure 10-8 shows the frequency of the major complications found in this study.

Hypotension

Hypotension, defined as a systolic blood pressure of less than 90 mmHg, can occur before or after hospitalization and can contribute to a poor outcome.[93] Prehospital hypotension occurred in 34.6 percent of the Traumatic Coma Data Bank patients and doubled the mortality. Hypotension in the posthospitalization period occurred in between 20 and 25 percent of these patients. Elimination of this complication would have resulted in a 9.3 percent reduction in unfavorable outcome. The adequacy of the volume status of the patients must be ensured, and hypotension must be corrected rapidly if it occurs. Fluid restriction to reduce "brain swelling" does not appear justified, particularly if electrolytes are normal.

Pneumonia

Pneumonia is common in severely head-injured patients, occurring in 41 percent in two recent studies and usually several days after injury.[93,94] The diagnosis can be established according to the following criterion: a new or

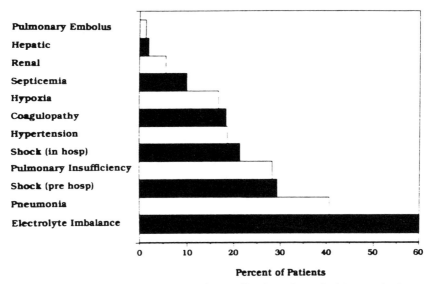

Figure 10-8 Incidence of extracranial complications from the Traumatic Coma Data Bank.[93]

progressing pulmonary infiltrate on chest roentgenograms in addition to two of the following findings: (1) new fever >38.5°C, (2) leukocyte count >12,000/mm^3, and (3) new purulent tracheobronchial secretions.[94]

Pneumonia can prolong ICU and hospital stay.[94] The Traumatic Coma Data Bank study estimated that a poor outcome could be avoided in 2.9 percent of all patients if pneumonia was eliminated as a complication.[93]

Coagulopathy

The coagulation abnormality that is most commonly encountered after head injury is disseminated intravascular coagulation (DIC).[95] The pathogenesis of DIC can be directly due to brain injury when brain material, which is highly thrombogenic, enters the circulation. This condition is often associated with extensive basal skull fractures and dural sinus injury and may contribute to the pathogenesis of intracranial bleeding.[96] Systemic injury can also cause DIC as a result of multisystem injury, hypothermia, massive transfusion, and fat embolism. The diagnosis of DIC is suggested by abnormally increased prothrombin time; partial thromboplastin time; and decreased platelets, plasma fibrinogen level, and hematocrit level; in addition to increased fibrin-split products. Confirmation of DIC can be obtained by using the plasma protamine test or ethanol gelation test.[97–99] Treatment of DIC is reversal of the underlying cause. If the cause is brain injury alone, the process usually spontaneously reverses itself. The correction of systemic abnormalities, such as hypothermia, shock, sepsis, and other primary causes will help to reverse the process. Blood components, such as platelets, fresh frozen plasma, red cells, and whole blood should be used as needed until the DIC resolves.[99]

Sepsis

The prevalence of sepsis was approximately 10 percent in the group of patients studied by the Traumatic Coma Data Bank. It was estimated that 1.5 percent of poor outcomes could have been eliminated if sepsis had not occurred.[93] Multiple sources of infection can occur in head-injured patients, particularly those with polytrauma, but special considerations should include the meticulous care of intravenous catheters and ventricular drains in addition to an awareness of sinus infections and meningitis.

SEIZURE PROPHYLAXIS

Seizures following head injury have been the topic of much study and controversey. Jennett and coworkers[100] classified seizures into "early" and "late" and early seizures were considered to be the result of acute reactions to trauma. Conversely, late seizures are considered to be the result of formation of an epileptic focus, and, therefore, are considered to be posttraumatic epilepsy. Others have further categorized seizures into (1) immediate (occurring within 24 h after injury), (2) delayed early (occurring during the remainder of the first week, and (3) late (occurring more than 1 week after the trauma).[101] The prevalence of delayed early seizures is estimated to be between 8 and 18 percent[101] in patients with risk factors for seizures and between 18 and 48 percent for late seizures. Risk factors include GCS score <10, hematoma, contusion, penetrating injury, early seizures, and depressed skull fracture. A major controversy regarding posttraumatic seizures has been the involvement of prophylactic anticonvulsants. Previous studies have been inconclusive because of the study design and the failure to document adequate drug levels. A recent prospective randomized double blind study on phenytoin for posttraumatic seizures concluded that this drug reduced seizures during the first week after head injury but did not prevent the development of late seizures.[101,102] We currently treat head-injured patients, who are at risk for seizures, with phenytoin after admission, maintain treatment for 1 week, and then discontinue the drug.

CONCLUSIONS

The ultimate outcome in the head-injured patient depends upon many factors. These include the premorbid condition of the patient, the severity of the initial injury, and the effectiveness of the treatment on reversing and preventing further secondary injury, including the effects of complications and the length of the recovery. Effective intensive care management is essential in promoting the optimal recovery. Avoidance of secondary injury, particularly ischemia, is a primary consideration because of the high incidence of this complication.[103] Of the various monitoring methods considered, each has its own unique capabilities, advantages, and disadvantages depending on the clinical situation. The recognition of secondary deterioration in head-injured patients requires the vigilance of the nursing staff and physicians who must rely on clinical judgment as well as the results of monitoring information and repeated radiographic studies. Prompt treatment of secondary deterioration is essential. Newer medications that provide cerebral protection against ischemia and brain injury are undergoing intensive investigation and clinical trials. The many factors which may promote neural recovery are also being investigated. In the future there will, no doubt, be many new clinical trials to evaluate these newer treatments.

REFERENCES

1. Chestnut RM, Marshall LF: Treatment of abnormal intracranial pressure. In Eisenberg HM, Aldrich EF (eds): *Neurosurgery Clinics of North America*, vol. 2. Philadelphia, WB Saunders, 1991:267–284.

2. Marmarou A, Tabaddor K: Intracranial pressure: Physiology and pathophysiology. In Cooper PR (ed): *Head Injury*, 3rd ed. Baltimore, Williams & Wilkins, 1993:203–224.

3. Marmarou A, Shulman K, Rosende RM: A non-linear analysis of the cerebrospinal fluid system and intracranial pressure dynamics. *J Neurosurg* 48:332, 1978.

4. Crutchfield JS, Narayan RK, Robertson CS, et al: Evaluation of a fiberoptic intracranial pressure monitor. *J Neurosurg* 71:482, 1990.

5. Guillaume J, Janny P: Monometric intracranienne continue; Interet physiopathologique et clinique de la méthode. *Presse Med* 59:953, 1951.

6. Lundberg N: Continuous recording and control of ventricular fluid pressure in neurosurgical practice. *Acta Psychiatr Scand (Suppl)* 149:1, 1960.

7. Risberg J, Lundberg N, Ingvar DH: Regional cerebral blood volume during acute transient rises of the intracranial pressure (plateau waves). *J Neurosurg* 31:303, 1969.

8. Lundberg N, Cronqvist S, Kjallquist A: Clinical investigation on interrelations between intracranial pressure and intracranial hemodynamics. *Prog Brain Res* 30:70, 1968.

9. Rosner MJ, Becker DP: Origin and evolution of plateau waves: Experimental observations and a theoretical model. *J Neurosurg* 60:312, 1984.

10. Auer LM, Sayama I: Intracranial pressure oscillations (B-waves) caused by oscillations in cerebrovascular volume. *Acta Neurochir* 68:93, 1983.

11. Newell DW, Aaslid R, Stooss R, et al: The relationship of blood flow velocity fluctuations to intracranial pressure B waves. *J Neurosurg* 76:415, 1992.

12. Higashi S, Yamamoto S, Hashimoto M, et al: The role of vasomotor center and adrenergic pathway in B-waves, In Hoff, JT, Betz AL (eds): *Intracranial Pressure VII*. Berlin, Springer-Verlag, 1989:220–224.

13. Maeda M, Takahashi K, Miyazaki M, et al: The role of the central monoamine system and the cholinoceptive pontine area on the oscillation of ICP "pressure waves". In Miller JD, Teasdale GM, Rowan JO, et al (eds): *Intracranial Pressure VI*. Berlin, Springer-Verlag, 1986:151–155.

14. Narayan RK, Kishore PRS, Becker DP, et al: Intracranial pressure: To monitor or not to monitor. *J Neurosurg* 56:650, 1982.

15. Ekstedt J: CSF hydrodynamic studies in man. II. Normal hydrodynamic variables related to CSF pressure and flow. *J Neurol Neurosurg Psychiatry* 41:345, 1978.

16. Marshall LF, Smith RW, Shapiro HM: The outcome with aggressive treatment in severe head injuries. I. The significance of intracranial pressure monitoring. *J Neurosurg* 50:20, 1979.

17. Enevoldsen EM, Jensen FT: Autoregulation and CO_2 responses of cerebral blood flow in patients with acute severe head injury. *J Neurosurg* 48:689, 1978.

18. Strandgaard S, Paulson OB: Cerebral autoregulation. *Stroke* 15:413, 1984.

19. Rosner MJ, Daughton S: Cerebral perfusion pressure management in head injury. *J Trauma* 30:933, 1990.

20. Miller JD, Becker DP, Ward JD, et al: Significance of intracranial hypertension in severe head injury. *J Neurosurg* 47:503, 1977.

21. Marmarou A, Anderson RL, Ward JD, et al: Impact of ICP instability and hypotension on outcome in patients with severe head trauma. *J Neurosurg* 75:S59, 1991.

22. Durward QJ, Amacher AL, DelMaestro RF, et al: Cerebral and cardiovascular responses to changes in head elevation with intracranial hypertension. *J Neurosurg* 59:938, 1983.

23. Feldman Z, Kanter MJ, Robertson CS, et al: Effect of head elevation on intracranial pressure, cerebral perfusion pressure, and cerebral blood flow in head-injured patients. *J Neurosurg* 76:207, 1992.

24. Rosner MJ, Coley IB: Cerebral perfusion pressure, intracranial pressure, and head elevation. *J Neurosurg* 60:636, 1986.

25. Cold GE: Does acute hyperventilation provoke cerebral oligaemia in comatose patients after acute head injury? *Acta Neurochir (Wein)* 96:100, 1989.

26. Sutton LN, McLaughlin AC, Dante S, et al: Cerebral venous oxygen content as a measure of brain energy metabolism with increased intracranial pressure and hyperventilation. *J Neurosurg* 73:927, 1990.

27. Cruz J, Miner ME, Allen SJ, et al: Continuous monitoring of cerebral oxygenation in acute brain injury: Injection of mannitol during hyperventilation. *J Neurosurg* 73:725, 1990.

28. Muizelaar JP, van der Poel HG, Li ZC, et al: Pial arteriolar vessel diameter and CO_2 reactivity during prolonged hyperventilation in the rabbit. *J Neurosurg* 69:923, 1988.

29. Muizelaar JP, Marmarou A, Ward JD, et al: Adverse effects of prolonged hyperventilation in patients with severe head injury: A randomized clinical trial. *J Neurosurg* 75:731, 1991.

30. Bell BA, Smith MA, Kean CM, et al: Brain water measured by magnetic resonance imaging. *Lancet* 1:66, 1987.

31. Nath F, Galbraith S: The effect of mannitol on cerebral white matter water content. *J Neurosurg* 65:41, 1986.

32. Muizelaar JP, Wei EP, Kontos HA, et al: Mannitol causes compensatory cerebral vasoconstriction and vasodilatation in response to blood viscosity changes. *J Neurosurg* 59:822, 1983.

33. Shapiro HM, Galindo A, Wyte SR, et al: Rapid intraoperative reduction of intracranial pressure with thiopentone. *Br J Anaesth* 45:1057, 1973.

34. Shapiro HM: Intracranial hypertension: Therapeutic and anesthetic considerations. *Anesthesiology* 43:445, 1975.

35. Nordstrom CH, Messeter K, Sundbarg G, et al: Cerebral blood flow, vasoreactivity, and oxygen consumption during barbiturate therapy in severe traumatic brain lesions. *J Neurosurg* 68:424, 1988.

36. Eisenberg H, Frankowski R, Contant C, et al: Comprehensive Central Nervous System Trauma Centers: High-dose barbiturate control of elevated intracranial pressure in patients with severe head injury. *J Neurosurg* 69:15, 1988.

37. Schwartz M, Tator C, Rowed D, et al: The University of Toronto Head Injury Treatment Study: A prospective, randomized comparison of pentobarbital and mannitol. *Can J Neurol Sci* 11:434, 1984.

38. Ward J, Becker D, Miller J, et al: Failure of prophylactic barbiturate coma in the treatment of severe head injury. *J Neurosurg* 62:383, 1985.

39. Winer JW, Rosenwasser RH, Jimenez F: Electroencephalographic activity and serum and cerebrospinal fluid pentobarbital levels in determining the therapeutic end point during barbiturate coma. *Neurosurgery* 29:739, 1991.

40. Chestnut RM, Marshall LF, Marshall SB: Medical management of intracranial pressure. In Cooper PR (ed): *Head Injury,* 3rd ed. Baltimore, Williams & Wilkins, 1993:225–246.

41. Cushing H: The establishment of cerebral hernia as a decompressive measure for inaccessible brain tumors; with the description of intermuscular methods of making the bone defect in temporal and occipital regions. *Surg Gynecol Obstet* 1:297, 1905.

42. Kjellberg RN, Prieto A: Bifrontal decompressive craniotomy for massive cerebral edema. *J Neurosurg* 34:488, 1971.

43. Clark K, Nash TM, Hutchison GC: The failure of circumferential craniotomy in acute traumatic cerebral swelling. *J Neurosurg* 29:367, 1968.

44. Ransohoff J, Benjjamin MV, Gage, EL, Jr, et al: Hemicraniectomy in the management of acute subdural hematoma. *J Neurosurg* 34:70, 1971.

45. Morantz RA, Abad RM, George AE, et al: Hemicraniectomy for acute extracerebral hematoma: An analysis of clinical and radiographic findings. *J Neurosurg* 39:622, 1973.

46. Britt RH, Hamilton RD: Large decompressive craniotomy in the treatment of acute subdural hematoma. *Neurosurgery* 2:195, 1978.

47. Cooper PR, Rovit RL, Ransohoff J: Hemicraniectomy in the treatment of acute subdural hematoma: A re-appraisal. *Surg Neurol* 5:25, 1976.

48. Elliott JP, LeRoux PD, Howard MA, et al: Outcome following decompressive craniectomy for acute intraoperative brain swelling associated with blunt head trauma. *Surgical Forum*, Vol XLIII, American College of Surgeons, 1992:548–550.

49. Hase U, Reulen H-J, Meinig G, et al: The influence of the decompressive operation on the intracranial pressure and the pressure-volume relation in patients with severe head injuries. *Acta Neurochir* 45:1, 1978.

50. Hatashita S, Hoff JT: The effect of craniectomy on the biomechanics of normal brain. *J Neurosurg* 67:573, 1987.

51. Rosner MJ, Becker DP: Experimental brain injury: Successful therapy with the weak base, tromethamine. With an overview of CNS acidosis. *J Neurosurg* 60:961, 1984.

52. Gaab MR, Seegers K, Goetz C: THAM (tromethamine, "tris-buffer"): Effective therapy of traumatic brain swelling. In Hoff JT, Betz AL (eds): *Intracranial Pressure VII*, Berlin, Springer-Verlag, 1989:616–619.

53. Wolf AL, Levi L, Marmarou A, et al: Effect of THAM upon outcome in severe head injury: A randomized prospective clinical trial. *J Neurosurg* 78:54, 1993.

54. Cooper P, Moody S, Clark W, et al: Dexamethasone and severe head injury. A prospective double blind study. *J Neurosurg* 51:307, 1979.

55. Dearden NM, Gibson JS, McDowal DG, et al: Effect of high-dose dexamethasone on outcome from severe head injury. *J Neurosurg* 64:81, 1986.

56. Gudeman SK, Miller JD, Becker DP: Failure of high-dose steroid therapy to influence intracranial pressure in patients with severe head injury. *J Neurosurg* 51:301, 1979.

57. Saul T, Ducker T, Salman M, et al: Steroids in severe head injury. A prospective, randomized clinical trial. *J Neurosurg* 54:596, 1981.

58. Marshall L, King J, Langfitt T: The complications of high-dose corticosteroid therapy in neurosurgical patients: A prospective study. *Ann Neurol* 1:201, 1977.

59. Hall ED: The neuroprotective pharmacology of methylprednisolone. *J Neurosurg* 76:13, 1992.

60. Olsen KS, Videback C, Agerlin N, et al: The effect of Tirilazed Mesylate (M74006F) on cerebral oxygen consumption and reactivity of cerebral blood flow to carbon dioxide in healthy volunteers. *Anesthesiology* 79:666, 1993.

61. Obrist WD, Langfitt TW, Jaggi JL, et al: Cerebral blood flow and metabolism in comatose patients with acute head injury. Relationship to intracranial hypertension. *J Neurosurg* 61:241, 1984.

62. Koshu K, Hirota S, Sonobe M, et al: Continuous recording of cerebral blood flow by means of a thermal diffusion method using a peltier stack. *Neurosurgery* 21:693, 1987.

63. Meyerson BA, Gunasekera L, Linderoth B, et al: Bedside monitoring of regional cortical blood flow in comatose patients using laser Doppler flowmetry. *Neurosurgery* 29:750, 1991.

64. Newell DW, Seiler RW, Aaslid R: Head injury and cerebral circulatory arrest. In Newell DW, Aaslid R (eds): *Transcranial Doppler*, New York, Raven Press, 1992:109–121.

65. Bouma GJ, Muizelaar JP, Stringer WA, et al: Ultra-early evaluation of regional cerebral blood flow in severely head-injured patients using xenon-enhanced computerized tomography. *J Neurosurg* 77:360, 1992.

66. Langfitt TW, Obrist WD: Cerebral blood flow and metabolism after intracranial trauma. *Prog Neurol Surg* 10:14, 1981.

67. Robertson CS, Contant CF, Gokaslan ZL, et al: Cerebral blood flow, arteriovenous oxygen difference, and outcome in head injured patients. *J Neurol, Neurosurg, Psychiatry* 55:594, 1992.

68. Aaslid R, Lindegaard KF, Sorteberg W, et al: Cerebral autoregulation dynamics in humans. *Stroke* 20:45, 1989.

69. Aaslid R, Newell DW, Stooss R, et al: Assessment of cerebral autoregulation dynamics from simultaneous arterial and venous transcranial Doppler recordings in humans. *Stroke* 22:148, 1991.

70. Newell DW, Aaslid R: Transcranial Doppler clinical and experimental uses. *Cerebrovasc Brain Metab Rev* 4:122, 1992.

71. Chan K-H, Miller JD, Dearden NM: Intracranial blood flow velocity after head injury: Relationship to severity of injury, time, neurological status and outcome. *J Neurol Neurosurg Psychiatry* 55:787, 1992.

72. Compton JS, Teddy PJ: Cerebral arterial vasospasm following severe head injury: A transcranial Doppler study. *Br J Neurosurg* 1:435, 1987.

73. Weber M, Grolimund P, Seiler RW: Evaluation of posttraumatic cerebral blood flow velocities by transcranial Doppler ultrasonography. *Neurosurgery* 27:106, 1990.

74. Martin NA, Doberstein C, Zane C, et al: Posttraumatic cerebral arterial spasm: Transcranial Doppler ultrasound, cerebral blood flow, and angiographic findings. *J Neurosurg* 77:575, 1992.

75. Newell DW, Eskridge J, Mayberg M, et al: Endovascular treatment of intracranial aneurysms and cerebral vasospasm. In Selman W (ed): *Clinical Neurosurgery*, Baltimore, Williams & Wilkins, 1992:348–360.

76. Cruz J, Miner ME, Allen SJ, et al: Continuous monitoring of cerebral oxygenation in acute brain injury: Assessment of cerebral hemodynamic reserve. *Neurosurgery* 29:743, 1991.

77. Garlick R, Bihari D: The use of intermittent and continuous recordings of jugular venous bulb oxygen saturation in the unconscious patient. *Scand J Clin Lab Invest Suppl* 47:47, 1987.

78. Sheinberg M, Kanter MJ, Robertson CS: Continuous monitoring of jugular venous oxygen saturation in head-injured patients. *J Neurosurg* 76:212, 1992.

79. Robertson CS, Narayan RK, Gokaslan ZL, et al: Cerebral arteriovenous oxygen difference as an estimate of cerebral blood flow in comatose patients. *J Neurosurg* 70:222, 1989.

80. Cohen RJ, Henry CE: The electroencephalogram in head injury. In Becker DP, Gudeman SK (eds): *Textbook of Head Injury*. Philadelphia, WB Saunders, 1989, pp 265–277.

81. Hume AL, Cant BR, Shaw NA: Central somatosensory conduction time in comatose patients. *Ann Neurol* 5:379, 1979.

82. Hume AL, Cant BR: Central somatosensory conduction after head injury. *Ann Neurol* 10:411, 1981.

83. Garcia-Larrea L, Artru F, Bertrand O, et al: The combined monitoring of brain stem auditory-evoked potentials and intracranial pressure in coma. A study of 57 patients. *J Neurol Neurosurg Psychiatry* 55:792, 1992.

84. Houlden DA, Li C, Schwartz ML, et al: Median nerve somatosensory-evoked potentials and the Glasgow Coma Scale as predictors of outcome in comatose patients with head injuries. *Neurosurgery* 27:701, 1990.

85. Lindsay K, Pasaoglu A, Hirst D, et al: Somatosensory and auditory brain stem conduction after head injury: a comparison with clinical features in prediction of outcome. *Neurosurgery* 26:278, 1990.

86. Firsching R, Frowein RA: Multimodality-evoked potentials and early prognosis in comatose patients. *Neurosurg Rev* 13:141, 1990.

87. Facco E, Baratto F, Munari M, et al: Sensorimotor central conduction time in comatose patients. *Electroencephalogr Clin Neurophysiol* 80:469, 1991.

88. Zentner J, Rohde V: The prognostic value of somatosensory- and motor-evoked potentials in comatose patients. *Neurosurgery* 3:429, 1992.

89. Facco E, Munari M, Baratto F, et al: Somatosensory-evoked potentials in severe head trauma. *Electroencephalogr Clin Neurophysiol Suppl* 41:330, 1990.

90. Goodwin SR, Friedman WA, Bellefleur M: Is it time to use evoked potentials to predict outcome in comatose children and adults? *Crit Care Med* 19:518, 1991.

91. Moulton R, Kresta P, Ramirez M, et al: Continuous automated monitoring of somatosensory-evoked potentials in posttraumatic coma. *J Trauma* 31:676, 1991.

92. Lam AM: Do evoked potentials have any value in anesthesia? *Anesthesiology Clin North Am* 10:657, 1992.

93. Piek J, Chestnut RM, Marshall LF, et al: Extracranial complications of severe head injury. *J Neurosurg* 77:901, 1992.

94. Hsieh AH, Bishop MJ, Kubilis PS, et al: Pneumonia following closed head injury. *Am Rev Respir Dis* 146:290, 1992.

95. Olson JD, Kaufman HH, Moake J, et al: The incidence and significance of hemostatic abnormalities in patients with head injuries. *Neurosurgery* 24:825, 1989.

96. Chan K-H, Mann KS, Chan TK: The significance of thrombocytopenia in the development of postoperative intracranial hematoma. *J Neurosurg* 71:38, 1989.

97. Feinstein DI: Diagnosis and management of disseminated intravascular coagulation: The role of heparin therapy. *Blood* 60:284, 1982.

98. Vecht CJ, Sibinga CT, Minderhoud JM: Disseminated intravascular coagulation and head injury. *J Neurol Neurosurg Psychiatry* 38:567, 1975.

99. Chestnut RM: Medical complications of the head-injured patient. In Cooper PR (ed): *Head Injury,* 3rd ed. Baltimore, Williams & Wilkins, 1993:459–501.

100. Jennett B: *Epilepsy after nonmissile injuries,* 2d ed Chicago, Year Book Medical Publishers 1975.

101. Temkin NR, Dikmen SS, Winn HR: Posttraumatic seizures. In Eisenberg HM, Aldrich EF (eds): *Neurosurgery Clinics of North America,* vol 2. Philadelphia, WB Saunders, 1991:425–435.

102. Temkin NR, Dikmen SS, Wilensky AJ, et al: A randomized, double-blind study of phenytoin for the prevention of post-traumatic seizures. *N Engl J Med* 323:497, 1990.

103. Graham DI, Adams JH, Doyle D: Ischaemic brain damage in fatal non-missile head injuries. *J Neurol Sci* 39:213, 1978.

Brain Death

David W. Newell

Physicians are often asked to make a medical determination of death. In-hospital death requires pronouncement by a physician and, most frequently, occurs as a result of cardiorespiratory failure. It is only relatively recently with the advent of cardiorespiratory support that the determination of brain death has become necessary. In patients not supported by a respirator, failure of the central nervous system invariably leads to failure of the medullary respiratory center, with subsequent respiratory arrest and progressive hypoxia followed by cardiac arrest. In patients who are supported by artificial respiration, progression to brain death is not followed by respiratory and cardiac arrest, and therefore, a determination of brain death is necessary. Many patients, however, who have respiratory support when brain function ceases, if allowed to follow their natural course, will progress to cardiovascular collapse. This is due to the loss of sympathetic activity and the subsequent loss of vasomotor tone and neurohypophyseal failure, which results in massive diabetes insipidus and electrolyte disturbance and ultimately leads to cardiac arrest. In such patients, however, a considerable time may elapse between the cessation of all brain functions and cardiovascular collapse due to its consequences. In this situation, a physician is often required to make the diagnosis of brain death, which has become medically and legally accepted as a criteria for death.[1]

The President's Commission for the Study of Ethical Problems in Medicine has established a definition of death that states that an individual who has sustained either (1) irreversible cessation of circulatory and respiratory functions or (2) irreversible cessation of all functions of the entire brain including the brain stem is dead. The determination of death must be made in accordance with accepted medical standards.[2] The need to make the determination of brain death arises when either the interval between cessation of brain function and cardiovascular collapse is prolonged or organ donation for transplant purposes is being considered. It is necessary to make the determination of brain death for several reasons. First, it is important to the patient's family members to be informed of the occurrence of brain death and not to have the family undergo a prolonged interval between the patient's brain death and cessation of cardiovascular function. The time of pronouncement of brain death is recorded in the medical records as the actual time of death despite the fact that cessation of cardiac function has not occurred. Second, in order to expedite the processing of the remains of the patient in addition to allowing the family to proceed with funeral arrangements, it is advisable to make a prompt diagnosis of brain death once it has occurred and then discontinue respiratory support. Third, when organ donation is not planned, it is advisable not to delay the diagnosis of brain death so that hospital staff will not continue to provide cardiorespiratory and other support after the diagnosis is clear. Finally, in cases of organ donation, the unequivocal diagnosis of brain death must be established before organ removal is undertaken. In this situation, however, careful attention must be paid to maintaining adequate cardiac and respiratory function for the optimal preservation of organ function.

GUIDELINES FOR THE DETERMINATION OF BRAIN DEATH

After the development of respiratory support, the need for determination of brain death became obvious. One of the first comprehensive attempts to establish uniform criteria was published in 1968 after the formation and report of the Ad Hoc Committee of the Harvard Medical School to examine the definition of brain death.[3] Before this report, there were individual reports on the utility of EEG in helping to make the diagnosis of brain death, but there was no uniformly accepted criteria.[4,5] Similarly, reports from other countries began to surface to try to establish uniformly accepted guidelines. By 1978, more than thirty sets of criteria for the determination of brain death had been published. Although these were in agreement on many aspects, there was no uniform consensus on the involvement of EEG and other ancillary tests, the specific clinical criteria to be included, and the timing.[6] In 1981, the guidelines for the determination of death were published by the President's Commission in an attempt to provide a more up-to-date consensus of leading physicians studying this problem.[2] The report of the President's Commission is intended to provide guidelines and emphasizes that these guidelines are only advisory. The guidelines are illustrated in Fig. 11-1.

The guidelines provided by the President's Commission are designed to assist qualified physicians in making the determination of brain death. Most states allow considerable leeway in allowing the physician to make the determination of death and only require that a qualified physician make this determination. Professional organizations have also aided by setting forth criteria. The American Medical Association by its judicial counsel has stated that "deaths shall be determined by the clinical judgment of the physician. In making this judgment the ethical physician will use all available currently accepted scientific tests."[7] There are many legal precedents now recognizing the diagnosis of brain death as a determination of death in many states. The American Bar Association has passed a resolution that recognizes that the physician should be allowed to decide the adequate criteria for death by prevailing standards, and the resolution also makes clear that brain death is a legal as well as medical entity and should fulfill the criteria for death. The resolution states "For all legal purposes, a human body with irreversible cessation of brain function according to usual and customary standards of medical practice shall be considered dead."[8,9]

HISTORY AND CLINICAL EXAMINATION

It is essential to obtain an adequate history of events in patients who are being evaluated for brain death. A clear history of injury or sudden ictal event that is consistent with conditions known to cause massive brain destruction

THE CRITERIA
FOR DETERMINATION OF DEATH

An individual presenting the findings in *either* section A (cardiopulmonary) *or* section B (neurological) is dead. In either section, a diagnosis of death requires that *both* cessation of functions, as set forth in subsection 1, *and* irreversibility, as set forth in subsection 2, be demonstrated.

A. An individual with irreversible cessation of circulatory and respiratory functions is dead.

1. Cessation is recognized by an appropriate clinical examination.

Clinical examination will disclose at least the absence of responsiveness, heartbeat, and respiratory effort. Medical circumstances may require the use of confirmatory tests, such as an ECG.

2. Irreversibility is recognized by persistent cessation of functions during an appropriate period of observation and/or trial of therapy.

In clinical situations where death is expected, where the course has been gradual, and where irregular agonal respiration or heartbeat finally ceases, the period of observation following the cessation may be only the few minutes required to complete the examination. Similarly, if resuscitation is not undertaken and ventricular fibrillation and standstill develop in a monitored patient, the required period of observation thereafter may be as short as a few mintues. When a possible death is unobserved, unexpected, or sudden, the examination may need to be more detailed and repeated over a longer period, while appropriate resuscitative effort is maintained as a test of cardiovascular responsiveness. Diagnosis in individuals who are first observed with rigor mortis or putrefaction may require only the observation period necessary to establish that fact.

B. An individual with irreversible cessation of all functions of the entire brain, including the brain stem, is dead. The "functions of the entire brain" that

are relevant to the diagnosis are those that are clinically ascertainable. Where indicated, the clinical diagnosis is subject to confirmation by laboratory tests, as described in the following portions of the text. Consultation with a physician experienced in this diagnosis is advisable.

1. Cessation is recognized when evaluation discloses findings of a and b:

a. Cerebral functions are absent, and . . .

There must be deep coma, that is, cerebral unreceptivity and unresponsivity. Medical circumstances may require the use of confirmatory studies such as an EEG or blood-flow study.

b. brain stem functions are absent.

Reliable testing of brain stem reflexes requires a perceptive and experienced physician using adequate stimuli. Pupillary light, corneal, oculocephalic, oculovestibular, oropharyngeal, and respiratory (apnea) reflexes should be tested. When these reflexes cannot be adequately assessed, confirmatory tests are recommended.

Adequate testing for apnea is very important. An accepted method is ventilation with pure oxygen or an oxygen and carbon dioxide mixture for ten minutes before withdrawal of the ventilator, followed by passive flow of oxygen. (This procedure allows $Paco_2$ to rise without hazardous hypoxia.) Hypercarbia adequately stimulates respiratory effort within 30 seconds when $Paco_2$ is greater than 60 mm Hg. A ten-minute period of apnea is usually sufficient to attain this level of hypercarbia. Testing of arterial blood gases can be used to confirm this level. Spontaneous breathing efforts indicate that part of the brain stem is functioning.

Peripheral nervous system activity and spinal cord reflexes may persist after death. True decerebrate or decorticate posturing or seizures are inconsistent with the diagnosis of death.

2. Irreversibility is recognized when evaluation discloses findings of a and b and c:

a. The cause of coma is established and is sufficient to account for the loss of brain functions, and . . .

Most difficulties with the determination of death on the basis of neurological criteria have resulted from inadequate attention to this basic diagnostic prerequisite. In addition to a careful clinical examination and investigation of history, relevant knowledge of causation may be acquired by computed tomographic scan, measurement of core temperature, drug screening, EEG, angiography, or other procedures.

b. the possibility of recovery of any brain functions is excluded, and . . .

The most important reversible conditions are sedation, hypothermia, neuromuscular blockade, and shock. In the unusual circumstance where a sufficient cause cannot be established, irreversibility can be reliably inferred only after extensive evaluation for drug intoxication, extended observation, and other testing. A determination that blood flow to the brain is absent can be used to demonstrate a sufficient and irreversible condition.

c. the cessation of all brain functions persists for an appropriate period of observation and/or trial of therapy.

Even when coma is known to have started at an earlier time, the absence of all brain functions must be established by an experienced physician at the initiation of the observation period. The duration of observation periods is a matter of clinical judgment, and some physicians recommend shorter or longer periods than those given here.

Except for patients with drug intoxication, hypothermia, young age, or shock, medical centers with substantial experience in diagnosing death neurologically report no cases of brain functions returning following a six-hour cessation, documented by

Figure 11-1 Guidelines for the determination of death as established by the President's Commission for the Study of Ethical Problems in Medicine and Biomedical and Behavioral Research. This set of guidelines was compiled after an extensive study of brain death and has been forth as a guide for practicing physicians to make the determination of brain death.

is helpful in establishing a working diagnosis. If there is a history of drug ingestion or hypothermia and no evidence of brain destruction on CT scanning, the physician must be more circumspect in reaching the diagnosis of brain death and must ensure that irreversibility is present. Equally important are the results of imaging studies, particularly CT, which has had a major

clinical examination and confirmatory EEG. In the absence of confirmatory tests, a period of observation of at least 12 hours is recommended when an irreversible condition is well established. For anoxic brain damage where the extent of damage is more difficult to ascertain, observation for 24 hours is generally desirable. In anoxic injury, the observation period may be reduced if a test shows cessation of cerebral blood flow or if an EEG shows electrocerebral silence in an adult patient without drug intoxication, hypothermia, or shock.

Confirmation of clinical findings by EEG is desirable when objective documentation is needed to substantiate the clinical findings. Electrocerebral silence verifies irreversible loss of cortical functions, except in patients with drug intoxication or hypothermia. (Important technical details are provided in "Minimal Technical Standards for EEG Recording in Suspected Cerebral Death" [*Guidelines in EEG 1980*. Atlanta, American Electroencephalographic Society, 1980, section 4, pp 19-24].) When joined with the clinical findings of absent brain stem functions, electrocerebral silence confirms the diagnosis.

Complete cessation of circulation to the normothermic adult brain for more than ten minutes is incompatible with survival of brain tissue. Documentation of this circulatory failure is therefore evidence of death of the entire brain. Four-vessel intracranial angiography is definitive for diagnosing cessation of circulation to the entire brain (both cerebrum and posterior fossa) but entails substantial practical difficulties and risks. Tests are available that assess circulation only in the cerebral hemispheres, namely radioisotope bolus cerebral angiography and gamma camera imaging with radioisotope cerebral angiography. Without complicating conditions, absent cerebral blood flow as measured by these tests,

in conjunction with the clinical determination of cessation of all brain functions for at least six hours, is diagnostic of death

COMPLICATING CONDITIONS

A. Drug and Metabolic Intoxication.—Drug intoxication is the most serious problem in the determination of death, especially when multiple drugs are used. Cessation of brain functions caused by the sedative and anesthetic drugs, such as barbiturates, benzodiazepines, meprobamate, methaqualone, and trichloroethylene, may be completely reversible even though they produce clinical cessation of brain functions and electrocerebral silence. In cases where there is any likelihood of sedative presence, toxicology screening for all likely drugs is required. If exogenous intoxication is found, death may not be declared until the intoxicant is metabolized or intracranial circulation is tested and found to have ceased.

Total paralysis may cause unresponsiveness, areflexia, and apnea that closely simulates death. Exposure to drugs such as neuromuscular blocking agents or aminoglycoside antibiotics, and diseases like myasthenia gravis are usually apparent by careful review of the history. Prolonged paralysis after use of succinylcholine chloride and related drugs requires evaluation for pseudocholinesterase deficiency. If there is any question, low-dose atropine stimulation, electromyogram, peripheral nerve stimulation, EEG, tests of intracranial circulation, or extended observation, as indicated, will make the diagnosis clear.

In drug-induced coma, EEG activity may return or persist while the patient remains unresponsive, and therefore the EEG may be an important evaluation along with extended observation. If the EEG shows electrocerebral silence, short latency auditory or somatosensory-evoked po-

tentials may be used to test brain stem functions, since these potentials are unlikely to be affected by drugs.

Some severe illnesses (eg, hepatic encephalopathy, hyperosmolar coma, and preterminal uremia) can cause deep coma. Before irreversible cessation of brain functions can be determined, metabolic abnormalities should be considered and, if possible, corrected. Confirmatory tests of circulation or EEG may be necessary.

B. Hypothermia.—Criteria for reliable recognition of death are not available in the presence of hypothermia (below 32.2 °C core temperature). The variables of cerebral circulation in hypothermic patients are not sufficiently well studied to know whether tests of absent or diminished circulation are confirmatory. Hypothermia can mimic brain death by ordinary clinical criteria and can protect against neurological damage due to hypoxia. Further complications arise since hypothermia also usually precedes and follows death. If these complicating factors make it unclear whether an individual is alive, the only available measure to resolve the issue is to restore normothermia. Hypothermia is not a common cause of difficulty in the determination of death.

C. Children.—The brains of infants and young children have increased resistance to damage and may recover substantial functions even after exhibiting unresponsiveness on neurological examination for longer periods compared with adults. Physicians should be particularly cautious in applying neurological criteria to determine death in children younger than 5 years.

D. Shock.—Physicians should also be particularly cautious in applying neurological criteria to determine death in patients in shock because the reduction in cerebral circulation can render clinical examination and laboratory tests unreliable.

Figure 11-1 (*Continued*)

impact in allowing an accurate diagnosis to be made in cases of brain death. The CT scan often reveals many important details about the structural pathology in the brain that led to extensive brain destruction. Many cases of brain death will be the result of trauma, gunshot wounds, or spontaneous intracerebral hemorrhage from aneurysms or other causes, and these conditions are accurately revealed by CT scanning. The physician can proceed with the diagnosis of brain death more confidently when there is CT evidence of massive brain destruction.

The clinical examination for brain death should be performed by experienced physicians who are thoroughly familiar with the complete neurologic examination and also with the accepted criteria established for the determination of brain death. The testing should also be performed when the core body temperature is greater than 32.2°C. It should be established that reversible causes of coma, such as alcohol, barbiturate, or other sedative toxicity, are not present. Neuromuscular blockade or other causes of peripheral nerve dysfunction must also be eliminated. The President's Commission advises that the determination of death must be recognized by the cessation of function as well as by irreversibility. Brain death is recognized when the irreversible cessation of all the functions of the entire brain including the brain stem is determined. Cessation of brain function is recognized when the cerebral functions and the brain stem functions are both absent. To determine the absence of cerebral function, there must be deep coma, unreceptiveness, and unresponsiveness. Absence of brain stem function is recognized when cranial nerve function and respiratory drive are both absent. When certain cranial nerves cannot be tested because of injury or other factors, it is recommended that confirmatory tests be undertaken. Testing of the cranial nerves includes testing of the pupillary light reflexes, corneal reflex, oculocephalic or oculovestibular reflexes and gag reflexes. In addition to these nerve tests, apnea testing should also be performed. Performance of these tests is discussed in the following sections.

Pupillary Light Reflexes

To perform this examination, the physician should dim the lights, direct a bright flashlight toward each pupil, and then observe both pupils. The ipsilateral pupil is observed for the direct response, and the contralateral pupil is observed for the consensual response. The process should be repeated on the opposite side. Drugs that can produce pupillary dilatation include scopolamine, atropine, and glutethimide.

Corneal Reflexes

Corneal reflexes are tested by applying a wisp of cotton to the cornea on each side while observing for contraction of the *orbicularis oculi* muscles. No contact lenses must be present during this examination.

Oculocephalic Reflexes

The oculocephalic reflexes are tested by forceful turning of the head from a neutral position to 60° off midline to each side while observing the alignment of the eyes. Any deviation of the eyes toward midline with this maneuver indicates the presence of the oculocephalic reflex.

Oculovestibular Reflexes

The oculovestibular reflex can be tested by elevating the head 30° above horizontal and instilling a solution of ice water in the ear with a syringe while the eyelids are held open for 30 s to 1 min to observe any tonic deviation of the eyes, which should be turned toward the cold stimulus in an unconscious patient. The process is then repeated on the opposite side after a waiting period of several minutes.

Gag Reflex

Oropharyngeal reflexes are tested by stimulating the oropharynx with a cotton swab while observing for any gag reflex or oropharyngeal contractions.

Apnea Test

When the testing of the cranial nerves is complete, apnea testing should then be undertaken. The objective of the apnea test is to allow the carbon dioxide level to increase to the point where the respiratory center should be maximally stimulated if it is still functional.[10] When performing this test, adequate oxygenation must be provided, and therefore, an accepted method is to preoxygenate with 100 percent oxygen before beginning the test. Usually a 10-min period of apnea is sufficient to attain a Pa_{CO_2} greater than 60 mmHg, which should stimulate the respiratory center. During this time oxygen is administered at 6 to 12 liters/min through an intratracheal catheter. It is usual to obtain blood gas confirmation of Pa_{CO_2} during the test. If the patient breathes during the apnea test, this indicates that the brain stem is still functioning. If the patient's history suggests chronic lung disease with dependence on a hypoxic stimulus for ventilation, then the Pa_{O_2} should be allowed to fall to less than 50 mmHg. It has been noted during testing in some patients that peripheral movements may occur that may indicate reflex activity but are still consistent with cerebral unresponsiveness. The "Lazarus sign" has been described in patients undergoing apnea testing, which consists of vigorous flexion of the arms to the chest either unilaterally or bilaterally in brain-dead patients.[11] Elicitation of movements of the arms by neck flexion as well as lower extremity flexor responses to stimulation have also been noted but do not invalidate the diagnosis of brain death.

PERFORMANCE OF ANCILLARY TESTS

One of the earliest ancillary tests to be used in the diagnosis of brain death was the electroencephalogram.[4,5] Some of the first reports of brain death included an EEG as one of the criteria. Subsequent to numerous reports, however, it is recognized that an EEG can sometimes be difficult to perform in the setting of a ventilated patient in the intensive care unit because of the multiple artifacts that can occur. It has also been recognized that there have been false positive and false negative EEG findings in cases of brain death.[12-15] It has subsequently been relegated by both the President's Commission and also by other criteria to an ancillary test rather than a primary requirement for the establishment of the diagnosis of brain death.[2,6]

The other major category of ancillary tests is cerebral blood flow studies. The gold standard for cerebral blood flow studies to determine the arrest of the cerebral circulation is four-vessel cerebral angiography.[1,16,17] This procedure has been commonly used in Europe, and the criteria for nonfilling of the intracranial circulation are well defined. Because this test is invasive and time consuming, other methods of cerebral blood flow determination have also been utilized in the determination of brain death. Radioisotope scanning using technetium 99 has been used, and the results of this technique have compared favorably with cerebral angiography.[17-20] This technique has the advantage of using portable equipment that can be brought to the intensive care unit. The study is relatively rapidly and easily performed, and criteria have been established for the interpretation of intracranial flow cessation to confirm the diagnosis of brain death (see Fig. 11-2). Transcranial Doppler has also emerged as a useful technique for determining the arrest of the cerebral circulation.[16,19,21-26] Initially, before the development of transcranial Doppler, characteristic waveforms of the velocity tracing were demonstrated by carotid Doppler[27] in patients with cerebral circulatory arrest. Subsequently,

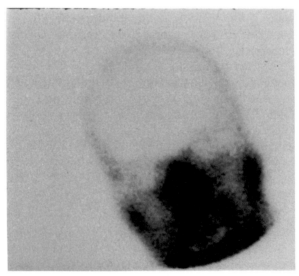

Figure 11-2 Radioisotope scan demonstrating lack of intracerebral blood flow and preservation of blood flow in the face and scalp.

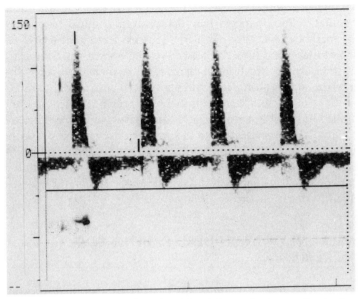

Figure 11-3 Example of reverberating blood flow velocity tracing in the middle cerebral artery using transcranial Doppler. This characteristic waveform correlates with arrest of the cerebral circulation due to obstruction of flow at the microcirculatory level with continued patency of the conducting arteries.

similar waveforms have been described using the transcranial Doppler. Reverberating flow velocity patterns found in the middle cerebral arteries have been correlated with radioisotope scanning as well as cerebral angiography in demonstrating a lack of supratentorial cerebral blood flow[16,19,23] (see Fig. 11-3). An advantage of the transcranial Doppler technique is its portability and the short time required for testing. As with all techniques, however, the results must be interpreted by experienced examiners, and under these circumstances, arrest of the cerebral circulation can be reliably documented.

All the ancillary testing methods that measure cerebral blood flow have been useful in confirming the diagnosis of brain death in suspicious circumstances or under circumstances where examination of the cranial nerves is made difficult. It must be emphasized, however, that although cerebral blood flow studies in most patients confirm brain death, some cases have been reported where confirmatory tests are at variance with the clinical findings of brain death. In such instances, the findings may be due to selective massive destruction of the brain stem from brain stem hemorrhage or posterior fossa lesions that render the patient clinically brain dead by causing impairment of all the cranial nerves and the respiratory center as well as interruption of all descending pathways. However, the supratentorial blood flow may be left intact, and therefore, because the cortical activity can persist, the EEG may not be flat.[26] Such patients may demonstrate residual blood flow by any of the methods of testing. Similarly, patients have been reported in which supratentorial blood flow has ceased, yet the patient still demonstrates weak brain stem activity, such as slight residual respiratory drive.[19] In these instances, the supratentorial structures have been destroyed, but minor residual blood flow to the brain stem probably is present, which accounts for the continued minimal function. These cases, given sufficient time, will all ultimately result in brain death, but at the time of testing, arrest of the cerebral circulation and clinical brain death are not always synonymous. With these caveats in mind, the confirmatory tests can be used intelligently in suspect cases to confirm the diagnosis of brain death or shorten the observation time required to determine irreversibility.[2]

MANAGEMENT OF BRAIN-DEAD PATIENTS FOR ORGAN RETRIEVAL

Once the diagnosis of brain death has been established, the time of this diagnosis can be legally recorded as the time of death, and all support may be discontinued. In cases which qualify for organ donation, however, a significant time may elapse between declaration of brain death and the harvest of organs. As mentioned previously, after cessation of all brain and brain stem functions, failure of the sympathetic tone and the neuroendocrine axis often lead to systemic instability and cardiac arrhythmia followed by cardiac arrest. When the objective is to preserve the central organ functions, such as the heart, kidneys, and lungs for transplant purposes, physiologic function must be maintained. Some of the normal sequelae of cessation of brain function include hypotension, arrhythmia, bradycardia, hypoxemia, diabetes insipidus, hypothermia, anemia, and infection.[28] It is necessary to develop a management strategy to preserve organ function when this cascade begins to occur. Hypotension will often ensue suddenly following brain death, and this is usually due to neurogenic shock from failure of sympathetic tone and may be aggravated by hypovolemia from diabetes insipidus. If hypotension is due mainly to neurogenic shock, clinically the patients are usually not tachycardic; they have either a normal pulse rate or bradycardia, and the extremities are usually warm. This is in contrast to hypovolemic shock where peripheral vasoconstriction is present, generally accompanied by tachycardia.

TREATMENT STRATEGIES FOR THE SEQUELAE OF BRAIN DEATH

Hypotension

Central monitoring, such as central venous pressure monitoring or pulmonary artery pressure monitoring, is helpful in guiding hemodynamic management. The initial strategy is to ensure that intravascular volume is adequate and after this, ionatropic agents can be used. Dopamine or dobutamine can be used initially followed by epinephrine or norepinephrine infusions. When using these agents the physician should have some knowledge of the total peripheral resistance and not be overly vigorous to the point where end organ damage occurs. Intravascular volume expansion can be accomplished with isotonic fluids (normal saline or lactated Ringers solution) in bolus infusions. A reasonable objective is to keep the mean arterial pressure greater than 70 mmHg.

Cardiac Arrhythmias

Electrolyte disturbances can be responsible for arrhythmias, and therefore, should be checked regularly. Bradycardia can be treated with atropine, and in refractory cases, transvenous pacing can be used.

Pneumonia and Hypoxemia

In patients who have been under intensive care for a prolonged period, pneumonia may ensure the onset of hypoxemia. Patients must then be treated with appropriate antibiotics, and adequate oxygenation must be maintained to prevent organ damage.

Diabetes Insipidus

This condition is usually due to neuroendocrine dysfunction secondary to interruption of the hypothalamic pituitary axis and can result in sudden large increases in urine output. Treatment consists of volume replacement and administration of vasopressin, 0.1 unit/min infusion or DDAVP, 0.3 μg/kg intravenously, to maintain a urine output of 1.5 to 3 ml/kg per hour. The electrolytes must also be checked frequently.

Hypothermia

Hypothermia can rapidly ensue after central nervous system failure, and if the central temperature drops too low, the coagulation system may fail. Therefore, the patient's temperature should be maintained at a level greater than 34°C with warming blankets.

Severe Anemia

In patients with multiple injuries or disseminated intravascular coagulation, severe anemia can occur and compromise organ function. As mentioned previously, maintenance of body temperatures is important and a transfusion may be necessary in order to maintain an adequate intravascular volume and keep the hematocrit above 30 percent.

SUMMARY AND CONCLUSIONS

Since the advent of artificial respiration it has become necessary for physicians to make the determination of brain death. Brain death is recognized both medically and legally as being synonymous with death of the patient. The accurate determination of brain death must be made to allow discontinuation of respiratory and cardiovascular support and also to serve as a prerequisite to organ donation for transplant purposes. Many organizations have attempted to reach a consensus on the criteria for determination of brain death. The most comprehensive set of guidelines has been established by the President's Commission, which was formed to establish specific guidelines for the determination of brain death. These guidelines not only state that the irreversible cessation of brain function including the brain stem is synonymous with brain death, but they also set forth the criteria for determining the absence of function as well as irreversibility. Under these guidelines also, clinical criteria are the main determinants of brain death, and EEG and cerebral blood flow studies are considered confirmatory tests. If continued cardiovascular support is necessary for organ donation in patients who have been declared dead, a recognized set of complications and physiologic events are described. The proper recognition and treatment of these physiologic responses will usually result in adequate organ function at the time of removal for transplantation.

REFERENCES

1. Black PMcL: Brain death. I, II, *N Engl J Med* 299:338, 393, 1978.

2. President's Commission: Guidelines for the determination of brain death. *JAMA* 246:2184, 1981.

3. A definition of irreversible coma: Report of the Ad Hoc Committee of the Harvard Medical School to examine the definition of brain death. *JAMA* 205:337, 1968.

4. Adams A: Studies on the flat electroencephalogram in man. *Electroencephalogr Clin Neurophysiol* 11:35, 1959.

5. Hamlin H: Life or death by EEG. *JAMA* 190:112, 1964.

6. Selby R: The medical determination of death. In Wilkins RH, Rengachary SS (eds): *Neurosurgery, vol III.* New York, McGraw Hill, 1985:2585–2597.

7. American Medical Association Judicial Council Opinions and Reports. Chicago, AMA Press, 1977, p 23.

8. American Bar Association: Report of the Committee on Medicine and Law. Forum 11:300, 1975.

9. The House of Delegates redefines death, urges redefinition of rape, and undoes the Houston Amendment. *Am Bar Assoc J* 61:463, 1975.

10. Earnest MP, Beresford HR, McIntyre HB: Testing for apnea in suspected brain death: Methods used by 129 clinicians. *Neurology* 36:542, 1986.

11. Ropper AH: Unusual spontaneous movements in brain-dead patients. *Neurology* 34:1089, 1984.

12. Alderete JF, Jeri FR, Richardson EP Jr, et al: Irreversible coma: A clinical electro-encephalographic and neuropathological study. *Trans Am Neurol Assoc* 93:16, 1968.

13. Hughes JR: Limitations of the EEG in coma and brain death. *Ann N Y Acad Sci* 315:121, 1978.

14. Silverman D, Masland RL, Saunders MG, et al: Irreversible coma associated with electrocerebral silence. *Neurology* 20:525, 1970.

15. Silverman D, Saunders MG, Schwab RS, et al: Cerebral death and the electroencephalogram: Report of the Ad Hoc Committee of the American Electroencephalographic Society on EEG Criteria for Determination of Cerebral Death. *JAMA* 209:1505, 1969.

16. Hassler W, Steinmetz H, Pirschel J: Transcranial Doppler study of intracranial circulatory arrest. *J Neurosurg* 71:195, 1989.

17. Korein J, Braunstein P, George A, et al: Brain Death: I. Angiographic correlation with the radioisotopic bolus technique for evaluation of critical deficit of cerebral blood flow. *Ann Neurol* 2:195, 1977.

18. Pearson J, Korein J, Harris JH, et al: Brain death: II. Neuropathological correlation with the radioisotopic bolus technique for evaluation of critical deficit of cerebral blood flow. *Ann Neurol* 2:206, 1977.

19. Newell DW, Grady S, Sirotta P, et al: Evaluation of brain death using transcranial Doppler. *Neurosurgery* 24:509, 1989.

20. Goodman JM, Heck LL, Moore BD: Confirmation of brain death with portable isotope angiography: A review of 204 consecutive cases. *Neurosurgery* 16:492, 1985.

21. Velthoven W, Calliauw L: Diagnosis of brain death. Transcranial Doppler sonography as an additional method. *Acta Neurochir* 95:57, 1988.

22. Bode H, Sauer M, Pringsheim W: Diagnosis of brain death by transcranial Doppler sonography. *Arch Dis Child* 63:1474, 1988.

23. Powers AD, Graeber MC, Smith RR: Transcranial Doppler ultrasonography in the determination of brain death. *Neurosurgery* 24:884, 1989.

24. Kirkham FJ, Levin SC, Padayachee TS, et al: Transcranial pulsed Doppler ultrasound findings in brain stem death. *J Neurol Neurosurg Psychiatry* 50:1504, 1987.

25. Petty GW, Mohr JP, Pedley TA, et al: The role of transcranial Doppler in confirming brain death: Sensitivity, specificity, and suggestions for performance and interpretation. *Neurology* 40:300, 1990.

26. Ropper AH, Kehne SM, Wechsler L: Transcranial Doppler in brain death. *Neurology* 37:1733, 1987.

27. Yoneda S, Nishimoto A, Nukada T, et al: To and fro movement and external escape of carotid arterial blood in brain death cases. A Doppler ultrasonic study. *Stroke* 5:707, 1974.

28. Robertson KM, Cook DR: Perioperative management of the multiorgan donor. *Anesth Analg* 70:546, 1990.

12

Experimental Head Injury and New Horizons

Yoram Shapira and Arthur M. Lam

HEAD TRAUMA MODELS

The pathophysiologic characteristics of the manifestations of traumatic brain injury (TBI) are highly variable and protean. Thus, many animal models of TBI emphasize only one aspect, or a combination of these manifestations.

Animal models of TBI are difficult to create. The data obtained should be reproducible and as relevant as possible to human head injury. For example, animal models in which the animal's body is accelerated and the freely moving head strikes a fixed object have been described.[1] Although many biomechanical features of human injury are closely approximated in such models, these techniques have typically provided variable results. In contrast, some models produce reliable data but bear no resemblance to situations associated with trauma in humans.[2-4] Another problem is the choice of species. The subhuman primates represent the ideal animal to study cerebral contusion because of their similarity to humans in terms of both their physiology and their skull configuration. However, the expense and the ethical concerns involved increasingly make such studies economically and ethically unfeasible.

The advantages of experimental models are obvious: there are some features of TBI that are difficult or impossible to investigate in injured humans. In human TBI, patients are usually seen more than 30 min to several hours after injury. Moreover, because human TBI frequently involves insults of multiple etiology, including hypoxia, ischemia, and hypotension, it is difficult to isolate the influence of any single variable, whereas laboratory models are more controllable. In addition, animal models allow the use of histopathologic, electrophysiologic, and biochemical techniques to study variables that are not applicable to human research. They can be used to examine pathophysiologic mechanisms at the chemical and cellular level and provide an opportunity for pre- and postinjury assessments in the same species. This chapter will discuss the different models of TBI and their relevance to human TBI, evaluate physiologic responses considered important to the outcome of TBI, and evaluate pharmacologic therapy to TBI based on experimental models.

Models of TBI fall into four general categories represented by acceleration-deceleration injury, compression injury, cryogenic injury, and penetrating injury. These categories are discussed further in the following sections:

Acceleration-Deceleration Injury

In 1982, Gennarelli and coworkers proposed a classification system[5] (Table 12-1) and demonstrated in a multicenter study different types of head trauma. Moreover, within each lesion category, patients were subdivided by their initial Glasgow Coma Scale (GCS) scores into less serious (GCS score of 6 to 8), and more serious injuries (GCS score of 3 to 5). Each of the lesion categories showed a consistently higher mortality rate as the severity of injury increased (Fig. 12-1). They demonstrated that immediate, prolonged uncon-

Table 12-1 Head-Injury Classification in 1107 Patients

Classification	No. of Patients
Focal injuries (total)	620
Extradural hematoma with operation	96
Acute subdural hematoma with operation	319
Other focal lesions (total)	205
With operation	71
Without operation	134
Diffuse injuries (total)	487
Coma for 6 to 24 h	92
Coma for longer than 24 h (total)	395
Not decerebrate	219
Decerebrate	176

SOURCE: From Gennarelli TA et al: Influence of the type of intracranial lesion on outcome from severe head injury. *J Neurosurg* 56:26, 1982.

sciousness unaccompanied by mass lesions occurs in almost half of severely head-injured patients (GCS score of 3 to 5), and is associated with 35 percent of all deaths from injury. Although coma in such injuries has been regarded in the past as the result of the primary brainstem injury, evidence gained from human postmortem material fails to support the presence of brainstem

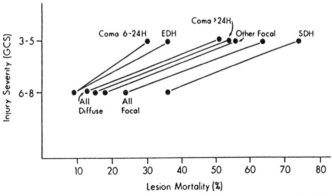

Figure 12-1 This depiction of injury severity, as judged by the Glasgow Coma Scale (GCS) scores, and lesion mortality rate for each of the lesion categories shows consistently higher mortality as injury severity increases. The similar slope of these plots demonstrate that severity has the same effect on mortality rate for each type of lesion. (*From Gennarelli TA, et al: Influence of the type of intracranial lesion on outcome from severe head injury. J Neurosurg 56:26, 1982, with permission.*)

injury in the absence of hemispheric damage.[6,7] The more common neuropathologic pattern includes diffuse microscopic damage to innumerable axons through the brain as well as focal lesions in the corpus callosum and in the dorsolateral quadrant of the rostral brainstem.[8-11] The cause of this axonal injury has been proposed, but not proved, to be due to shear strain.[12-14] The term "shear," however, connotes a specific injury mode to the biomechanician, and the more descriptive term "diffuse axonal injury" (DAI) is preferred.

Gennarelli concluded that acceleration-deceleration forces impart to the head high momentum, rotational and shear forces but with relatively low kinetic energy. This mechanism classically occurs in road traffic accidents. Acceleration models include all those that produce movement of the intact cranium either by impact or by accelerating the helmet enclosing the head without impact.

Acceleration Model

The most thoroughly characterized model of cranial acceleration is the primate model of Ommaya and coworkers,[15] which has been modified by Gennarelli and coworkers.[16] In this later "Penn II" device, the animal's head is placed in a form-fitting helmet. The helmet is attached by mechanical linkages to a pneumatically activated, piston-driven device, which can move the head in a plane horizontal to the ground (transitional movement) (Fig. 12-2).[17,18] The pneumatic activator is internally programmed to provide a reproducible acceleration-time waveform.

Other linkages can rotate the head in a whiplash-like fashion through a 45° angle (rotational movement) while simultaneously translating. Magnitudes of acceleration can be quantified (g's or rad/s^2) and related to differing physiologic and neurologic responses. The acceleration of the animal's head, encased in a helmet and not accompanied by impact, certainly does not accurately simulate the event associated with clinical head injury, but it is reproducible. Conversely, models in which the freely moving head strikes a fixed object may have variable pathologic results according to the impact velocity.[1] This procedure faithfully replicates many features of the clinical head injury seen in contact sports, such as football.[19]

Repetitive Acceleration

In this model a repetitive traumatic insult is produced in cats by rapidly shaking the head, whereas a single insult failed to produce satisfactory results.[20]

Ommaya and coworkers[15] and Gennarelli and coworkers[16] showed that translation of the head in the horizontal plane produces focal effects only, resulting in well-circumscribed cerebral contusions and intracerebral hemato-

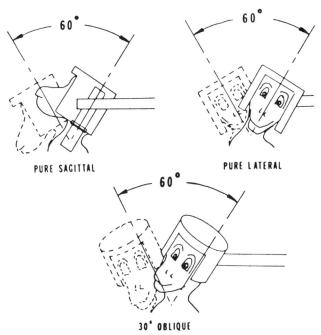

60°   60°

PURE SAGITTAL   PURE LATERAL

60°

30° OBLIQUE

Figure 12-2 Model of acceleration/deceleration injury. Examples of three types of head motion imparted by the Penn II device used to produce experimental concussion in primates. Note that the head is encased in a helmet and the cranium accelerated without impact to the skull. In all cases shown here, the amount of movement (60°) and the center of rotation are the same. [*Reproduced from Textbook of Head Injury. Becker DP, Gludeman SK (eds): Philadelphia, WB Saunders, with permission.*]

mas; such effects on the brain were evident at head acceleration levels up to 1400 g's in the squirrel monkey.

Although this model mimics only about 35 percent of the closed head injury, its effects encompass the entire spectrum of traumatic unconsciousness described in human beings.[17-21] By manipulation of the magnitude, duration, and direction of acceleration, Gennarelli and coworkers could create coma of varying length and depth, which was very similar to the clinical situation. Pathologically, Gennarelli and coworkers demonstrated axonal damage and formation of retraction balls and assumed that the shear strain of the injury physically injured axons.[1] Moreover, postmortem examination of victims of severe head injury consistently revealed the presence of axon retraction balls believed by most researchers to have been formed through the physical shearing or tearing of axons with the subsequent extrusion of their exoplasm, thereby forming large reactive swelling.[10,11,22-26]

Compression Injury

Compression models include all those in which the head is maintained in a fixed position during impact. There are two types of compression models. With the first type, the cranium remains intact. Injury models of this type use weight drop devices,[27] blasting caps,[28] and humane stunners.[29] With the second type, the impact is delivered directly to the dura through an opening in the skull. Injury models of this type include those created by fluid percussion,[30,31] and by a contusing device.[32]

Intact Cranium

WEIGHT-DROP DEVICE IN RATS[27] This experimental model is designed to deliver a standard blow in order to elicit a controlled TBI. The impact imparted to the cranium of the rat is proportional to the momentum of the platform at the end of its free fall. The momentum is determined by the height from which the mass (weight) is allowed to fall; manipulating this height affects the momentum of the blow. In this model the reproducibility of the standard blow is tested by measuring the velocity developed during the free fall of the mass and the change in velocity on collision with the target. There is a linear correlation between the change in velocity during collision and the height from which the tip falls, as long as the tip falls more than 3 cm (Fig. 12-3). The weight-drop device enables gradation of the degree of insult according to the momentum of impact that is applied to the skull. Only part of the energy is transferred to the brain itself because of its dissipation by the bony skull. However, by altering the height from which the moving plate is dropped (i.e., momentum of the impact), the resultant injury can range from no observable ill effect to immediate death of all the animals. The reproducibility of this model is high as demonstrated by the degree of brain edema, water content, and blood-brain barrier (BBB) permeability defect, as well as the histopathologic studies. The advantages of this model include its resemblance to human traumatic brain injury and its provision of a normalized baseline neurologic status for valid comparison of brain protection therapy (this is accomplished by determining the neurologic status 1 h after head trauma).

BLASTING CAPS With this model a closed head injury is produced by detonating an electric blasting cap secured to the head. The detonation results in a scalp wound, an intact skull, and a uniform neurologic syndrome. The advantage of this model is the production of the uniform neurologic syndrome in the survivors. However, the injury is generally associated with a high immediate mortality. Moreover, the gross pathology findings of the brains showed a lack of uniformity, and small hemorrhages into the brainstem were found in half of the brains. The symptoms of the resulting neurologic syndrome, characterized by somnolence, inability to stand and ataxia, were thus attributed to damage to the labyrinth system.[28] This model therefore bears little resemblance to human traumatic brain injury.

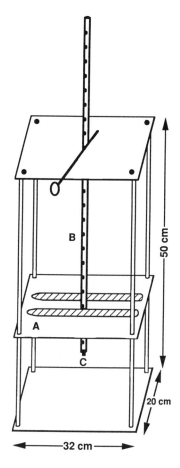

Figure 12-3 Model of closed cranium/impact injury. The figure depicts a weight-drop device used to produce closed head trauma in rat. The impact imparted to the cranium of the rat is proportional to the momentum of the platform at the end of its free fall. The momentum is determined by the height from which the platform is allowed to fall and the mass (1600 g) of the falling platform (A + B + C). Manipulating this height affects the momentum of the blow. (*Redrawn from Shapira et al.: Experimental closed head injury in rats: Mechanical, pathophysiologic, and neurologic properties. Crit Care Med 16:258, 1988.*)

HUMANE STUNNER This device is used to combine impact energy and acceleration. Tornheim and coworkers used a humane stunner manufactured by Remington to deliver a blow to the exposed feline skull.[29] This device involves increasing rotation of the head following the impact. It consists of a barrel housing a series of viscoelastic springs and a piston assembly fitted at one end with a stainless steel impact disc. The stunner is held rigidly in an acrylic and aluminum frame. The head is positioned under the striking disc, rotated approximately 20° counterclockwise. The animal is injured by detonation of the impact disc with a blank cartridge.

In these models the impact is influenced by the ratio of the head to brain mass, which varies between different species. The resultant injury is a complex one that involves both impact to the skull and acceleration of the head.[33] The proponents suggest that these are the prime mechanisms of blunt intracranial injury in humans.

Direct Dural Impact

FLUID PERCUSSION This model was originally described in rabbits by Lindgren and Rinder,[34] and subsequently modified by Sullivan and coworkers[30] for use in cats and by Vink and coworkers[31] to use in rats. The apparatus causes injury by producing displacement of neural tissue by a sudden input of extradural fluid. A weighted pendulum strikes a cork-tipped piston at the end of a saline-filled reservoir. The device is connected to the cat's skull by a hollow central injury shaft. The shaft is placed above the dura of the brain, which is exposed by craniotomy and affixed to the skull with acrylic. A fixed volume of fluid is displaced into the cranial cavity, producing deformation of neural tissue (Fig. 12-4). Pressure transients associated with fluid loading of the brain are recorded by a pressure transducer located extracranially. An increased volume of fluid, introduced into the dura by varying the height from which the weight is dropped, is associated with large pressure transients and increased brain pathology. This device produces a pulse of increased intracranial pressure of fairly constant duration (21 to 23 ms). This pressure transient is associated with distortion and deformation of brain tissue. Because the duration of the pulse is constant, the amplitude of the increased intracranial pressure is used as a measure of the magnitude of the brain injury.

The advantages of this model include its reproducibility and close control of the trauma quality and quantity. However, at the time of impact the cranium is not intact, and therefore, it does not perfectly mimic human TBI.

CONTUSIVE DEVICE This device is held in place by means of an electrode carrier mounted on a stereotaxic apparatus.[32] The base of the device consists of a stainless steel circular footplate. After removal of a small bone flap, the footplate is placed so that it rests upon the surface of the intact dura. The falling weight is guided by a stainless steel tube that is placed at a right angle to the footplate. A string is used to lower the weight to the proper height. This model results in a highly reproducible injury but not one that resembles human TBI.

Cryogenic Injury

This model consists of a penetrating injury that is caused by a 9 mm diameter cylindrical copper probe filled with liquid nitrogen.[35,36] By means of a small craniectomy, the cylinder is held against the intact dura for a cold exposure time of 60 s. This model also results in a reproducible injury, but one that is substantially different from human TBI.

Penetrating Injury

Cerebral Missile Injury

This model is characterized by high focal kinetic energy and relatively low momentum. A major problem with penetrating TBI is the difficulty in separat-

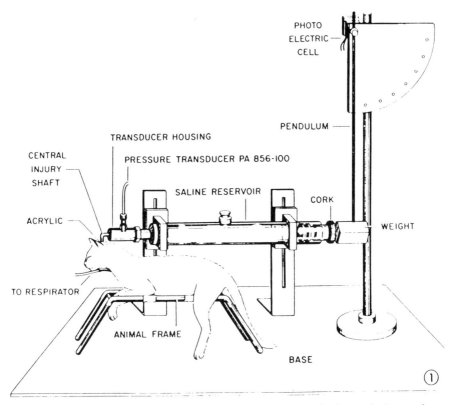

PHOTO
ELECTRIC
CELL

PENDULUM

TRANSDUCER HOUSING

CENTRAL
INJURY
SHAFT

PRESSURE TRANSDUCER PA 856-100

SALINE RESERVOIR

CORK

ACRYLIC

WEIGHT

TO RESPIRATOR

ANIMAL FRAME

BASE

Figure 12-4 Model of fluid-percussion injury. The figure depicts a device used to produce fluid-percussion injury to the brain of a cat. A weighted pendulum strikes a cork-tipped piston at the end of a saline-filled reservoir. The device is connected to the cat's skull by a hollow central injury shaft. The shaft is placed above the dura of the brain exposed by a craniotomy and affixed to the skull with acrylic. A fixed volume of fluid is displaced into the cranial cavity, producing deformation of neural tissue. Pressure transients associated with fluid loading of the brain are recorded by a pressure transducer located extracranially. Increased volumes of fluid, introduced by varying the angle through which the weight is dropped, are associated with larger pressure transients (expressed in atmospheres) and increased brain pathology. [*Reproduced from Textbook of Head Injury. Becker DP, Gludeman SK (eds): Philadelphia, WB Saunders, with permission.*]

ing the focal effect of direct damage by the missile on specific brain centers from the more generalized results of the explosive forces released by the bullet. The missile pathway varies among animals, and major intracranial vessels may or may not be damaged. Such additional damage can aggravate the initial injury. Therefore, although these models are very similar to human penetrating TBI (gunshot wounds), the injuries are not reproducible.

To overcome the problem of reproducibility, Crockard and coworkers[37] drilled a hole in the cranium through which the impact is delivered. The bullets were fired through the exposed dura. As the missile came to rest within the tissue, all the energy was absorbed by the brain and its covering, and the quantity absorbed could be calculated. However, such an external interference with the skull integrity reduces the similarity to human TBI.

Focal Laceration and Contusion

Cortical injury in gerbils has been produced with an electric drill directed along a determined path to a distance of 4 mm.[38] This model results in a reproducible injury due to the stereotaxic head frame in which the animal is placed. However, the injury it simulates is not commonly seen in human TBI.

PHYSIOLOGIC CONSIDERATIONS

The Role of Osmolarity, Oncotic Pressure, and Brain Edema in TBI

Patients suffering severe TBI traditionally are treated with restriction of fluid intake. The stated reasons for fluid restriction is to reduce brain water content, prevent cerebral edema, and decrease intracranial pressure (ICP).[39] Collins and coworkers advocated that fluid be restricted to 75 ml/h for adults,[40] whereas McComish and Bodley suggested that no more than 60 ml/h should be administered[41]; however, the efficacy of fluid restriction has been questioned. Thomas and Gurdjian recommended moderate fluid restriction during the first 24 h only.[42] Safar[43] and Becker[44] suggested an infusion rate of 125 ml/h of 5% dextrose in 0.45% saline for adults; they claimed that overhydration per se will not cause brain edema if the serum sodium concentration remains normal. Moreover, head trauma patients frequently suffer from multiple injuries, necessitating large volumes of intravenous fluids for resuscitation. Experimental studies by others indicated that vigorous fluid resuscitation after fluid percussion injury,[45] cryogenic injury,[46] or brain ischemia,[47] independent of the type of fluid used, did not have major adverse effects on either the injured or noninjured brain in the posttrauma period.

Acute Cerebral Effects of Changes in Plasma Osmolarity and Oncotic Pressure on the Noncontused Brain

Colloid-containing solutions have traditionally been used in neurosurgery because of concern that reduction in oncotic pressure will cause brain edema, just as it causes peripheral edema. However, recent evidence indicated that water content in the brain following colloid administration is not significantly different from that following crystalloid administration.[45,47,48] The key determinant of water movement across the intact BBB is plasma osmolarity, rather than colloid oncotic pressure.

In a study in rabbits with no brain injury, plasma was removed and replaced with solutions of different osmolarity or oncotic pressure, and then brain edema was determined by measuring tissue specific gravity. Decrease of plasma osmolarity by 13 ± 6 mosmol/kg (from a baseline value of 295 ± 5 mosmol/kg) resulted in a significant increase in cortical water content (about 0.5 percent), whereas a 65 percent reduction in oncotic pressure (from 20 ± 2 mmHg to 7 ± 1 mmHg) failed to produce any change.[49] Tommasino and coworkers studied rabbits without brain injury; in one group, plasma was removed and replaced with solutions of different osmolarity (lactated Ringer's) or oncotic pressure (6% hetastarch), and in the other group, rabbits received iso-osmolar solution at the rate of 4 ml/kg per h without hemodilution. In the first group, large volumes of lactated Ringer's (approximately 3 times more) were required to maintain normovolemia as compared with hetastarch. In the lactated Ringer's group, muscle and brain water content increased, and tissue specific gravity decreased. No change was observed in the second group of animals receiving iso-osmolar solutions.[50] Moreover, when plasma is removed and replaced with hypertonic saline (480 mosmol/kg), Todd and coworkers demonstrated in uninjured rabbits that there was a decrease in water content and an increase in specific gravity.[51] The results of these studies suggest that administration of isotonic colloids and crystalloids have similar effects on ICP and brain water content in normal brain. A reduction in oncotic pressure alone is inadequate to result in a net water movement into the brain tissue, as colloid oncotic pressure forms only a small fraction of total osmolarity, whereas a significant change in osmolarity, after administration of hyper- or hypo-osmolar solution, will affect the brain water content.

Acute Cerebral Effects of Changes in Plasma Osmolarity and Oncotic Pressure after Brain Injury

In the injured brain, where the blood-brain barrier is disrupted, oncotic and osmotic gradients cannot be maintained, and edema formation is dependent on hydrostatic forces. Therefore, administration of isotonic colloid and crystalloid solutions exert similar effects on edema formation and ICP in brain injury.[2,45,47] In most of these studies, the cryogenic injury model was used. Zornow and coworkers investigated the acute cerebral effect of 3 commonly used isotonic fluids (0.9% saline, 6% hetastarch, and 5% human albumin) on ICP and brain water content in cryogenic-injured rabbits[2]; plasma was removed and replaced with these solutions, and no significant difference was observed between the groups in osmolarity, ICP and brain edema. Although oncotic pressure was changed significantly in the hetastarch and human albumin groups, the specific gravity was not affected.

Kaieda and coworkers[52] also investigated this issue in the same model. They used plasmapheresis to separate the plasma from the blood. They then replaced the plasma by one of 3 solutions: (1) 6% hetastarch in hypoosmolar lactated Ringer's (LR), (2) isoosmotic LR, and (3) 6% hetastarch in iso-osmolar LR. They demonstrated that in the acute phase of brain injury, reduction of colloid oncotic pressure is not important in brain edema formation, and changes in osmolarity alter water content in relatively normal brain regions.

Zornow and coworkers also examined brain water content and ICP when hypertonic LR (469 mosmol/kg) or isotonic LR was used for isovolemic hemodilution in rabbits with cryogenic brain injury.[3] Although there was a blood osmolarity difference of 19 mosmol/kg between the groups, no decrease in water content was seen in the injured hemisphere as determined by the wet/dry weight method. However, a small but statistically significant increase in specific gravity was found in the noninjured hemisphere. Similarly, Shapira and coworkers, using the direct impact closed head injury model in rats, administered either no fluid, a large volume (3 times more than the oral intake) of isotonic solution, or a hypertonic solution after head trauma. They found no statistically significant difference in neurologic outcome or brain edema between the groups.[53]

When the BBB is intact, water is known to move rapidly across it (half time of 3 min), whereas sodium moves more slowly (half life for equilibration is 1 to 4 h), and albumin and mannitol are excluded from the brain by the intact BBB. When the BBB becomes disrupted, the movement of water across the BBB then becomes a function of hydrostatic pressure rather than osmotic gradients. At the same time, the permeability to sodium, albumin, and mannitol are all markedly increased.

The Role of Mannitol and Hypertonic Solution Usage to Reduce ICP: Brain Tissue Water Content, Cerebral Blood Volume, and Cerebrospinal Fluid Dynamics

The cranial cavity is generally considered to be a rigid box containing the brain volume, blood volume (CBV), and the cerebrospinal fluid (CSF) volume. Since the report of Weed and McKibben,[54] the effect of hypertonic solution on intracranial pressure has been attributed to reduction in intracellular water content, leading to a reduction in brain volume.

INFLUENCE OF MANNITOL ON BRAIN VOLUME In 1962 it was confirmed by Reed and Woodbury[55] that hypertonic solutions reduce ICP and decrease brain volume. It is well established that water movement across the BBB is dependent primarily upon the osmotic gradient between plasma and brain.[56] Water is removed from the brain interstitial space when plasma osmotic pressure is increased, just as with mannitol or hypertonic saline. Intracellular water then moves into the relatively hyperosmolar interstitium. Administration of 5% dextrose in water is similar to giving free water and causes brain edema, because the uptake and metabolism of glucose is rapid. McManus recently demonstrated in vitro that the effect of osmotic gradient on glial cell volume is very transient as the osmoreceptors of the cell regulate its internal environment, such that the cell volume is returned to normal within 15 min.[57]

INFLUENCE OF MANNITOL ON INTRACRANIAL BLOOD VOLUME Using the cranial window technique, Muizelaar and coworkers measured the change in the pial arteriolar diameter in cats after administration of mannitol.[58] They demonstrated an immediate decrease in blood viscosity after an IV bolus of 1 g/kg of mannitol. The decrease in blood viscosity (23 percent), vessel diameter (12 percent), and ICP (28 percent) peaked at 10 min after mannitol administration. They concluded that the vasoconstriction is a reflex response to the decrease in viscosity and that this action is responsible for the reduction in ICP. However, Ravussin and coworkers demonstrated that rapid infusion of mannitol of 2 g/kg for 2 min caused an increase in cerebral blood volume in dogs that was associated with an increased ICP.[59] The CBV peaked (increase of 25 percent) at 2 min, then declined to a 15 percent increase at 15 min and lasted for 90 min. This study showed that ICP returned to baseline value 5 min after mannitol administration and then continued to decrease further, while CBV remained at 10 to 17 percent above baseline. Thus, despite the work of Muizelaar and coworkers, it is conceivable that cerebral blood volume is not the major reason for decrease in ICP after mannitol administration.

INFLUENCE OF MANNITOL ON CSF VOLUME In 1978 Sahar and Tsipstein studied the effect of mannitol and furosemide on the rate of CSF formation in cats by the method of ventriculocisternal perfusion.[60] They showed that mannitol decreased the rate of CSF formation by 89 percent when serum osmolarity was increased by 25 mosmol/kg, while furosemide, in a dose-dependent manner, reduced the rate of CSF formation by up to 94 percent. Another group of animals was studied with ventriculocisternal perfusion of furosemide at a constant rate of 0.1448 ml/min at a concentration of 0.11 mg/ml. The rate of CSF formation was reduced by 75 percent without causing saluresis or diuresis. Takagi and coworkers injected cats with an intravenous bolus of 1 g/kg of mannitol and determined the rate of CSF formation with a pressure-volume method.[61] Brain water content was measured by specific gravity technique in both the normal hemisphere and the edematous hemisphere (caused by extracellular microinjection of water) after mannitol treatment. Mannitol had minimal effects on the specific gravity and water content at various times up to 1 h after treatment. Intracranial pressure, serum osmolarity, and the pressure-volume index increased while CSF outflow resistance decreased. They concluded that the main factor in reducing ICP associated with vasogenic edema by direct administration of mannitol is not due to the decrease of brain volume by the dehydrating action, but is due, instead, to the decrease of CSF volume.

Donato and coworkers studied the same issue using a ventriculocisternal perfusion model in rabbits and administered mannitol in the following 3 doses: 0.25, 0.75, and 2 g/kg.[62] They observed that ICP and the rate of CSF formation decreased while osmolarity increased in a dose-dependent manner. Resistance to reabsorption increased at a dose of 0.75 g/kg but was not different from the baseline at 2 g/kg. However, they also found that water content significantly decreased.

Summarizing the literature, although the classic action of osmotic diuretics (mannitol, hypertonic saline, or urea) on ICP and brain bulk is believed to be mediated through extraction of water from the interstitial and intracellular space, CSF dynamics may play a more important role than is traditionally considered.

THE ROLE OF CEREBROSPINAL FLUID DYNAMICS AND BRAIN TISSUE WATER IN BRAIN INJURY When hypertonic saline (HS) 3 to 7.5% was used to resuscitate dogs from hemorrhagic[63,64] or endotoxic shock,[65] it was reported that ICP was lowered.[63-65] Furthermore, hypertonic crystalloid solution has been shown to improve ICP, cerebral edema, and CBF in a variety of experimental models. Todd and coworkers reported that HS decreased ICP and brain water content and increased CBF when used for isovolemic hemodilution in rabbits.[51]

Zornow and coworkers demonstrated in cryogenic-injured rabbits that hyperosmolar saline (3%) can be an alternative to mannitol, 2 g/kg, for controlling increased ICP after brain injury.[4] Both drugs resulted in a similar increase in blood osmolarity and central venous pressure as well as a similar decrease in ICP. Wilson and coworkers reported that HS (5.8%) decreased ICP in dogs when an increase in ICP was produced by infusion of 5% glucose.[66] Zornow and coworkers evaluated brain water content and ICP when hypertonic lactated Ringer's solution (469 mosmol/kg) or isotonic lactated Ringer's solution was used for isovolemic hemodilution in rabbits with a cryogenic brain injury.[3] Both brain water content in the nonlesioned hemisphere and ICP were lower with hypertonic than with isotonic lactated Ringer's solution.

Intracranial pressure is determined by intracranial volume-pressure relationship, brain tissue volume, cerebral blood volume and cerebrospinal fluid volume. Foxworthy and Artru administered 3% HS at 7 ml/h to rabbits and evaluated its effect on brain water content and CSF dynamics.[67] Although osmolality increased by 18 mosmol/kg, cerebral edema and ICP were not reduced whereas the rate of CSF formation decreased significantly.

The reason for the decrease in the rate of CSF formation with an increase in plasma osmolarity is not clear. Normally, the osmolarity of the CSF is greater than that of plasma. This osmolarity gradient favors the movement of fluid from the plasma across brain tissue and into the CSF (i.e., "passive" formation of CSF), accounting for 30 to 60 percent of the total rate of CSF formation.[68] It has been suggested that an increase in plasma osmolarity reduces that gradient and therefore, by reducing the "passive" formation of CSF, decreases the total rate of CSF formation.[69] An alternative explanation is that a change in plasma osmolarity may alter fluid movement at the level of the choroid plexus. Normally, 40 to 70 percent of the total rate of CSF formation results from "active," energy-dependent processes that move fluid from the choroidal stroma across the epithelial cells of the choroid plexus.[68] An increase in plasma osmolarity opposes this movement of fluid from plasma into the choroidal stroma, thereby reducing the fluid available for "active," energy-dependent "secretion" by choroid plexus epithelial cells. If one considers that the CSF space acts as a sink for the removal of brain edema, the administration of high-dose hyperosmolar saline might favor a reduction in cerebral edema and decreased ICP, if the rate of CSF formation were decreased. Fisher and coworkers recently reported promising results from the use of hypertonic saline in pediatric head injury.[70]

Osmotic and Osmotic-Loop Diuresis in TBI

The most commonly used osmotic and osmotic-loop diuretics are mannitol and furosemide, respectively, either as sole agents or in combination. The relative efficacy of these two agents and their combination for control of ICP has been studied under a variety of experimental conditions. Important considerations are discussed in the following sections:

RATE OF MANNITOL ADMINISTRATION Mannitol is usually not administered rapidly for fear of increasing ICP. Cottrell and coworkers treated humans with no evidence of increased ICP with mannitol, 1 g/kg by bolus intravenous injection, and determined that mannitol significantly increased ICP at the onset of diuresis and significantly decreased ICP at the completion of diuresis.[71] They also observed a significant increase in serum osmolarity at the onset of diuresis. In contrast, they observed a significant decrease in ICP after intravenous injection of furosemide, 1 mg/kg, whereas osmolality remained unchanged. Recently, Abou-Madi and coworkers showed that in dogs with normal ICP, the rapid infusion of mannitol, 2 g/kg for 5 min, resulted in a significant increase in ICP, whereas in dogs with induced intracranial hypertension, it resulted in an immediate decrease in ICP.[72] Similar results were also obtained by Zornow and coworkers.[4] They treated rabbits with mannitol, 2 g/kg, 45 min after cryogenic injury, and observed a decrease in ICP and an increase in osmolality. In a dose response study, Marshall and coworkers administered boluses of 0.25, 0.5, or 1 g/kg mannitol to humans who suffered intracranial hypertension after acute head trauma.[73] They also observed no increase in ICP after mannitol administration.

Summarizing these studies, it appears that the potential danger of exacerbation of intracranial hypertension by the rapid infusion of mannitol may be overstated, and such cautions may not be warranted.

DOSAGE OF MANNITOL In the dose response study mentioned previously, Marshall and coworkers observed no difference in ICP response in brain-injured patients to 0.25, 0.5, or 1 g/kg mannitol.[73] They concluded that smaller and more frequent doses are as effective in reducing ICP as higher doses, while at the same time, avoiding the risk of osmotic disequilibrium and severe dehydration. However, these observations are at variance with other studies. McGraw and coworkers observed in humans (mostly head-injured patients) a linear dose-response curve after mannitol administration.[74]

Similarly, Roberts and coworkers observed that in dogs with normal intracranial hemodynamics, the response of ICP to mannitol was dose-dependent, whether mannitol was administered as a bolus or as an infusion.[75]

To summarize, the dose response of ICP to mannitol appears to be complex, and no conclusive statement can be made. A higher dose should certainly be given if the response to a low dose should prove unsatisfactory. The preexisting ICP before mannitol administration may have significant influence on the response to mannitol both in animals and humans.

FUROSEMIDE IN COMBINATION WITH MANNITOL In 1977 Cottrell and coworkers demonstrated that, in humans with normal ICP, furosemide, 1 mg/kg, is more effective than mannitol, 1 g/kg, in reducing ICP.[71] Moreover, because they observed that electrolytes (sodium and potassium) and osmolality changes were less with furosemide than with mannitol, they recommended that furosemide could replace mannitol in neurosurgery management. However, Pollay and coworkers demonstrated in dogs that the combination of mannitol and furosemide produced a greater and more sustained decrease in ICP than mannitol or furosemide alone.[76] This finding correlated with a prolongation of the reversal of blood-brain osmotic gradient and the rate of urine formation. No significant decrease in serum sodium was noted with the combined treatment. Roberts and coworkers evaluated different combinations of furosemide and mannitol in dogs with increased ICP (30 to 40 mmHg), and determined that the most profound and sustained reduction in ICP was achieved in animals receiving a mannitol bolus followed by furosemide 15 min later as compared with simultaneous mannitol/furosemide administration or furosemide followed by mannitol 15 min later.[75] Thus, it would appear that mannitol followed by furosemide in 15 min may be the optimal regimen.

Glucose Administration in TBI

Animal studies provide convincing evidence that dextrose administration, with or without marked hyperglycemia, increases neurologic damage in global cerebral ischemia[77-79] and spinal cord ischemia.[80] An increase in blood glucose levels also appears to exacerbate or indicate severe neurologic damage in humans after stroke,[81] cardiac arrest,[82] and traumatic brain injury.[83-85] Glucose administration is believed to increase ischemic neurologic damage by increasing the production of lactic acid by the anaerobic metabolism of brain glucose. Lactic acid decreases neuronal pH and increases postischemic injury.[86]

The threshold level of blood glucose above which ischemic neurologic damage is increased is not known. Some studies suggest that a threshold may not exist and that exacerbation of neurologic injury is noted even with mild hyperglycemia.[79,84] Lanier and coworkers demonstrated that monkeys treated with 50 ml IV of D5/0.45 saline (equivalent to 1 liter/70 kg, blood glucose = 180 mg/dl), before global cerebral ischemia, had a significantly greater neurologic deficit than monkeys who received lactated Ringer's solution (glucose = 140 mg/dl).

However, whereas most animal studies demonstrating the deleterious effects of hyperglycemia have used global ischemia models,[77-80] human TBI is associated with both focal and global ischemia. Indeed, results from the experimental studies are not always consistent. When focal ischemia data are evaluated, it appears that the exacerbation by hyperglycemia[87,88] and the protective effect of insulin treatment[89,90] are evident primarily in reperfusion injuries. In the case of permanent focal ischemia without reperfusion, hyperglycemia improved neuronal damage,[91] infarct size,[92,93] and neurologic outcome.[94] Similar observations were made by Prado and coworkers, who studied the correlation between infarct size and hyperglycemia in collaterally perfused versus end arterial vascular territories.[95] Their results suggest that infarcted regions with collateral circulation are vulnerable to the deleterious effects of hyperglycemia, whereas regions of nonanastomosing (end aterial) vascular supply are not. They showed that the harmful effects of elevated plasma glucose in stroke appear to be complex and may depend critically on the degree to which collateral perfusion is available to the specific brain regions affected, as well as the extent to which local blood flow is reduced and the timing of glucose administration.

Nedergaard perhaps offers the best explanation as to why hyperglycemia has a more damaging effect in transient than permanent focal ischemia.[96] He observed that the vessel degradation was increased by hyperglycemia[97] and that cerebral blood flow was better preserved in fasted animals than in animals given glucose.[98] The endothelial cells showed a progressive swelling during recirculation in hyperglycemic animals, but only minor vascular changes were seen in normoglycemic animals.[99] Nedergaard thus concluded that hyperglycemia induced capillary destruction, leading to profound brain hypoperfusion after transient ischemia.[96] This could explain why the predominant injury in a hyperglycemic condition is infarction and not selective neuronal injury. Because less lactic acid is produced during ischemia when plasma glucose is low, the infarcts are smaller in hypoglycemic rats. However, hyperglycemia may have a salutary effect on spreading depression, a phenomenon that represents the generalized response of the cerebral cortex to a variety of noxious influences and is accompanied by marked changes in extracellular ion concentrations.[100] There is a possibility that hyperglycemia exacerbates selective neuronal injury to infarction in transient ischemia but attenuates selective neuronal injury around an infarct in permanent ischemia.

Perhaps because of this mixed effect, Shapira and coworkers in their closed head trauma model in rats did not observe any difference in brain edema or neurologic outcome between animals with or without 5% dextrose administration 18 h after TBI.[53]

In summary, although the influence of hyperglycemia on neurologic outcome is complex and a cause-effect relationship has not been firmly established in clinical studies, there is a general consensus that hyperglycemia worsens the tolerance of the brain to transient ischemia. Therefore, glucose-containing solutions should not be administered to patients suffering from TBI unless there are specific indications.

Hypothermia

In 1944 Field and coworkers showed that hypothermia decreased cerebral oxygen consumption.[101] Since the late 1950s physiologists and clinicians have used hypothermia as a potent nonpharmacologic means of reducing brain and whole body metabolism, limited only by the degree of hypothermia achieved. It had also found a variety of applications in the operating room.[102] These earlier applications were entirely dependent on the cerebral metabolic depression attributed to profound hypothermia, whereas more recent studies are concerned with the suppression of neurotransmitters with mild and moderate hypothermia.

Effect of Hypothermia on Cerebral Metabolic Rate

The effects of profound hypothermia on cerebral metabolic rate have been clarified by Michenfelder.[103] The relationship of temperature to metabolic rate is commonly expressed as the Q10 value, which is simply the ratio of two metabolic rates separated by 10°C difference. It defines a simple exponential relationship. Thus, if the Q10 value is 2.0, it means that a 10° C decrease in temperature will result in a 50 percent decrease in metabolism (Fig. 12-5).

Based on the analysis of published studies,[104–107] Michenfelder concluded that, for the functioning brain, the relationship between temperature and metabolic rate is not a simple exponential.[103] Thus, between 37° and 28°C the calculated Q10 was 2.4, whereas between 28° and 18°C it was 5.8, and below 18°C it was again 2.3. The striking increase in Q10 between 28° and 18°C is accounted for by the cessation of cerebral function (as evidenced by an isoelectric EEG) that characteristically occurs between 18° and 21°C. This is the classic explanation for the protective effect of hypothermia.

Suppression of Toxic Neurotransmitter Release by Hypothermia

Recent studies have suggested that decreased metabolism is not the only mechanism by which hypothermia can protect the brain. This hypothesis stems from studies reporting that similar degrees of metabolic suppression such as hypothermia, caused by barbiturates or isoflurane, fail to show consistent benefits.[108] Moreover, recent studies have shown that while modest hypothermia (33°C) does not preserve high-energy phosphates (e.g., adenosine triphosphate phosphocreatine) or prevent the accumulation of metabolic wastes (e.g., lactate),[109] it does confer histopathologic protection from ischemia.[110]

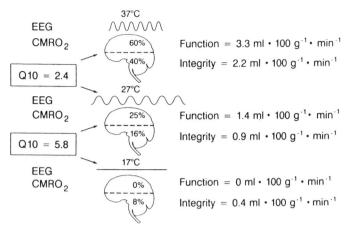

EEG

CMRO$_2$ 60% 40%   Function = 3.3 ml · 100 g^{-1}· min^{-1}

Q10 = 2.4   Integrity = 2.2 ml · 100 g^{-1}· min^{-1}

EEG

CMRO$_2$ 25% 16%   Function = 1.4 ml · 100 g^{-1}· min^{-1}

Q10 = 5.8   Integrity = 0.9 ml · 100 g^{-1}· min^{-1}

EEG

CMRO$_2$ 0% 8%   Function = 0 ml · 100 g^{-1}· min^{-1}

     Integrity = 0.4 ml · 100 g^{-1}· min^{-1}

Figure 12-5 Change in cerebral metabolic rate with temperature. This figure depicts the theoretical interaction of temperature, brain function, CMRO$_2$, and calculated Q10 values. In reducing the temperature from 37° to 27°C, function is maintained, and both of the energy-consuming processes (i.e., function and integrity) are presumed to be affected equally with a slightly more than 50 percent reduction in CMRO$_2$, thus generating a Q10 value of about 2.4. With a further 10°C reduction in temperature to 17°C, function is abolished, thus resulting in a step decrease in CMRO$_2$ such that the calculated Q10 value is 5.0 or greater. At this point the total oxygen consumed by the brain is reduced to less than 8 percent of the normothermic value. [*From Anesthesia and The Brain. JD Michenfelder (ed): New York, Churchill Livingstone, with permission.*]

Considerable evidence has now accumulated from both in vitro studies with neuronal cultures and in vivo experiments that excitatory amino acids (particularly glutamate and aspartate) are important in the evolution of ischemic brain damage[111–113] (see the section headed Excitatory Amino Acids Antagonist), and hypothermia suppresses the release of these amino acids.[109] Indeed, the cerebroprotective effect of the NMDA receptor antagonist MK-801, or dizocilpine, has been attributed to the simultaneous occurrence of hypothermia.[114]

Busto and coworkers had shown that a small decrease (33°C) in brain temperature alone while the rest of the body is maintained normothermic can decrease neuronal injury as evidenced by histopathology.[110] More recently, Baker and coworkers demonstrated that hypothermia of 29°C afforded almost complete protection from 10 min of global cerebral ischemia in rabbits.[115] Outcome was assessed by both neurologic and neuropathologic criteria. Ischemia-induced increases in the concentrations of glutamate (3 times baseline), aspartate (12 times baseline), and glycine (3 times baseline) in the normothermic group were strikingly attenuated in the hypothermic group. In addition, the prolonged postischemic elevation of glycine levels seen in the normothermic group was absent in the hypothermic group. These results suggest that the neuroprotective properties of hypothermia may reside, partly, in their ability to prevent increases in the extracellular concentrations of excitatory amino acids that increase the activity of the N-methyl-D-aspartate receptor complex. The data of Baker and coworkers also confirm the observation that the extracellular concentration of glutamate returns quickly to baseline levels during reperfusion. The ability of glycine to facilitate the actions of glutamate at the NMDA receptor and its persistent elevation during the postischemic period may help to explain the apparent ongoing toxicity of glutamate. The ability of hypothermia to block a sustained elevation of the extracellular glycine concentration in response to ischemia may reflect an important component of the protective mechanism of hypothermia. It may be speculated that the ability of hypothermia to decrease glycine levels may be at least as important as its effect on glutamate concentrations. The importance of this mechanism is emphasized by the recent observation that glutamate levels are increased in the cerebrospinal fluid of patients suffering TBI.[116]

Relevant to the study of experimental TBI is the recent recognition that the brain temperature is consistently lower than the rectal temperature in the fluid percussion model, and some of the previously reported efficacy of experimental brain protection therapy may be due to the incidental mild hypothermia rather than the therapy itself.[117] Paradoxically, intraoperative recording of brain (intraventricular) temperature in patients undergoing neurosurgical procedures has registered higher brain temperature than the nasopharyngeal temperature.[118] These studies have underscored the importance of brain temperature and suggest that mild to moderate hypothermia may provide cerebral protection due more to the suppression of the release of excitotoxic neurotransmitters than to the reduction of cerebral metabolic rate. Preliminary clinical trials for human TBI are promising,[119,120] but more investigations are required.

Induced Hypertension

Although induced hypertension has never been used for treatment of TBI, in view of the data from the National Traumatic Coma Data Bank indicating that systemic hypotension is an independent factor contributing to poor outcome,[121] its use may be a worthwhile consideration. In experimental cerebral ischemia (middle cerebral artery occlusion in rats), increasing the arterial blood pressure by about 40 percent (phenylephrine-induced hypertension) above the preocclusion levels has been shown to impove local cerebral blood flow in an area of focal ischemia.[122] In the clinical setting, it is well known that the neurologic status of patients with symptomatic vasospasm after aneurysmal subarachnoid hemorrhage can improve with induced hypertension.[123] However, the situation is far more complex in TBI; i.e., increase in blood pressure may improve perfusion, but it may also increase the risk of hemorrhage and favor the development of vasogenic edema, particularly if the BBB is impaired. Thus, carefully planned investigations should be performed before clinical trials are undertaken. Nevertheless systemic hypotension should be treated aggressively in patients with TBI.

PHARMACOLOGIC TREATMENTS FOR EXPERIMENTAL TBI

Pharmacologic approach to experimental TBI is predicated on the current understanding of the pathophysiology of TBI that leads to ultimate neuronal death. Although this is a rapidly evolving field, a simple schematic is useful to illustrate the potential actions of various pharmacologic treatments. This is shown in Fig. 12-6.

Glucocorticoid and Nonglucocorticoid Lipid Antioxidants

Glucocorticoid (GC) treatment was initiated in brain injury and ischemia after encouraging results were obtained with such therapy in the treatment of brain edema secondary to the presence of tumors and intracerebral abscesses.

The benefits of GC were initially attributed to inhibition of the production of prostaglandins. The role of prostaglandins in causing cerebral edema and ischemia had been established by several experimental studies,[124,125] and Weidenfeld and coworkers demonstrated that dexamethasone can decrease prostaglandin production.[126] They observed that different areas of the brain are differentially affected by dexamethasone, and the maximum effect is observed in the cortex. Ohers have shown that GC acts mainly to decrease the permeability of the BBB and not brain edema itself.[127,128] Demopolous and coworkers observed that dexamethasone stabilizes membranes and does not inhibit prostaglandin synthesis.[129] Similarly, Hall found that the administration of a high dose of GC immediately after head trauma in mice improved neurologic recovery.[130] He hypothesized that the steroids act to protect the integrity of the cell membranes, inhibit free radicals and oxidation of lipids, but do not inhibit prostaglandin synthesis.

In a model of closed head injury in rats developed in our laboratory, neither dexamethasone[131] nor methylprednisolone[132] affected the specific gravity of traumatized brain, the neurologic condition of the animal, or the tissue prostaglandin levels. However, dexamethasone, when administered as the nonionic base, significantly inhibited prostaglandin synthesis.[131] This effect was not seen when the sodium phosphate form of dexamethasone was used. The failure of dexamethasone sodium phosphate to inhibit prostaglandin synthesis may have been due to four reasons:

(1) The dose or timing was inappropriate.
(2) The derivative may have affected the membrane lipophilic characteristics and may have lacked the ability to penetrate the BBB.

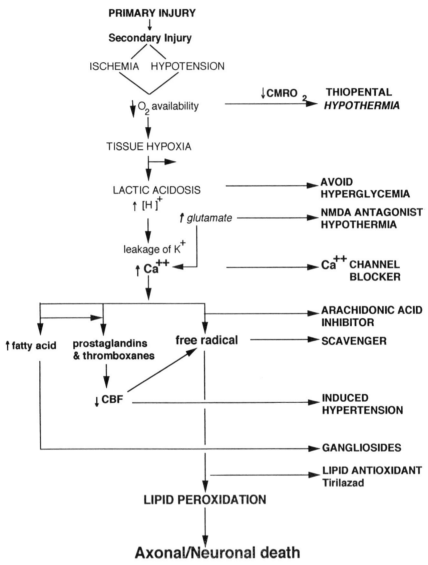

Figure 12-6 A proposed schematic summarizing the functional abnormalities of traumatic brain injury and illustrating the potential therapeutic approaches using pharmacologic means.

(3) The hydrolysis of ester to free dexamethasone needed a specific enzyme.

(4) A different route of administration may have been required.

These results do not support the use of GC in head trauma, even though GC may depress prostaglandin synthesis considerably. Other investigators claim that GC may even cause deterioration in the outcome of injury. McEwen and coworkers demonstrated that GC administration during stress may injure neurons in the hippocampus, which is a major target organ for steroids.[133,134] GC may impair the energy metabolism of these neurons.[135] The neurons of the hippocampus, which usually die either of old age or of ischemic injury due to vasoconstriction or convulsions, may be discharged by the steroids.[136-139]

Sapolsky and coworkers demonstrated in tissue culture that the addition of GC decreased the cell's viability after neurotoxin administration, when compared with the control cells.[140] The addition of glucose to the cultures that contained both the toxin and GC increased the viability; however, the initial viability was not changed when glucose was added to cultures containing toxin alone.

Excision of the adrenal gland decreased the damage observed in the hippocampus after hypoxia or ischemia.[141,142] Sapolski and coworkers suggest that the GC action on neurons is mediated through the inhibition of glucose utilization and energy formation in these cells.[140] The resultant hyperglycemia may also aggravate the ischemic injury.

Thus, the action of GC is complex, and its beneficial effect of inhibition of lipid oxidation is balanced by other undesirable effects attributed to the glucocorticoid action. The role of GC in both clinical and experimental TBI, therefore, remains controversial, and despite early enthusiasm with promising results,[143-149] many subsequent clinical trials failed to demonstrate any beneficial effect of steroids in central nervous system trauma.[150-153] Because of these conflicting results, it was assumed that the drug was effective but might not have been administered in either the optimal dose or by the proper pathway.

More recently, with the demonstration that high-dose methylprednisolone is effective in improving outcome after acute spinal cord injury,[154,155] there is renewed interest in the use of steroids in TBI. More potent lipid antioxidants devoid of glucocorticoid action (21-aminosteroids) are now available and appear promising.[156,157] One of these steroids, Tirilazad mesylate, has been shown recently to have no direct effect on cerebral blood flow and metabolism in healthy humans[158] and is currently undergoing clinical trials in TBI as well as subarachnoid hemorrhage.

Excitatory Amino Acids Antagonists

There is considerable evidence that excitatory amino acids are important in the development of delayed neuronal necrosis.[159-162] Energy depletion after brain ischemia or head trauma results in synaptic release of glutamate and the failure of cellular reuptake of glutamate[163-166] in addition to intracellular calcium accumulation by voltage-dependent channels.[159,161] High concentrations of extracellular glutamate stimulate glutamate receptors of the kainate- and quisqualate-preferring subtypes, causing a massive influx of sodium, chloride, and water, and also stimulate glutamate receptors of the N-methyl-D-aspartate (NMDA)-preferring subtype, causing substantial calcium influx.[159-162,167-169] Intracellular calcium accumulation activates enzymes that catalyze the breakdown of proteins, lipids, and nucleic acids, leading to neuronal death.[168,170-172] Stimulation of NMDA receptors appears to be a crucial step in glutamate-induced neuronal death, because blockade of NMDA receptors with specific antagonists or noncompetitive ion channel blockers provides protection against glutamate neurotoxicity.[166,173]

Certain NMDA receptor antagonists have been reported to improve neurologic outcome in experimental models of brain ischemia, head trauma, and other forms of cerebral injury. Competitive NMDA antagonists include 2-amino-5-phosphonovalerate (APV), 2-amino-7-phosphonoheptanoate (APH), 1-(cis-2-carboxypiperidine-4-yl) methyl-1-phosphonate (CGS 19755), and 3-[(C-)-2-carboxypiperazine-4-yl] propyl-1-phosphonate (CPP).[174] These compounds reduce brain infarct volume and/or improve abnormal tissue in ischemia and/or focal brain injury.[175-180] Noncompetitive NMDA antagonists include (+)-5-methyl-10,11-dihydro-5H-dibenzo [a,d] cyclohepten-5,10-amine, maleate (MK-801, or dizocilpine), phencyclidine (PCP), dextrophan, and dextromethorphan.[174] These have been reported to improve cerebral blood flow, brain edema, energy state, damaged tissue, infarct volume and/or neurologic status in cerebral ischemia, head trauma, hypoxia and/or anoxia.[164,176,178,181-190] Dizocilpine also produces prolonged sedation[182,191] that extends beyond 24 h after ischemia or head trauma.

Thus, NMDA receptor antagonists that can penetrate the BBB have potential therapeutic use in the treatment of brain injury. One of the most investigated drugs is dizocilpine maleate (MK-801), which is a noncompetitive antagonist for glutamate receptor of the NMDA subtype. Most studies determined that this compound is efficacious in transient focal cerebral ischemia but not in severe or global ischemia. Ozyurt and coworkers, using a model of focal cerebral ischemia (middle cerebral artery occlusion), demonstrated that pretreatment with dizocilpine significantly reduced the volume of the ischemic damage.[181] In contrast, in many animal models of global ischemia NMDA antagonists often were not effective. Michenfelder and coworkers observed no improvement after dizocilpine treatment in a model of complete cerebral ischemia.[191] In experimental TBI, Faden and coworkers found that noncompetitive NMDA receptor antagonists improved the neurologic status of the animals, the bioenergy state, and increased intracellular free magnesium.[164] Similarly Shapira and coworkers[182] and McIntosh and coworkers[183] observed improvement in both neurologic status and brain edema in a brain injury model.

Ketamine, as a noncompetitive NMDA antagonist, is of considerable interest to the anesthesiologist.[192] In a dose-dependent manner, ketamine reduced swelling of cultured astrocytes after incubation with glutamate.[193] Moreover, the neurodegenerative effect of ibotenic acid, quinolate and NMDA injection into the rat hippocampus was substantially blocked by high-dose ketamine (150 to 180 mg/kg intraperitoneally).[194,195] Similarly, ketamine has been observed to increase survival rate and increase the density of the pyramidal cells in the hippocampus after bilateral carotid occlusion in gerbils.[196]

In experimental TBI (closed head impact model), Shapira and coworkers observed that ketamine significantly improved neurologic outcome and reduced cerebral infarct volume.[197] In an additional study ketamine was found to reduce the increase in tissue calcium and the decrease in tissue magnesium level normally seen after brain injury.[198] In the only study of cerebral metabolic rate after administration of ketamine to patients, Takeshita and coworkers reported no change in metabolic rate ($CMRO_2$) despite a 62 percent increase in cerebral blood flow (CBF).[199]

Previous recommendations against the use of ketamine in head-injured patients were based on reports that ketamine increased CBF, $CMRO_2$ and ICP.[200–204] Although pretreatments with thiopental, hypocapnia, benzodiazepines, or opioids may reverse ketamine-induced increases of $CMRO_2$, CBF, and ICP in animals or patients without intracranial pathology,[205,206] these treatments may not be completely effective in patients with intracranial tumors, hydrocephalus, or other intracranial pathology. Although ketamine increases systemic blood pressure and ICP, because its potential value for brain protection, its role in neuroanesthesia needs to be reevaluated.

Magnesium is another noncompetitive NMDA antagonist that may be useful in the treatment of TBI. Brain injury is associated with an immediate decline in intracellular magnesium, which is maximal at the site of injury, and the magnitude of magnesium depletion directly correlates with the severity of the injury.[207,208] This depletion of tissue magnesium appears to be a common feature of brain injury.[209] Treatment with magnesium 30 min after experimental TBI has been shown to be effective in reducing neurologic deficits.[210]

Nonspecific Inhibitors of Arachidonic Acid Metabolic Pathway (Nonsteroidal Anti-Inflammatory Drugs)

The increased production of arachidonic acid metabolites in the injured brain suggested the use of prostaglandin inhibitors to improve outcome. Shapira and coworkers evaluated the effect of indomethacin on closed head TBI.[131] Despite a decrease in prostaglandin (Pg) levels this treatment (10 mg/kg 1 h before and 7 h after head trauma) neither reduced brain edema nor improved the neurological condition of the rats. Chan and coworkers obtained similar results in their study.[124] They induced brain edema by administering arachidonic acid intracranially and determined that treatment with 10 mg/kg of indomethacin did not reduce edema formation. These results suggest that whereas decreasing Pg production does not improve edema, these compounds are not important in edema formation.[211,212] However, this statement may not be entirely true because it is difficult to predict the effect of the various Pg blockers. Other researchers have reported that prostacyclin was effective in decreasing brain edema. In our study, indomethacin did lower levels of all Pgs including prostacyclin (PGI_2), however, we could observe no effect on brain edema.[131]

Another explanation for the ineffectiveness of indomethacin in reducing edema is that indomethacin specifically blocks the cyclooxygenase pathway. There is evidence that leukotrienes, which are the products of the lipoxygenase pathway, are involved in brain edema formation.[213–216] Dempsey and others found that indomethacin blocked the cyclooxygenase pathway but also elevated leukotriene levels.[215] This effect may be explained by the increased availability of the substrate arachidonic acid to the lipoxygenase pathway. These results were supported by Black and coworkers,[216] who injected arachidonic acid directly into the brain and demonstrated increased BBB permeability. This increase in BBB permeability, which indomethacin failed to inhibit, was prevented by a specific lipooxygenase inhibitor. It was concluded that vasogenic edema formation is mainly dependent on formation of leukotrienes and not on Pg.

However, these findings are in direct contrast to those of Yen and Lee, who recorded decreased brain edema (induced by a freeze lesion) in rats treated with indomethacin, but only when the drug was given 48 h before injury.[217] In a clinical study, Jensen and coworkers administered 30-mg bolus intravenously followed by a continuous infusion of 30 mg/h for 7 h to head-injured patients with elevated ICP. They observed a decrease in ICP within 5 to 7 s, and during the next 4 h, ICP remained well controlled.[218] The decrease in ICP, however, was secondary to a decrease in CBF, not to a decrease of edema formation.

Specific Inhibitors in the Arachidonic Acid Metabolic Pathway

Arachidonic acid affects the regulation of cerebral blood flow under both normal and ischemic conditions.[219] A selective increase in thromboxane B_2 synthesis was demonstrated by Shohami and coworkers in an incomplete ischemia model in the rat.[220] Dempsey and coworkers showed that, after 10 min of ischemia in gerbils followed by reperfusion of 50 min, a slow lasting decrease in cerebral blood flow results that causes hypoperfusion.[221] At the same time a significant increase in thromboxane concentration (420 percent) and a lesser increase in 6-keto-$PGF_1\alpha$ concentration (220 percent) were observed in the brain tissue.[221] Thromboxane synthetase inhibition by imidazole was shown by Roy and coworkers to increase the blood flow in the penumbra region of the ischemic cat's brain.[222] The penumbra region is the area close to the primary injury where the cells are not dead but are at risk of dying. In ischemia models it is the area adjacent to the infarction zone, and similarly in experimental TBI, it is the area adjacent to the traumatic region where permanent damage has not occurred and the pathologic changes are potentially reversible. The penumbra area is, thus, the prime target for pharmacologic therapy because of this potential reversibility.

Ishihara and coworkers showed thromboxane synthetase inhibitors and prostacyclin (PGI_2) synthetase stimulants to be effective in the treatment and prevention of thromboembolic events.[223] Preventive treatment with thromboxane inhibitors prevented energy failure and the disappearance of sensory-evoked responses in the brain during platelet thromboembolism.[224] Nihei and coworkers reported improved blood flow in white matter, but not in grey matter, after treatment with a thromboxane synthetase inhibitor.[225] Moufarrij and coworkers, conversely, succeeded in significantly decreasing the concentration of thromboxane in the tissues after ischemia with these inhibitors, but failed to reduce the injury.[226] Thromboxane synthetase inhibitors may also prevent injury in other target organs, such as in acute tubular necrosis after renal ischemia. Treatment with a thromboxane receptor antagonist significantly reduced mortality and prevented expansion of myocardial infarction.[227] The role of thromboxane synthetase inhibitors in treatment of head injury remains to be clarified.

Calcium Channel Blockers

Intracellular calcium concentration is regulated by voltage-dependent and receptor-operated ionic channels (mainly NMDA receptors). The voltage-dependent channels are classified into L-type, N-type, and T-type.[228] The importance of the Ca channels is underscored by the recognition that the intracellular influx of calcium represents the final common pathway signifying the onset of cellular death in central nervous system injury. Calcium channel blockers prevent the Ca influx through voltage-dependent channels activated in excitable cells. By this mechanism, these drugs lower the availability of free, intracellular Ca ions that are necessary for cell function. In brain tissue these drugs have two main functions:

(1) They prevent arterial vasoconstriction in the brain. Smooth vascular muscle cells depend for constriction on transmembranal Ca ions fluxes supplied from the extracellular spaces for contraction.[229]

(2) They decrease Ca influx into neuronal cells and thus prevent the tissue damage arising from calcium accumulation.

Nimodipine is a cerebrovascular selective Ca channel blocker that blocks dihydropyridine-sensitive, voltage-dependent L-type channels.[230] This has been demonstrated in isolated blood vessels as well as in animal studies. One important advantage of nimodipine is that, when given at the appropriate doses, it has no significant cardiovascular effect, i.e., it does not cause marked hypotension clinically.[231]

Nimodipine has been investigated extensively and is used clinically to treat vasospasm secondary to subarachnoid hemorrhage. In experimental ischemia its maximal effect on cerebral blood flow was found in areas where perfusion was especially impaired.[232] It may also prevent "steal phenomenon," in which diffuse dilation of cerebral blood vessels may detour blood away from ischemic-injured areas. Although pretreatment with nimodipine improves the neurologic outcome, it has not been shown to alter either the incidence or the severity of vasospasm.

The use of nimodipine as cerebroprotective therapy has been investigated in both acute cerebral ischemia[233] and brain trauma.[234] Kostron and coworkers reported eight patients with severe head trauma and vasospasm who were treated with nimodipine and showed better than average improvement in their conditions.[235] However, a multicenter randomized trial of nimodipine for head injury did not find any significant improvement in outcome.[236]

In a model of global cerebral ischemia, Steen and coworkers observed neurologic and neuropathologic improvement with nimodipine treatment initiated 5 min after ischemia.[237] This effect was attributed to improvement in blood flow from vasodilation secondary to Ca-channel blockade in the smooth muscles of the blood vessel. It is well established in animal models that, after complete cerebral ischemia, an initial brief hyperemic phase is succeeded by a prolonged period of delayed hypoperfusion.[232,233] In dogs, this period lasts for more than 6 h, with cerebral blood flow often decreased to 20 percent of normal.[237,238] In patients, after cardiac arrest, a low-flow state has been observed in the initial 2 to 6 h after resuscitation with restoration of normal cerebral blood flow after 24 h. This hypoperfusion state, which is due in part to Ca-induced cerebral vasospasm, might be partly responsible for the brain damage frequently seen after cardiac arrest.[232]

Kass and coworkers studied the effect of nimodipine on evoked responses after anoxic damage in rat hippocampal slice and observed that, although it did not restore ATP levels to normal as compared with the control groups, it did improve the evoked responses.[239] Similar results were also obtained with cobalt and magnesium treatment. The release of Ca ions during ischemia triggers a chain of events leading to membrane destruction, while at the same time, causing a drastic reduction in ATP levels (which prevents the regeneration of the membrane). Even though the presence of Ca channel blockers does not prevent the release of calcium ions, they may reduce their number. Moreover, dilation of injured blood vessels by Ca channel blockers may improve blood flow to the area, thus reducing the cellular ischemia. Unfortunately, no mechanism has been found to prevent the intracellular release of calcium ions.

As mentioned previously, another mechanism by which calcium ions may accumulate in cells is mediation by receptor-operated channels. Activation of some receptors by agonists (e.g., excitatory amino acids) opens voltage-insensitive Ca channels. The Ca channel blocker, nifedipine, has been shown to attenuate neurotoxicity produced by excitatory amino acids in neuronal cultures.[240]

In summary, intracellular calcium ion influx through both voltage-sensitive and insensitive channels is probably the final common pathway in neuronal injury, and more than one class of drugs is probably required to effect a complete blockade. More central nervous system-specific calcium channel antagonists are currently being investigated.[241]

Free Radical Scavengers

Most molecules have paired electrons in their electron orbits. The two electrons spin in opposite directions, thereby canceling each other's magnetic field, resulting in a low-energy state. A free radical is a molecule with an unpaired electron in an outer orbital, which has a magnetic field that produces a high energy state, thus, making the molecule extremely reactive and unstable with a very short half-life. Oxygen-derived free radicals impair capillary endothelial cell mechanisms that help to maintain homeostasis of electrolytes and water in the brain, cause peroxidation of membrane phospholipids, and attack neuronal membranes. Free radicals can be produced by energy transfer, such as irradiation by gamma or x-rays, or thermal homolysis of bonds, or by chemical agents known as inhibitors.[242] Because of their very short half life and their production in special conditions, they are usually present in very low concentrations and do not frequently travel from their site of formation.

Free radical reactions do not occur only in pathologic states, but are also part of normal cellular metabolism. Normally, during the production of ATP, the mitochondrial cytochrome oxidase enzyme system is linked to the reduction of molecular oxygen to water and generates free radicals. Usually all four electrons are gained at once. If the electrons are acquired singly, a series of radical intermediates are formed: superoxide ($\cdot O_2^-$) hydrogen peroxide (H_2O_2) and the hydroxyl radical ($OH\cdot$)[243] Because of their potential for severe damage, a chemical reaction occurs where the free radicals are scavenged by superoxide dismutase (SOD) to form hydrogen peroxide and oxygen (Eq. 1).

$$\cdot O_2^- + \cdot O_2^- + 2H + SOD \rightarrow H_2O_2 + O_2 \qquad (1)$$

To prevent further damage the free radicals usually remain tightly bound within mitochondrial membrane so they can donate electrons further down the chain. The free radicals that leak out are controlled by the scavenging system.

During ischemia and reperfusion free radicals are produced from dissociation of the mitochondrial electron transport chain because of the lack of oxygen as a terminal electron acceptor. Another potential source results from breakdown of arginine and the consequent production of nitric oxide radicals. The most important free radical is the superoxide radical, ($\cdot O_2^-$). Ischemia activates xanthine oxidase, which in the presence of calcium ions, converts hypoxanthine to xanthine, reducing superoxide to the superoxide radical,

$\cdot O_2^-$ in the process.[244,245] The superoxide radical, $\cdot O_2^-$, attacks proteins, polyunsaturated phospholipids in membranes and disrupts the cellular function, thereby leading to cellular injury.[246,247] As in the physiological process, the scavenger SOD catalyzes the reaction of $\cdot O_2^-$ to form hydrogen peroxide (H_2O_2).[248] Further reaction by other enzymes convert the hydrogen peroxide to water and oxygen as indicated in Eq. 2

$$2H_2O_2 + \text{catalase and peroxidase} \rightarrow 2H_2O + O_2 \text{ (Ref 245)} \qquad (2)$$

However, when H_2O_2 exceeds the normal intracellular level, the catalase and peroxidase concentration would be insufficient to eliminate them. The highly reactive hydroxyl radical $(OH\cdot)$ is then generated from reaction between $\cdot O_2^-$ and H_2O_2. Moreover, there is no scavenging system for the $OH\cdot$ radical, whose level is totally dependent on H_2O_2 and $\cdot O_2^-$ concentrations.[249]

The previous theories suggest that administration of free radical scavengers may be therapeutic in brain injury. Cerchiari and coworkers treated dogs at the beginning of cardiopulmonary resuscitation after apnea-induced cardiac arrest of 7 min with a combination of SOD and deferoxamine.[250] They demonstrated elimination of the initial cerebral reactive hyperemia in addition to improvement of delayed postischemic CBF and increased normalization of somatosensory-evoked responses. Both drugs were equally effective when given separately. Ikeda and coworkers demonstrated that deferoxamine given after cryogenic injury in cats can decrease brain edema,[251] and similar observations were made by Schettini and coworkers administering SOD in a decompressive hypoperfusion model in dogs.[252] Moreover, vitamin E, mannitol and glucocorticoids have been shown to work as free radical scavengers.[253,254] Although the main interest currently in cerebroprotective therapy does not focus on free radicals and their scavengers, the hypothesis that free radicals are heavily involved in producing brain damage after ischemia and trauma remains attractive. The safety and potential benefits of SOD were recently confirmed in a clinical trial.[255]

Endogenous Opioid Peptide Antagonists

Endogenous opioids are released after spinal cord injury and have been shown to contribute to the pathophysiology of injury by decreasing the microcirculatory blood flow, a process that can be treated with an opiate antagonist.[256] More recently it has been suggested that the k-opioid receptors may contribute to the pathophysiology of secondary injury after TBI.[257] This sparked an interest in using opioid antagonists to treat central nervous system trauma. The discovery of thyrotropin-releasing hormone (TRH), which can physiologically antagonize the effects of endogenous opioid peptides without altering analgesia, has made it therapeutically possible to treat TBI without causing pain; however, the results from experimental studies are inconsistent and the mechanism of action remains in doubt.[257]

Gangliosides (Sialoglycosphingolipids)

Gangliosides are sialic acid-containing glycosphingolipids found in abundance in the lipid bilayer of the neuronal plasma membrane.[258] Recent findings suggest that these compounds may promote neuronal sprouting and growth and enhance recovery. Although the mechanism of action of gangliosides remains unknown, its purported effects include reduction of the release of excitatory amino acids and attenuation of NMDA-induced neurotoxicity.[257] Recently, in a small clinical trial, the administration of monosialoganglioside has been shown to improve neurologic function after acute spinal cord injury.[259] The therapeutic effect of gangliosides in TBI has not yet been investigated.

SUMMARY

This chapter has reviewed the different models used in experimental TBI and has outlined the various pharmacologic approaches to this difficult problem. Because the injury mechanism is complex with multiple pathways and cascades, it follows that there are many potential ways of attacking the problem of secondary injury after TBI. One obvious potential therapeutic approach is to combine several drugs to increase their individual actions. Although such studies are underway, preliminary results caution against optimism because the interaction between these compounds and, hence the outcome, are not always predictable.[260]

Although none of the compounds discussed in this chapter represents the panacea to the treatment of TBI, we are hopeful that, with better characterization of the mechanism of secondary injury, there will exist not only a "golden hour" for resuscitation, but also a golden "therapeutic window" for the administration of appropriate pharmacologic agents.

REFERENCES

1. Nilsson B, Pont'en U, Voigt G: Experimental head injury in the rat. *J Neurosurg* 47:241, 1977.

2. Zornow MH, Scheller MS, Todd MM, et al: Acute cerebral effects of isotonic crystalloid and colloid solutions following cryogenic brain injury in the rabbit. *Anesthesiology* 69:180, 1988.

3. Zornow MH, Scheller MS, Shackford SR: Effect of a hypertonic lactated Ringer's solution on intracranial pressure and cerebral water content in a model of traumatic brain injury. *J Trauma* 29:484, 1989.

4. Zornow MH, Oh YS, Scheller MS: A comparison of the cerebral and hemodynamic effects of mannitol and hypertonic saline in a rabbit model of brain injury. *Anesthesiology* 69:623, 1988.

5. Gennarelli TA, Spielman GM, Langfitt TW, et al: Influence of the type of intracranial lesion on outcome from severe head injury. *J Neurosurg* 56:26, 1982.

6. Mitchell DE, Adams JH: Primary focal impact damage to the brainstem in blunt head injuries: does it exist? *Lancet* 2:215, 1973.

7. Rosenblum WI, Greenberg RP, Seelig JM, et al: Midbrain lesions: frequent and significant prognostic feature in closed head injury. *Neurosurgery* 9:613, 1981.

8. Adams JH: The neuropathology of head injuries. In Vinken PJ, Bruyn GW (eds): *Handbook of Clinical Neurology,* Vol 23. *Injuries of the Brain and Skull. Part I.* New York, American Elsevier, 1975, pp 35–65.

9. Adams JH, Graham DI, Murray LS, et al: Diffuse axonal injury due to nonmissile head injury in humans: An analysis of 45 cases. *Ann Neurol* 12:557, 1982.

10. Adams JH, Graham DI, Scott G, et al: Brain damage in fatal nonmissile head injury. *J Clin Pathol* 33:1132, 1980.

11. Adams JH, Mitchell DE, Graham DI, et al: Diffuse brain damage of immediate impact type. *Brain* 100:489, 1977.

12. Holbourn AHS: Mechanics of head injuries. *Lancet* 2:438, 1943.

13. Holbourn AHS: The mechanics of brain injuries. *Br Med Bull* 3:147, 1945.

14. Strich SJ: Lesions in the cerebral hemispheres after blunt head injury. *J Clin Pathol* 23(suppl 4):166, 1970.

15. Ommaya AK, Gennarelli TA: Cerebral contusion and traumatic unconsciousness: Correlation of experimental and clinical observations on blunt head injuries. *Brain* 97:633, 1974.

16. Gennarelli TA, Adams JH, Graham DI: Acceleration induced head injury in the monkey: Neuropathology. *Neuropathol Appl Neurobiol* 6:234, 1980.

17. Gennarelli JA, Thibault LE, Adams JH, et al: Diffuse axonal injury and traumatic coma in the primate. *Ann Neurol* 12:564, 1982.

18. Gennarelli TA: Head injury mechanisms. In Torg JS (ed): *Athletic Injuries to the Head, Neck and Face.* Philadelphia, Lea & Febiger, 1982:65–73.

19. Gosch H, Gooding E, Scheider RC: Cervical spinal cord hemorrhages in experimental head injuries. *J Neurosurg* 33:640, 1970.

20. Nelson LR, Bourke RS, Popp AJ, et al: Evaluation of treatment modalities in severe head injuries using an animal model. In: Popp AJ, et al., (eds): *Neural Trauma.* New York, Raven Press, 1979:297–311.

21. Rimel RW, Giordani B, Barth JT, et al: Disability caused by minor head injury. *Neurosurgery* 9:221, 1981.

22. Nevin NC: Neuropathological changes in the white matter following head injury. *J Neuropathol Exp Neurol* 26:77, 1967.

23. Oppenheimer DR: Microscopic lesions in the brain following head injury. *J Neurol Neurosurg Psychiatry* 31:299, 1968.

24. Peerless SJ, Newcastle NB: Shear injuries of the brain. *Can Med Assoc J* 96:577, 1967.

25. Siesjo BK: Cell damage in the brain: A speculative synthesis. *J Cereb Blood Flow Metab* 2:155, 1981.

26. Strich SJ: Shearing of nerve fibers as a cause of brain damage due to head injury. *Lancet* 2:443, 1961.

27. Shapira Y, Shohami E, Sidi A, et al: Experimental closed head injury in rats: Mechanical, pathophysiologic, and neurologic properties. *Crit Care Med* 16:258, 1988.

28. Govons SR: Experimental head injury produced by blasting cap: An experimental study. Surgery 15:606, 1944.

29. Tornheim PA, Liwnicz BH, Hirsch CS, et al: Acute responses to blunt head trama: Experimental model and gross pathology. *J Neurosurg* 59:431, 1983.

30. Sullivan HG, Martinez J, Becker DP, et al: Fluid percussion model of mechanical brain injury in the cat. *J Neurosurg* 45:520, 1976.

31. Vink R, McIntosh TK, Weiner MW, et al: Effects of traumatic brain injury on cerebral high-energy phosphates and pH: A 31P magnetic resonance spectroscopy study. *J Cereb Blood Flow Metab* 7:563, 1987.

32. Feeney DM, Boyeson MG, Linn RT, et al: Responses to cortical injury. I. Methodology and local effects of contusion in the rat. *Brain Res* 211:67, 1981.

33. Ommaya AK, Hirsch AE: Tolerance of cerebral concussion from head impact and whiplash in primates. *J Biomech* 4:13, 1971.

34. Lindgren S, Rinder L: Production and distribution of intracranial and intraspinal pressure changes at sudden extradural fluid volume input in rabbits. *Acta Physiol Scand* 76:340, 1969.

35. Gazedam J, Go KG, van Zanten AK: Composition of isolated edema fluid in cold-induced brain edema. *J Neurosurg* 51:70, 1979.

36. Herrmann HD, Neurenfeldt D: Development and regression of a disturbance of the blood-brain barrier and of edema in tissue surrounding a circumscribed cold lesion. *Exp Neurol* 34:115, 1972.

37. Crockard HA, Brown FD, Johns LM, Mullan S: An experimental cerebral missile injury model in primates. *J Neurosurg* 46:776, 1977.

38. Crockard HA, Kang J, Ladds G: A model of focal cortical contusion in gerbils. *J Neurosurg* 57:203, 1982.

39. Shenkin HA, Bezier HS, Bowzarth WF: Restricted fluids intake: Rational management of the neurosurgical patient. *J Neurosurg* 45:432, 1976.

40. Collins WF, Vangilder JC, Vanes JL, et al: Neurologic surgery. In Schwartz

SI, Lillehei RC, Shires GI, et al: (eds): *Principles of Surgery*, 2d ed. New York, McGraw-Hill, 1974:1631.

41. McComish PB, Bodley PO: Head injury. In: McComish PB, Bodley PO (eds): *Anesthesia for Neurological Surgery*. London: Lloyd-Luke, 1971:304.

42. Thomas LM, Gurdjian ES: Cerebral contusion in closed head injury and nonoperative management of head injury. In Youmans JR (ed): *Neurological Surgery*. Philadelphia, WB Saunders, 1973:956.

43. Safar P, Bircher NG: *Cardiopulmonary cerebral resuscitation*. Philadelphia, WB Saunders, 1988:248.

44. Becker PD, Garner S: Intensive management of head injury. In Wilkins RH, Rengachary SS (eds): *Neurosurgery*. New York, McGraw-Hill, 1985:1593.

45. Wisner W, Busche F, Sturm J, et al: Traumatic shock and head injury: Effects of fluid resuscitation on the brain. *J Surg Res* 46:49, 1989.

46. Tommasino C, Todd MM, Shapiro HM: The effects of fluid resuscitation on brain water content. *Anesthesiology* 57:A109, 1982.

47. Warner DS, Boehland LA: Effects of iso-osmolal intravenous fluid therapy on post-ischemic brain water content in the rat. *Anesthesiology* 68:86, 1988.

48. Poole GV, Johnson JC, Prough DS, et al: Cerebral hemodynamics after hemorrhagic shock: Effects of the type of resuscitation fluid. *Crit Care Med* 14:629, 1986.

49. Zornow MH, Todd MM, Moore SS: The acute cerebral effects of changes in plasma osmolality and oncotic pressure. *Anesthesiology* 67:936, 1987.

50. Tommasino C, Moore SS, Todd MM: Cerebral effects of isovolemic hemodilution with crystalloid or colloid solutions. *Crit Care Med* 16:862, 1988.

51. Todd MM, Tommasino C, Moore S, et al: The effect of hypertonic saline on intracranial pressure, cerebral blood flow and brain water content. *Anesthesiology* 61:A123, 1984.

52. Kaieda R, Todd MM, Cook LN, et al: Acute effects of changing plasma osmolality and colloid oncotic pressure on the formation of brain edema after cyrogenic injury. *Neurosurgery* 24:671, 1989.

53. Shapira Y, Artru AA, Cotev S, et al: Brain edema and neurosurgical status following head trauma in the rat; no effect from large volumes of isotonic or hypertonic IV fluids, with or without glucose. *Anesthesiology* 77:79, 1992.

54. Weed LH, McKibben PS: Experimental alteration of brain bulk. *Am J Physiol* 48:531, 1919.

55. Reed DJ, Woodbury DM: Effect of hypertonic urea on cerebrospinal fluid pressure and brain volume. *J Physiol* 164:252, 1962.

56. Fenstermacher JD: Volume regulation of the central nervous system. In Staub NC, Taylor AE (eds): *Edema*. New York, Raven Press, 1984:383.

57. McManus ML, Strange K: Acute volume regulation of brain cells in response to hypertonic challenge. *Anesthesiology* 78:1132, 1993.

58. Muizelaar JP, Wei EP, Kontos HA, et al: Mannitol causes compensatory cerebral vasoconstriction and vasodilation in response to blood viscosity changes. *J Neurosurg* 59:822, 1983.

59. Ravussin P, Archer DP, Meyer E, et al: The effects of rapid infusions of saline and mannitol on cerebral blood volume and intracranial pressure in dogs. *Can Anaesth Soc J* 32:506, 1985.

60. Sahar A, Tsipstein E: Effects of mannitol and furosemide on the rate of formation of cerebrospinal fluid. *Exp Neurol* 60:584, 1978.

61. Takagi H, Saitoh T, Kitahara T: The mechanism of ICP reducing effect of mannitol. Fifth International Symposium on Intracranial Pressure, 1982.

62. Donato T, Shapira Y, Artru A, et al: Effect of mannitol on cerebrospinal fluid dynamics and brain tissue edema. *Anesth Analg* 78:58, 1994.

63. Gunnar WP, Merlotti GJ, Barrett J, et al: Resuscitation from hemorrhagic shock. *Ann Surg* 204:686, 1986.

64. Prough DS, Johnson JC, Poole GV, et al: Effects on intracranial pressure of resuscitation from hemorrhagic shock with hypertonic saline versus lactated Ringer's solution. *Crit Care Med* 13:407, 1985.

65. Prough DS, Johnson JC, Stullken EH, et al: Effects on cerebral hemodynamics of resuscitation from endotoxic shock with hypertonic saline versus lactated Ringer's solution. *Crit Care Med* 13:1040, 1985.

66. Wilson BJ, Jones RF, Coleman ST, et al: The effects of various hypertonic sodium salt solutions on cisternal pressure. *Surgery* 30:361, 1951.

67. Foxworthy JC, Artru AA: Cerebrospinal fluid dynamics and brain tissue composition following intravenous infusion of hypertonic saline in anesthetized rabbits. *J Neurosurg Anesth* 2:256, 1990.

68. Milhorat TH, Hammock MK: Cerebrospinal fluid as reflection of internal milieu of brain. In Wood JH (ed): *Neurobiology of Cerebrospinal Fluid*, vol 2. New York, Plenum Press, 1983:1.

69. Hochwald GM, Wald A, Dimattio J, et al: The effects of serum osmolarity on cerebrospinal fluid volume flow. *Life Sci* 15:1309, 1974.

70. Fisher B, Thomas D, Peterson B: Hypertonic saline lowers raised intracranial pressure in children after head trauma. *J Neurosurg Anesthesiol* 4:4, 1992.

71. Cottrell JE, Robstelli A, Post K, et al: Furosemide and mannitol induced changes in intracranial pressure and serum osmolality and electrolytes. *Anesthesiology* 47:28, 1977.

72. Abou-Madi M, Trop D, Abou-Madi N, et al: Does a bolus of mannitol initially aggravate intracranial hypertension? A study at various Pa_{CO_2} tensions in dogs. *Br J Anesth* 59:630, 1987.

73. Marshall LF, Smith RW, Rauscher LA, et al: Mannitol dose requirements in brain-injured patients. *J Neurosurg* 48:169, 1978.

74. McGraw CP, Alexander E, Howard G: Effect of dose and dose schedule on the response of intracranial pressure to mannitol. *Surg Neurol* 10:127, 1978.

75. Roberts PA, Pollay M, Engles C, et al: Effect on intracranial pressure of furosemide combined with varying doses and administration rates of mannitol. *J Neurosurg* 66:440, 1987.

76. Pollay M, Fullenwider C, Roberts PA, et al: Effect of mannitol and furosemide on blood brain osmotic gradient and intracranial pressure. *J Neurosurg* 59:945, 1983.

77. Pulsinelli WA, Waldman S, Rawlinson D, et al: Moderate hyperglycemia augments ischemic brain damage: A neuropathologic study in the rat. *Neurology* 32:1239, 1982.

78. D'alecy LG, Lundy EF, Barton KJ, et al: Dextrose-containing intravenous fluid impairs outcome and increases death after eight minutes of cardiac arrest and resuscitation in dogs. *Surgery* 100:505, 1986.

79. Lanier W, Stangland KJ, Scheithauer BW, et al: The effects of dextrose infusion and head position on neurologic outcome after complete cerebral ischemia in primates: Examination of a model. *Anesthesiology* 66:39, 1987.

80. Drummond JC, Moore SS: The influence of dextrose administration on neurologic outcome after temporary spinal cord ischemia in the rabbit. *Anesthesiology* 70:64, 1989.

81. Pulsinelli WA, Levy DE, Sigsbee B, et al: Increased damage after ischemic stroke in patients with hyperglycemia with or without established diabetes mellitus. *Am J Med* 74:540, 1983.

82. Longstreth WT, Inui TS: High blood glucose level on hospital admission and poor neurological recovery after cardiac arrest. *Ann Neurol* 15:59, 1984.

83. Young B, Ott L, Dempsey R, et al: Relationship between admission hyperglycemia and neurologic outcome of severely brain-injured patients. *Ann Surg* 210:466, 1989.

84. Lam AM, Winn HR, Cullen BF, et al: Hyperglycemia and neurological outcome in patients with head injury. *J Neurosurg* 75:545, 1991.

85. Michaud LJ, Rivara FP, Longstreth WT Jr, et al: Elevated initial blood glucose levels and poor outcome following severe brain injuries in children. *J Trauma* 31:1356, 1991.

86. Gardiner M, Smith ML, Kagstrom E, et al: Influence of blood glucose concentration on brain lactate accumulation during severe hypoxia and subsequent recovery of brain energy metabolism. *J Cereb Blood Flow Metab* 2:429, 1982.

87. Venables GS, Miller SA, Gibson G, et al: The effects of hyperglycemia on changes during reperfusion following focal cerebral ischemia in the cat. *J Neurol Neurosurg Psychiatry* 48:663, 1985.

88. Nedergaard M: Transient focal ischemia in hyperglycemic rats associated with increased cerebral infarction. *Brain Res* 408:79, 1987.

89. Voll CL, Auer RN: The effect of postischemic blood glucose levels on ischemic brain damage in the rat. *Ann Neurol* 24:638, 1988.

90. LeMay DR, Gehua L, Zelenock GB, et al: Insulin administration protects neurologic function in cerebral ischemia in rats. *Stroke* 19:1411, 1988.

91. Zasslow MA, Pearl RG, Shuer LM, et al: Hyperglycemia decrease acute neuronal ischemic changes after middle cerebral artery occlusion in cats. *Stroke* 20:519, 1989.

92. Rapp RP, Young B, Fargman D, et al: The favorable effect of early parenteral feeding on survival in head-injured patients. *J. Neurosurg* 58:906, 1983.

93. Ginsberg MD, Prado R, Dietrich WD, et al: Hyperglycemia reduces the extent of cerebral infarction in rats. *Stroke* 18:570, 1987.

94. Jernigan J, Evans OB, Kirshner HS: Hyperglycemia and diabetes improve outcome in rat model of anoxia/ischemia (abstr). *Neurology* 34(S1):262, 1984.

95. Prado R, Ginsberg MD, Dietrich WD, et al: Hyperglycemia increases infarct size in collaterally perfused but not end arterial vascular territories. *J Cereb Blood Flow Metab* 8:186, 1988.

96. Nedergaard M: Mechanisms of brain damage in focal cerebral ischemia. *Acta Neurol Scand* 77:81, 1987.

97. Nedergaard M, Diemer NH: Focal ischemia of the rat brain. With special reference to the influence of plasma glucose concentration. *Acta Neuropathol* 73:131, 1987.

98. Ginsberg MD, Welsh FA, Budd WW: Deleterious effect of glucose pretreatment on recovery from diffuse cerebral ischemia in the cat. Local cerebral blood flow and glucose utilization. *Stroke* 11:347, 1980.

99. Paljarvi L, Rehncrona S, Soderfeldt B, et al: Brain lactic acidosis and ischemic cell damage: quantitative ultrastructural changes in capillaries of rat cerebral cortex. *Acta Neuropathol (Berl)* 60:232, 1983.

100. Nedergaard M, Astrup J: Infarct Rim: effect of hyperglycemia on direct current potential and (^{14}C)2-deoxyglucose phosphorylation. *J Cereb Blod Flow Metab* 6:607, 1986.

101. Field J II, Shearman FA, Martin AW: Effect of temperature on oxygen consumption of brain tissue. *J Neurophysiol* 7:717, 1944.

102. Michenfelder JD, Terry HR, Jr., Daw EF, et al: Induced hypothermia: Physiologic effects, indications and techniques. *Surg Clin North Am* 45:889, 1965.

103. Michenfelder JD: *Anesthesia and the brain*. New York, Churchill Livingstone, 1988:23–34.

104. Michenfelder JD, Theye RA: Hypothermia: Effect of canine brain and whole body metabolism. *Anesthesiology* 29:1107, 1968.

105. Bering EA, Jr: Effect of body temperature change on cerebral oxygen consumption of the intact monkey. *Am J Physiol* 200:417, 1961.

106. Cohen PH, Wollman H, Alexander SC, Chase PE, Behar MG: Cerebral carbohydrate metabolism in man during halothane anesthesia: Effects of Pa_{CO_2} on some aspects of carbohydrate utilization. *Anesthesiology* 25:185, 1964.

107. Steen PA, Newberg LA, Milde JH, et al: Hypothermia and barbiturates: Individual and combined effects on canine cerebral oxygen consumption. *Anesthesiology* 58:527, 1983.

108. Drummond JC: Brain protection during anesthesia: A reader's guide. *Anesthesiology* 79:877, 1993.

109. Busto R, Globus MY, Dietrich WD, et al: Effect of mild hypothermia on ischemia-induced release of neurotransmitters and free fatty acids in rat brain. *Stroke* 20:904, 1989.

110. Busto R, Dietrich DW, Globus MY, et al: Small differences in intraischemic brain temperature critically determine the extent of ischemic neuronal injury. *J Cereb Blood Flow Metab* 7:729, 1987.

111. Rothman SM, Olney JW: Excitotoxicity and the NMDA receptor. *Trends Neurosci* 10:299, 1987.

112. Benveniste H, Jorgensen M, Sandberg M, et al: Ischemic damage in hippocampal CA1 is dependent on glutamate release and intact innervation from CA3. *J Cereb Blood Flow Metab* 9:629, 1989.

113. Choi DW, Koh J-Y, Peters S: Pharmacology of glutamate neurotoxicity in cortical cell culture: Attenuation by NMDA antagonist. *J Neurosci* 8:185, 1988.

114. Buchan A, Pulsinelli WA: Hypothermia but not the NMDA antagonist, MK-801, attenuates neuronal damage in gerbils subjected to transient global ischemia. *J Neurosci* 10:311, 1990.

115. Baker AJ, Zornow MH, Grafe MR, et al: Hypothermia prevents ischemia-induced increase in hippocampal glycine concentration in rabbits. *Stroke* 22:666, 1991.

116. Baker AJ, Moulton RJ, Macmillan VH, et al: Excitatory amino acids in cerebrospinal fluid following traumatic brain injury in humans. *J Neurosurg* 79:369, 1993.

117. Jiang JY, Lyeth BG, Clifton GL, et al: Relationship between body and brain temperature in traumatically brain-injured rodents. *J Neurosurg* 74:492, 1991.

118. Mellergard P, Nordstrom CH: Intracerebral temperature in neurosurgical patients. *Neurosurgery* 28:709, 1991.

119. Marion DW, Obrist WD, Carlier PM, et al: The use of moderate therapeutic hypothermia for patients with severe head injuries: a preliminary report. *J Neurosurg* 79:354, 1993.

120. Shiozaki T, Sugimoto H, Taneda M, et al: Effect of mild hypothermia on uncontrollable intracranial hypertension after severe head injury. *J Neurosurg* 79:363, 1993.

121. Marmarou A, Anderson RL, Ward JD, et al: Impact of ICP instability and hypotension on outcome in patients with severe head trauma. *J Neurosurg* 75:S59, 1991.

122. Drummond JC, Oh Y-S, Cole DJ, et al: Phenylephrine-induced hypertension reduces ischemia following middle cerebral artery occlusion in rats. *Stroke* 20:1538, 1989.

123. Awad IA, Carter LP, Spetzler RF, et al: Clinical vasospasm after subarachnoid hemorrhage: response to Hypervolemic hemodilution and arterial hypertension. *Stroke* 18:365, 1987.

124. Chan PH, Fishman RA, Caronna J, et al: Induction of brain edema following intracerebral injection of arachidonic acid. *Ann Neurol* 13:625, 1983.

125. Iannotti F, Crockard A, Ladds G, et al: Are prostaglandins involved in experimental ischemic edema in gerbils? *Stroke* 12:301, 1981.

126. Weidenfeld J, Lysy J, Shohami E: Effect of dexamethasone on prostaglandin synthesis in various areas of the rat brain. *J Neurochem* 48:1351, 1987.

127. Chan PH, Schmidley JW, Fishman RA, et al: Brain injury, edema and vascular permeability changes induced by oxygen-derived free radicals. *Neurology* 34:313, 1984.

128. Gamache DA, Ellis EF: Effect of dexamethasone, indomethacin, ibuprofen, and probenecid on carrageenan-induced brain inflammation. *J Neurosurg* 65:686, 1986.

129. Demopoulos HB, Milvy P, Kakari S, et al: Molecular aspects of membrane structure in cerebral edema. In Reulen HJ, Schurmann K (eds): *Steroids and Brain Edema.* Berlin, Springer-Verlag, 1972:29.

130. Hall ED: High-dose glucocorticoid treatment improves neurological recovery in head injured mice. *J Neurosurg* 62:882, 1985.

131. Shapira Y, Davidson E, Weidenfeld Y, et al: Dexamethasone and indomethacin do not affect brain edema following head injury in rats. *J Cereb Blood Flow Metab* 8:395, 1988.

132. Shapira Y, Artru AA, Yadid G, et al: Methylprednisolone does not decrease eicosanoid levels or edema in brain tissue or improve neurological outcome following head trauma in rats. *Anesth Analg* 75:238, 1992.

133. McEwen BS, Weiss JM, Schwartz LS: Selective retention of corticosterone by limbic structures in rat brain. *Nature* 220:911, 1968.

134. McEwen BS, De Kloet ER, Rostene W: Adrenal steroid receptors and actions in the nervous system. *Physiol Rev* 66:1121, 1986.

135. Sapolsky RM: Glucocorticoid toxicity in the hippocampus: Reversal by supplementation with brain fuels. *J Neurosci* 6:2240, 1986.

136. Landfield PW, Baskin RK, Pitler TA: Brain aging correlates: Retardation by hormonal-pharmacological treatments. *Science* 214:581, 1981.

137. Sapolsky R: Glucocorticoid toxicity in the hippocampus: Temporal aspects of neuronal vulnerability. *Brain Research* 339:300, 1985.

138. Sapolsky R, Krey L, McEwen B: The neuroendocrinology of stress and aging: the glucocorticoid cascade hypothesis. *Endocr Rev* 7:284, 1986.

139. Sapolsky RM, Pulsinelli WA: Glucocoticoids potentiate ischemic injury to neurons: Therapeutic implications. *Science* 229:1397, 1985.

140. Sapolsky RM, Packan DR, Vale WW: Glucocorticoid toxicity in the hippocampus: In vitro demonstration. *Brain Res* 453:367, 1988.

141. Sapolsky RM: Glucocorticoid toxicity in the hippocampus: Temporal aspects synergy with a kainic acid. *Neuroendocrinology* 43:440, 1986.

142. Sapolsky RM, Krey L, McEwen B: Prolonged glucocorticoid exposure reduces hippocampal neuron number: Implications for aging. *J Neurosci* 5:1221, 1985.

143. Yamaguchi M, Shirakata S, Taomoto K, et al: Steroid treatment of brain edema. *Surg Neurol* 4:5, 1975.

144. Korbine AI, Kempe LG: Studies in head injury. II. Effect of dexamethasone on traumatic brain swelling. *Surg Neurol* 1:38, 1973.

145. Means ED, Anderson DK, Waters TR, et al: Effect of methylprednisolone in compression trauma to the feline spinal cord. *J Neurosurg* 55:200, 1981.

146. Pappius HM: Dexamethasone and local cerebral glucose utilization in freeze-traumatized rat brain. *Ann Neurol* 12:157, 1982.

147. Hall ED, Wolf DL, Braughler JM: Effects of a single large dose of methylprednisolone sodium succinate on experimental posttraumatic spinal cord ischemia. Dose response and time action analysis. *J Neurosurg* 61:124, 1984.

148. Hall ED, Braughler JM: Glucocorticoid mechanisms in acute spinal injury: A review and therapeutic rationale. *Surg Neurol* 18:320, 1984.

149. Giannotta SL, Weiss MH, Apuzzo ML, et al: High-dose glucocorticoids in the management of severe head injury. *Neurosurgery* 15:497, 1984.

150. Braakman R, Schouten HJA, Blaauw van Dishoeck M, et al: Megadose steroids in severe head injury. Results of a prospective double blind clinical trial. *J Neurosurg* 58:326, 1983.

151. Cooper PR, Moody S, Clark WK, et al: Dexamethasone and severe head injury. A prospective double blind study. *J Neurosurg* 51:307, 1979.

152. Gudeman SK, Miller JD, Becker DP: Failure of high-dose steroids therapy to influence intracranial pressure in patients with severe head injury. *J Neurosurg* 51:301, 1979.

153. Dearden NM, Gibson JS, McDowall DG, et al: Effect of high-dose dexamethasone on outcome from severe head injury. *J Neurosurg* 64:81, 1986.

154. Bracken MB, Shepard MJ, Collins WF, et al: A randomized, controlled trial of methylprednisolone or naloxone in the treatment of acute spinal cord injury. *N Engl J Med* 322:1405, 1990.

155. Bracken MB, Shepard MJ, Collins WF Jr, et al: Methylprednisolone or naloxone treatment after acute spinal cord injury: 1-year follow-up data. *J Neurosurg* 76:23, 1992.

156. Hall ED, Yonkers PA, Andrus PK, et al: Biochemistry and pharmacology of lipid antioxidants in acute brain and spinal cord injury. *J Neurotrauma* 9:S425, 1992.

157. Thomas PD, Mao GD, Rabinovitch A, et al: Inhibition of superoxide generating NADPH oxidase of human neutrophils by lazaroids [21-aminosteroids and 2-methylaminochromans]. *Biochem Pharmacol* 45:241, 1993.

158. Olsen KS, Videbaek C, Agerlin N, et al: The effect of Tirilazad mesylate (U74006F) on cerebral oxygen consumption, and reactivity of cerebral blood flow to carbon dioxide in healthy volunteers. *Anesthesiology* 79:666, 1993.

159. Choi DW: Calcium-mediated neurotoxicity: Relationship to specific channel types and role in ischemic damage. *Trends Neurosci* 11:465, 1988.

160. Rothman SM, Oleney JW: Excitotoxicity and the NMDA receptor. *Trends Neurosci* 10:299, 1987.

161. Meyer FB: Calcium, neuronal hyperexcitability and ischemic injury. *Brain Res Rev* 14:227, 1989.

162. Albers GB, Goldberg MP, Choi DW: N-methyl-D-aspartate antagonists: Ready for clinical trial in brain ischemia? *Ann Neurol* 25:398, 1989.

163. Simon RP, Swan JH, Griffiths T, et al: Blockade of N-methyl-D-aspartate receptors may protect against ischemic damage in the brain. *Science* 226:850, 1990.

164. Faden AI, Demediuk P, Panter SS, et al: The role of excitatory amino acids and NMDA receptors in traumatic head injury. *Science* 244:798, 1989.

165. Beneviste H, Drejer J, Schousboe A, et al: Elevation of extracellular concentration of glutamate and aspartate in rat hippocampus during transient ischemia monitored by intracerebral microdialysis. *J Neurochem* 43:1369, 1984.

166. Cotman CW, Iverson LL: Excitatory amino acids in the brain—focus on NMDA receptors. *TINS* 10:263, 1987.

167. Stevens MK, Yaksh TL: Systemic studies on the NMDA receptor antagonist MK-801 on cerebral blood flow and responsivity, EEG, and blood brain barrier following complete reversible cerebral ischemia. *J Cereb Blood Flow Metab* 10:77, 1990.

168. Siesjo BK, Bengtsson F: Calcium fluxes, calcium antagonists, and calcium-related pathology in brain ischemia, hypoglycemia, and spreading depression: A unifying hypothesis. *J Cereb Blood Flow Metab* 9:127, 1989.

169. MacDermot AB, Mayer ML, Westbrook GL, et al: NMDA receptor activation increases cytoplasmic calcium concentration in cultured spinal cord neurons. *Nature* 321:519, 1986.

170. Desphande JK, Siesjo BK, Wieloch T: Calcium accumulation in the rat hippocampus following cerebral ischemia. *J Cereb Blood Flow Metab* 7:89, 1987.

171. Wieloch T, Harris RJ, Siesjo BK: Brain metabolism and ischemia: Mechanism of cell damage and principles of protection. *J Cereb Blood Flow Metab* 2:S5, 1982.

172. Cheung JY, Bonaventure JV, Malis CD, et al: Calcium and ischemic injury. *N Engl J Med* 314:1670, 1986.

173. Kohmura E, Yamada K, Hayakawa T, et al: Hippocampal neurons become more vulnerable to glutamate after subcritical hypoxia: An in vitro study. *J Cereb Blood Flow Metab* 10:877, 1990.

174. Diemer NH, Johansen FF, Jorgensen MB: *N*-methyl-D-aspartate and non-*N*-methyl-D-aspartate antagonists in global cerebral ischemia. *Stroke* 21(suppl 3):39, 1993.

175. Roman R, Bartkowski H, Simon R: The specific NMDA receptor antagonist AP-7 attenuates focal ischemic brain injury. *Neurosci Lett* 104:19, 1989.

176. Swan J, Meldrum BS: Protection by NMDA antagonists against selective cell loss following transient ischemia. *J Cereb Blood Flow Metab* 10:343, 1990.

177. Bullock R, Graham DI, Chen M-H, et al: Focal cerebral ischemia in the cat: Pretreatment with a competitive NMDA receptor antagonist, D-CPP-ene. *J Cereb Blood Flow Metab* 10:668, 1990.

178. Levy DI, Lipton SA: Comparison of delayed administration of competitive and uncompetitive antagonists in preventing NMDA receptor-mediated neuronal death. *Neurology* 40:852, 1990.

179. Simon R, Shiraishi K: *N*-methyl-D-aspartate antagonist reduces stroke size and regional glucose metabolism. *Ann Neurol* 27:606, 1990.

180. Bullock R, McCulloch J, Graham DI, et al: Focal ischemic damage is reduced by CPP-ene: Studies in two animal models. *Stroke* 21(suppl 3):32, 1990.

181. Ozyurt E, Graham DI, Woodruff GN, et al: Protective effect of glutamate antagonist, MK-801 in focal cerebral ischemia in the cat. *J Cereb Blood Flow Metab* 8:138, 1988.

182. Shapira Y, Yadid G, Cotev S, et al: Protective effect of MK-801 in experimental brain injury. *J Neurotrauma* 3:131, 1990.

183. McIntosh TK, Soares H, Hayes RL, et al: The *N*-methyl-D-aspartate receptor antagonist MK-801 prevents edema and improves outcome after experimental brain injury in rats (abstract). In Hoff and Betz (eds): *Seventh International Symposium on ICP and Brain Injury,* Ann Arbor, MI, University of Michigan Press, 1988, p. 199.

184. Steinberg GK, Jamshid S, Kunis D, et al: Protective effect of *N*-methyl-D-aspartate antagonist after focal cerebral ischemia in rabbits. *Stroke* 20:1247, 1989.

185. Ford LM, Sanberg PR, Norman AB, et al: MK-801 prevents hippocampal neurodegradation in neonatal hypoxic-ischemic rats. *Arch Neurol* 46:1090, 1989.

186. Nabeshima T, Yoshida S, Morinaka H, et al: MK-801 ameliorates delayed

amnesia, but potentiates acute amnesia induced by CO. *Neurosci Lett* 108:321, 1990.

187. Meyer FB, Anderson RE, Friedrich PF: MK-801 attenuates capillary bed compression and hypoperfusion following incomplete focal cerebral ischemia. *J Cereb Blood Flow Metab* 10:895, 1990.

188. Barth TM, Grant MA, Schallert T: Effects of MK-801 on recovery from sensory cortex lesions. *Stroke* 21(suppl 3):153, 1990.

189. Goldberg MP, Choi DW: Intracellular free calcium increases in cultural cortical neurons deprived of oxygen and glucose. *Stroke* 21(suppl):III-75, 1990.

190. Van-Rijen PC, Verheul HB, Van-Echteld CJA, et al: Effects of dextromethorphan on rat brain during ischemia and reperfusion assessed by magnetic resonance spectroscopy. *Stroke* 22:343, 1991.

191. Michenfelder JD, Lanier WL, Scheithauer BW, et al: Evaluation of the glutamate antagonist dizocilpine maleate (MK-801) on neurologic outcome in a canine model of complete cerebral ischemia: Correlation with hippocampal histopathology. *Brain Res* 481:228, 1989.

192. Olney JW, Price MT, Fuller TA, et al: The anti-excitotoxic effects of certain anesthetics, analgesics and sedative-hypnotics. *Neurosci Lett* 68:29, 1990.

193. Chan PH, Chu L: Ketamine protects cultured astrocytes from glutamate induced swelling. *Brain Res* 487:380, 1989.

194. Lees GJ: Halothane anaesthesia reverses the neuroprotective effect of ketamine against ibotenic acid toxicity in the rat hippocampus. *Brain Res* 502:280, 1989.

195. Lees GJ: Effects of ketamine on the in vivo toxicity of quinolinate and N-methyl-D-aspartate in the rat hippocampus. *Neurosci Lett* 78:180, 1987.

196. Marcoux FW, Goodrich JE, Probert AW, et al: Ketamine prevents glutamate-induced calcium influx and ischemia nerve cell injury. In Domino EF, Kamenka J (eds): *Sigma and Phencyclidine-like Compounds as Molecular Probes in Biology.* Ann Arbor, Domino and NPP Books, 1988:735.

197. Shapira Y, Artru AA, Lam AM: Ketamine decreases cerebral infarct volume and improves neurological outcome following experimental head trauma in rats. *J Neurosurg Anesth* 4:231, 1992.

198. Shapira Y, Lam AM, Artru AA, et al: Ketamine alters calcium and magnesium in brain tissue following experimental head trauma in rats. *J Cereb Blood Flow Metab* 13:962, 1993.

199. Takeshita H, Okuda Y, Sari A: The effects of ketamine on cerebral circulation and metabolism in man. *Anesthesiology* 36:69, 1972.

200. Fukuda S, Murakawa T, Takeshita H, et al: Direct effects of ketamine on isolated canine cerebral and mesenteric arteries. *Anesth Analg* 62:553, 1983.

201. Cavazutti M, Porro CA, Biral GP, et al: Ketamine effects on local cerebral blood flow and metabolism in the rat. *J Cereb Blood Flow Metab* 7:806, 1987.

202. Belopavlovic M, Buchthal A: Modification of ketamine-induced intracranial hypertension in neurosurgical patients by pretreatment with midazolam. *Acta Anaesthesiol Scand* 26:458, 1982.

203. Crosby G, Crane AM, Sokoloff L: Local changes in cerebral glucose utilization during ketamine anesthesia. *Anesthesiology* 56:437, 1982.

204. David DW, Mans AM, Biebuyck JF, et al: The influence of ketamine on regional brain glucose use. *Anesthesiology* 69:199, 1988.

205. Dawson B, Michenfelder JD, Theye RA: Effects of ketamine on canine cerebral blood flow and metabolism: Modification by prior administration of thiopental. *Anesth Analg* 50:443, 1971.

206. Artru AA, Katz RA: Cerebral blood volume and CSF pressure following administration of ketamine in dogs; Modification by pre- or posttreatment with hypocapnia or diazepam. *J Neurosurg Anesth* 1:8, 1989.

207. McIntosh TK, Vink R, Weiner MW, et al: Alterations in free magnesium, high-energy phosphates, and lactate following traumatic brain injury: Assessment by nuclear magnetic resonance spectroscopy. *J Cereb Blood Flow Metab* 7:S620, 1987.

208. Vink R, McIntosh TK, Demediuk P, et al: Decrease in total and free magnesium concentration following traumatic brain injury in rats. *Biochem Biophys Res Commun* 149:594, 1987.

209. Vink R, McIntosh TK: Pharmacological and physiological effect of magnesium on experimental traumatic brain injury. *Magnes Res* 3:163, 1990.

210. McIntosh TK, Vink R, Yamakami I: Magnesium protects against neurological deficit after brain injury. *Brain Res* 482:252, 1989.

211. Brouhard BH, Carvajal HF: Effect of inhibiting prostaglandin synthesis on edema formation and albumin leakage during thermal trauma in rat. *Prostaglandins* 17:939, 1979.

212. Pappius HM, Wolf LS: Some further studies on vasogenic edema. In Pappius HM, Feindel W, (eds): *Dynamics of Brain Edema*. Heidelberg: Springer-Verlag, 1976:138.

213. Lewis RA, Austen KF: The biologically active leukotrienes biosynthesis, metabolism, receptors, functions, and pharmacology. *J Clin Invest* 73:889, 1984.

214. Dempsey RJ, Roy MW, Cowen DE, et al: Lipoxygenase metabolites of arachidonic acid and the development of ischemic cerebral edema. *Neurol Res* 8:53, 1986.

215. Dempsey RJ, Roy MW, Meyer KC: Development of cyclooxygenase and lipoxygenase metabolites of arachidonic acid after transient cerebral ischemia. *J Neurosurg* 64:118, 1986.

216. Black KL, Hoff JT: Leukotrienes increase BBB permeability following intraparenchymal injections in rats. *Ann Neurol* 18:349, 1985.

217. Yen MH, Lee SH: Effects of cyclooxygenase and lipoxygenase inhibitors on

cerebral edema induced by freezing lesions in rats. *Eur J Pharmacol* 144:369, 1987.

218. Jensen K, Cold GE, Astrup J, et al: Indomethacin in severe head injury. *Lancet* 336:246, 1990.

219. Pickard JD, Walker V: *Current Concepts of the Role of Prostaglandins and Other Eicosanoids in Acute Cerebrovascular Disease.* L.E.R.S., vol. 2. Mackenzie ET et al (eds). New York, Raven Press, 1984:191.

220. Shohami E, Rosenthal J, Lavy S: The effect of incomplete cerebral ischemia on prostaglandin levels in rat brain. *Stroke* 13:494, 1982.

221. Dempsy RJ, Roy MW, Meyer K, et al: Development of cyclooxygenase and lipooxygenase metabolites of arachidonic acid after transient cerebral ischemia. *J Neurosurg* 64:118, 1986.

222. Roy MW, Dempsey RJ, Cowen DE, et al: Thromboxane synthetase inhibition with imidazole increases blood flow in ischemic penumbra. *Neurosurgery* 22:317, 1988.

223. Ishihara Y, Uchida Y, Kitamura S: Effect of thromboxane synthetase inhibitors (OKY-046,OKY-1580) on experimentally induced air embolism in anesthetized dogs. *Prostaglandins Leukot Med* 21:197, 1986.

224. Fredriksson K, Rosen I, Johansson BB, et al: Cerebral platelet thromboembolism and thromboxane synthetase inhibition. *Stroke* 16:800, 1985.

225. Nihei C, Metoki H, Shimanaka Y, et al: Clinical study on the effect of thromboxane A2 synthetase inhibitor (OKY-046) to clarify the regulation of cerebral blood flow in cerebral thrombosis. *Adv Prostaglandin Thromboxane Leukot Res* 17B:953, 1987.

226. Moufarrij NA, Little JR, Skrinska V, et al: Thromboxane synthetase inhibition in acute focal cerebral ischemia in cats. *J Neurosurg* 61:1107, 1984.

227. Hock CE, Brezinski ME, Lefer AM: Anti-ischemia action of a new thromboxane receptor antagonist, SQ-29548, in acute myocardial ischemia. *Eur J Pharmacol* 122:213, 1986.

228. Tsien RW, Lipscome D, Madison DV, et al: Multiple types of neuronal calcium channels and their selective modulators. *Trends Neurosci* 11:431, 1988.

229. McCalden TA, Bevan JA: Sources of activator calcium in rabbit basilar artery. *Am J Physiol* 241:129, 1981.

230. Kazda S, Hoffmeister F, Garthoff B, et al: Prevention of the postischemic impaired reperfusion of the brain by nimodipine (Bay e9736). *Acta Neurol Scand* 60(suppl 72):302, 1979.

231. Allen GS, Ahn HS, Preziosi TJ, et al: Cerebral arterial spasm—a controlled trial of nimodipine in patients with subarachnoid hemorrhage. *N Engl J Med* 17:619, 1983.

232. Steen PA, Gisvold SE, Milde JH, et al: Nimodipine improves outcome when given after complete cerebral ischemia in primates. *Anesthesiology* 62:406, 1985.

233. Gaab NR, Haubitz I, Brauranski A, et al: Acute effects of nimodipine on cerebral blood flow and intracranial pressure. *Neurochirurgia* 28:88, 1985.

235. Kostorn H, Rumpl E, Stampl E, et al: Treatment of cerebral vasospasm following severe head injury with the calcium influx blocker nimodipine. *Neurochirurgia* 28:103, 1985.

236. Teasdale G, Bailey I, Bell A, et al: The effect of nimodipine on outcome after head injury: A prospective randomized control trial. *Acta Neurochir Suppl (Wien)* 51:315, 1990.

237. Steen PA, Newberg LA, Milde JH, et al: Cerebral blood flow and neurologic outcome when nimodipine is given after complete cerebral ischemia in the dog. *J Cereb Blood Flow Metab* 4:82, 1984.

238. Steen PA, Milde JH, Michenfelder JD: Cerebral metabolic and vasculature effects of barbiturate therapy following complete global ischemia. *J Neurochem* 31:1317, 1978.

239. Kass IS, Cottrell JE, Chambers G: Magnesium and cobalt, not nimodipine, protect neurons against anoxic damage in the rat hippocampal slice. *Anesthesiology* 69:710, 1988.

240. Weiss JH, Hartley DM, Choi DW: The calcium channels blocker nifedipine attenuates slow EAA Neurotoxicity. *Science* 247:1474, 1990.

241. McBurney RN, Daly D, Fischer JB, et al: New CNS-specific calcium antagonists. *J Neurotrauma* 9:S531, 1992.

242. Steen PA, Michenfelder JD: Mechanisms of barbituate protection. *Anesthesiology* 53:183, 1980.

243. Clarck IA, Cowden WB, Hunt NH: Free radical-induced pathology. *Med Res Rev* 5:297, 1985.

244. McCord JM: Oxygen derived free radicals in post ischemic tissue injury. *N Engl J Med* 312:159, 1985.

245. Chambers DE, Parks DA, Patterson G, et al: Xanthine oxidase as source of free radical damage in myocardial ischemia. *J Mol Cell Cardiol* 17:145, 1985.

246. Freeman BA, Crapo JD: Biology of disease. Free radicals and tissue injury. *Lab Invest* 47:412, 1982.

247. Del maestro RF: An approach to free radicals in medicine and biology. *Acta Scand Suppl* 492:153, 1980.

248. Fridovich I: The biology of oxygen radicals. *Science* 201:875, 1978.

249. Thompson JA, Hees ML: The oxygen free radical system: A fundamental mechanism in the production of myocardial necrosis. *Prog Cardiovasc Dis* 28:449, 1986.

250. Cerchiari EL, Hoel TM, Safar P, et al: Protective effect of combined superoxide dismutase and deferoxamine on recovery of cerebral blood flow and function after cardiac arrest in dogs. *Stroke* 18:899, 1987.

251. Ikeda Y, Ikeda K, Long DM: Protective effect of iron chelator deferoxamine on cold-induced brain edema. *J Neurosurg* 71:233, 1989.

252. Schettini A, Lippman HR, Walsh EK: Attenuation of decompressive hypoperfusion and cerebral edema by superoxide dismutase. *J Neurosurg* 71:578, 1989.

253. Yoshida S: Brain injury after ischemia and trauma: The role of Vitamin E. *Ann N Y Acad Sci* 570:219, 1989.

254. Suzuki J, Imaizumi S, Kayama T, et al: Chemiluminescence in hypoxic brain-the second report: Cerebral protective effect of mannitol, vitamin E and glucocorticoid. *Stroke* 16:695, 1985.

255. Muizelaar JP, Marmarou A, Young HF, et al: Improving the outcome of severe head injury with the oxygen radical scavenger polyethylene glycol-conjugated superoxide dismutase: A phase II trial. *J Neurosurg* 78:375, 1993.

256. Fadem AI, Jacobs TP, Holaday JW: Opiate antagonist improves neurologic recovery after spinal injury. *Science* 211:493, 1981.

257. McIntosh TK: Novel pharmacologic therapies in the treatment of experimental traumatic brain injury: a review. *J Neurotrauma* 10:215, 1993.

258. Skaper SD, Leon A: Monosialogangliosides, neuroprotection, and neuronal repair processes. *J Neurotrauma* 9:S507, 1992.

259. Geisler FH, Dorsey FC, Coleman WP: Recovery of motor function after spinal-cord injury—a randomized placebo-controlled trial with GM-1 ganglioside. *N Engl J Med* 324:1829, 1991.

260. Faden AI: Comparison of single and combination drug treatment strategies in experimental brain trauma. *J Neurotrauma* 10:91, 1993.

I N D E X

ABCs of trauma care, 88–90, 104
Acceleration-deceleration injury,
 75–77, *100,* 286–289
Acceleration models, 288–289, *289*
Acute head injury. *See also* Intensive
 care management; Monitoring
anesthetic management, 199–200
initial resuscitation, 87–96, 127. *See
 also* Resuscitation
intensive care management, 243–263
monitoring, 243–263
pediatric, 223–235. *See also* Pediatric
 head injury
surgical management
 alternative and associated
  procedures, 136
 craniectomy for skull/meningeal
  lesions, 118–130
 craniofacial injuries, 130–134
 craniotomy for mass lesions,
  102–118. *See also* Craniotomy;
  Hematoma
 vascular injuries, 134–136
Adult respiratory distress syndrome. *See*
 ARDS
Advanced Trauma Life Support
 (ATLS), 92–94, 234

Age
 epidemiologic aspects, 4–5
 and mechanisms of injury, 12
 and outcome, 225–226, *228*
Airway management
 and complication rate, 230–231
 emergency care, 91–94, *93*
 in pediatric head trauma, 231–234
Alcohol-related accidents, 7–8
ALS (Advanced Trauma Life Support),
 92–94, 234
AMA (American Medical Association),
 273
American College of Surgeons ALS
 recommendations, 92–94, 93t
American Medical Association (AMA),
 273
American Society of Anesthesiologists
 *Practice Guidelines for
 Management of the Difficult
 Airway,* 94
Anemia in brain death, 281
Anesthetic agents. *See also* Anesthetic
 management
 and CO_2 reactivity, 197–198
 and CSF formation and absorption,
  198
 and hemodynamics/cerebral blood
  flow, 196–197
 for induction, 200–201
 inhalation, 197
 intravenous, 196